Praise For *Your Bones*

"*Your Bones* provides valuable, detailed information on the best balance of exercise (short bursts of vigorous walking and weight-bearing workouts), targeted diet (organic, vegetarian, and low-fat), and supplements needed to guard against crippling or fatal bone loss."

—*ForeWord*

"The information is presented in a straightforward and easy-to-read style that will be understandable to lay readers. Consumer(s) . . . looking for [a] book about the natural ways to prevent osteoporosis would do well to choose this title."

—*Library Journal*

"Your bones are under the constant stress of life, so it's best to take care of them. *Your Bones: How You Can Prevent Osteoporosis & Have Strong Bones for Life—Naturally* is a guide to greater bone health, as Lara Pizzorno advises women how to age with healthy bones, and dispel the myth that women have naturally fragile bones in old age. Warning against the dangers of osteoporosis drugs and the dangers they pose, she encourages old-fashioned diet and exercise for health into the gray years. *Your Bones* is a must for any active woman who wants to stay active."

— *Midwest Book Review*

"Lara Pizzorno emphatically raises the red flag on conventional bone medicine. . . . Highlighting natural prevention and treatment strategies for different situations, *Your Bones* offers uncomplicated scientific advice for bone health."

— *Spirit of Change Magazine*

"Osteoporosis is that sleeping giant that can sneak up on our aging population. Lara Pizzorno finally shines light on this hidden epidemic and what you can do about it. If you are over 50, read this book! Lara, thanks for writing this book. I have given it to my wife."

—WAYNE JONAS, MD, President and CEO, Samueli Institute

"This is a book filled with wisdom and information written in a style which is easy to understand and put to use. I heartily recommend it to all those who care about maintaining a healthy body."

—BERNIE SIEGEL, MD, author of *Faith, Hope & Healing* and *365 Prescriptions For The Soul*

"*Your Bones* is a down-to-earth guide to osteoporosis, one of the most common health challenges of modern life. If you are 30 or older, you cannot afford to ignore the wisdom in this book."

—LARRY DOSSEY, MD, author of *The Science of Premonitions, Healing Words, and Reinventing Medicine*

"This superb text explains the causes and solutions of osteoporosis, and its associated problems, comprehensively, clearly, and accurately. Despite the complexity of the condition, this is an easy read, with no dumbing down of the content—brilliantly highlighting safe, natural, and effective prevention and treatment strategies. Highly recommended."

—LEON CHAITOW, ND, DO, Honorary Fellow,
University of Westminster, London Editor-in-Chief,
Journal of Bodywork & Movement Therapies

"This is one of the best books ever written on bone health—absolutely fantastic! In this book, Lara Pizzorno, MA provides scientifically based advice for men and women of all ages to help them develop and maintain strong healthy bones. She makes a complex issue easily comprehensible and provides information that empowers the reader to take measures towards ensuring their own bone health. I highly recommend it."

—GEORGE MATELJAN, Philanthropist,
author of the book, *The World's Healthiest Foods*

"I found *Your Bones* by Lara Pizzorno to be highly readable, provocative and often persuasive. Do, please, read this book. It is full of startling insights into the nature of age-related bone loss."

—PETER D'ADAMO, ND, MIFHI

"Everything you need to know for healthy bones in one book. Packed with facts, this book is as easy to read as the tips and insights to bone-building living are easy to implement. Informative and inspiring."

—LANI LOPEZ, BHSc, Adv Dip Nat

Your Bones

Your Bones

*How **You** Can Prevent Osteoporosis
& Have Strong Bones For Life—
Naturally*

UPDATED AND EXPANDED EDITION

Lara Pizzorno, MA, LMT
with Jonathan V. Wright, MD

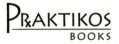

PRAKTIKOS
BOOKS

DISCLAIMER

Ideas and information in this book are based upon the experience and training of the authors and the scientific information currently available. The suggestions in this book are definitely not meant to be a substitute for careful medical evaluation and treatment by a qualified, licensed health professional. The author and publisher do not recommend changing or adding medication or supplements without consulting your personal physician. They specifically disclaim any liability arising directly or indirectly from the use of this book.

Praktikos Books
PO Box 457
Edinburg, VA 22824
888.542.9467   info@praktikosinstitute.org

Praktikos Books are produced in alliance with Axios Press.

Pilates photos © 2013 by Michael Carnagey.
Pilates text (pages 278-298) © 2013 by Nancy Brose and Kristi Quinn.

Library of Congress Cataloging-in-Publication Data

Pizzorno, Lara.
      Your bones : how you can prevent osteoporosis & have strong bones for life-naturally / Lara Pizzorno, MDiv, MA, LMT ; with Jonathan V. Wright, MD—Revised edition.
      pages cm
      Includes bibliographical references and index.
      ISBN 978-1-60766-013-2 (pbk.)
      1. Osteoporosis—Prevention—Popular works. 2. Osteoporosis—Diet therapy—Popular works. 3. Osteoporosis—Nutritional aspects—Popular works. 4. Osteoporosis—Exercise therapy—Popular works. I. Wright, Jonathan V. II. Title.

RC931.O73P53 2013
616.7'16—dc23

                                                                        2012047340

Contents

List of Tables

Preface

WOMEN TODAY ARE REINVENTING what "old age" looks like. You can have strong bones for life, naturally. The photo on the back cover

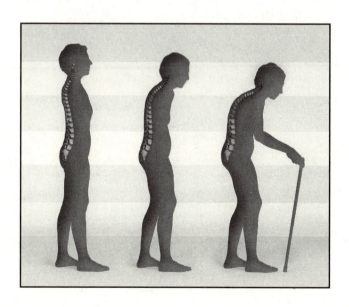

is of me, *Your Bones* co-author Lara, aged 60, on a 2009 Mother's Day hike in Stehekin, Washington. I was diagnosed with osteopenia in my very early 50s. Today, I have strong, healthy bones, which I credit to having done everything recommended in this book. I am genetically at very high risk for osteoporosis, but now I will be the first woman in my family in all the generations I know about not to die an osteoporosis-related death. You too can have strong, healthy bones for life.

PART 1

You Are at Risk for Osteoporosis

CHAPTER 1

If You Are a Woman, You're at High Risk for Osteoporosis

What Is Osteoporosis?

OSTEOPOROSIS—LITERALLY, "POROUS BONE" (OSTEO = bone, porosis = porous)—is a progressive loss of bone that results in bone thinning and increased vulnerability to fracture. Osteoporotic fractures—also called *fragility fractures* because they happen in thinned out, fragile bone—occur primarily in the wrist, rib, spine, and hip, often during daily activities, such as stepping off a curb, which should normally pose no risk for a fracture.[1]

WHY ARE WOMEN AT HIGHER RISK THAN MEN OF LOSING TOO MUCH BONE?

For Two Key Reasons:

First, women start out with less bone than men. Women's peak bone mass is naturally less than men's because women are smaller and have less muscle. When we use our muscles, the muscle contractions put stress on bone, to which it responds by becoming stronger. Men's larger muscles produce stronger contractions, resulting in more stress and approximately 35–40% larger bones.[2]

Secondly, the female hormones, estrogen and progesterone, play vital roles in bone remodeling, and levels of both hormones drop with menopause (medically defined as the last menstrual period); for most women in the Western world, the median age for menopause is 51, but the range for its onset is large—generally between ages 42 and 58. Estrogen prevents excessive action by *osteoclasts*, specialized bone cells that remove worn out or dead bone to make room for new bone. Progesterone is required by *osteoblasts*, the bone-forming cells that pull calcium, magnesium, and phosphorous from the blood to build new bone. Production of both hormones greatly declines during a woman's transition through menopause, resulting in increased bone resorption and decreased formation of new bone.

AM I REALLY AT RISK? HOW COMMON IS OSTEOPOROSIS?

If you are a woman, the answer is emphatically "Yes!" One in four women will develop osteoporosis after menopause. Lifetime risk for fragility fractures, an indicator of osteoporosis, is 50% in women versus 25% in men.[3] Twenty-five million Americans have osteoporosis or are at significant risk for it.[4] Osteoporosis is responsible for at least 1.5 million fractures each year, including 250,000 hip fractures.

MEN ARE NOT IMMUNE TO OSTEOPOROSIS

Although women are most at risk, 25–33% of men will experience an osteoporotic fracture in their lifetime. In men, however, the rapid increase in fracture risk begins later, at approximately age 70.[5]

WHAT ARE MY CHANCES OF RECOVERING FROM A HIP FRACTURE DUE TO OSTEOPOROSIS?

Nearly one-third of all women and one-sixth of all men will suffer an osteoporotic hip fracture. The most catastrophic of fractures, hip fracture leads to death in 12–20% of cases and long-term nursing home care for over 50% of those who survive.

Men fare even worse than women after a hip fracture: a woman's risk of death doubles, a man's risk more than triples.[6] For virtually everyone who suffers an osteoporotic hip fracture, life never returns to "normal."

This is something you definitely want to prevent, and fortunately you can, but *not* by relying on the patent medicines (also called "pharmaceuticals" and/or "drugs") prescribed to prevent osteoporosis.

PART 2

Why Conventional Medicine Is Not the Answer for Strong Bones

CHAPTER 2

The Bisphosphonate Patent Medicines Prescribed to Prevent Osteoporosis Should Be Your *Last* Choice for Healthy Bones

T'S TRUE, AS SALLY FIELD emphasizes in her TV ads for Boniva®, that you have only one body. It's *not* true that Boniva® or the other bisphosphonate patent medicines commonly prescribed to prevent osteoporosis offer the best way to take care of it!

PATENT MEDICINES

Patent medicines are not a "relic of the past"! They've been with us all our lives. The overwhelming number of prescriptions written in the United States for the entire 20th century and thus far in the 21st century have been for written for patented or formerly patented substances. Even though today's gigantic patent medicine companies try their best to disguise this obvious fact by calling their products "pharmaceuticals," they're still just patent medicines under another name.

All patent medicines have the same basic problem by law: a patent can only be "granted" for substances never, ever found in human bodies or anywhere else on planet Earth. Although it sounds strange, it's literally true to say that patent medicines are "extraterrestrial, space alien" substances!

Since our bodies were designed (or evolved) from entirely natural materials, patent medicines are fundamentally incompatible with the design of the human body. It's no wonder more than 100,000 Americans die from patent medications every year, and hundreds of thousands more experience serious adverse effects.[7] By contrast, according to the most recent report of the American Association of Poison Control Centers, not a single American died in 2008 from the use of vitamins, minerals, amino acids, essential fatty acids, hundreds of other supplemental nutrients, or any of thousands of herbal products.[8]

Given this enormous difference in safety, why aren't medical research and medical practice focused on safe and effective natural substances? You've heard of "follow the money"? Here it is again: Because of that patent, no competition is allowed, so patent medicines that cost 98¢ a unit to produce can be (and are) sold for $98 a unit (100 times their cost), or more. Natural substances are also sold at a profit, but competition limits the profit margin to 2 to 3 times cost of production. Predictably, the focus of patent medicine (pharmaceutical) companies is profit, first and foremost. Your health is a secondary goal.

In our opinion, patent medications should always be the last choice for treatment of illness, used only when "body-compatible" natural substances or energies are not available to do the job. Even then, patent medicines should be used with great caution and for the shortest time possible.

The Bisphosphonate Patent Medicines Prescribed for Osteoporosis (e.g., Fosamax®, Actonel®, Boniva®, Reclast®), Have Very Nasty Side Effects

Although prescribed to 30 million Americans each year, the bisphosphonate patent medicines (the oral forms, including Fosamax®, Boniva®, Actonel®, and the latest additions to the bisphosphonate arsenal, the once yearly IV-administered patent medicines Reclast® and Aclasta®), are well known to be dangerous.

An FDA alert, issued January 2008, warned physicians that all bisphosphonate patent medicines may cause "severe and sometimes incapacitating bone, joint, and/or muscle (musculoskeletal) pain . . . [which] may occur within days, months, or years" after starting the medication, and in some patients, may not resolve *even after discontinuing the patent medicine*.[9]

Even more alarming, these patent medicines have now been conclusively linked to a number of other serious adverse side effects including *osteonecrosis of the jaw* (jaw bone death, osteo = bone, necrosis = death), *atrial fibrillation* (irregular heartbeat), and increased risk of bone fragility leading to bone fracture—yes, that's right, an *increased risk of bone fracture from the very patent medicines prescribed to prevent it*!

BISPHOSPHONATES DON'T BUILD HEALTHY, NEW BONE—THEY CAUSE RETENTION OF OLD, BRITTLE BONE

The bisphosphonate patent medicines suppress the activity of *osteoclasts*, the body's specialized cells whose job it is to remove worn out, injured, or otherwise damaged bone. This is a task that must be taken care of before such weakened bone can be replaced with new strong bone.

Osteoclasts are the first phase of the bone renewal process. They take out the bone "trash" to make room for new bone. If osteoclasts are prevented from doing this necessary job—which they very effectively are by bisphosphonates, which work by literally poisoning osteoclasts—damaged bone is left in place rather than cleared out, so no room is made for new bone to be laid down. Eventually, the amount of unhealthy, compromised bone tissue accumulates to the point that bones become very fragile, and any trauma or insult heals poorly, if at all.

The bisphosphonates don't just inhibit, they virtually crush all new bone formation. Researchers at the University of Texas performed bone biopsies on nine women who had been taking Fosamax® for 3 to 8 years, but had nevertheless suffered non-spinal fractures (in the lower back, ribs, hip, or femur) while performing normal daily activities (walking, standing, turning around). New bone formation in these women was nearly *a hundred times lower* than that normally seen in postmenopausal women.[10]

BISPHOSPHONATES CAUSE OSTEONECROSIS OF THE JAW (ONJ)

In the jaw, bisphosphonates' prevention of normal bone remodeling results in the accumulation of dying bone and its eventual exposure to the inside of the mouth, along with greatly increased risk of oral infection—precisely what is seen in women taking bisphosphonates who develop ONJ.

More than 2,000 cases of bisphosphonate-induced ONJ have been reported since 2003. In August 2009, a class action suit was brought against Merck, the pharmaceutical company responsible for Fosamax®, the most widely prescribed of the bisphosphonates. Merck has been accused of failing to adequately warn that this patent medicine may cause ONJ—a highly significant failure for those who have developed ONJ after taking Fosamax® since the condition is extremely difficult to live with, persistent, and responds poorly, if at all, to conventional treatments.

No one, not even Merck, is disputing the growing numbers of reports of ONJ in individuals taking Fosamax® and other bisphosphonates. According to the Mayo Clinic, ONJ occurs in 1 out of every 1,000 women taking a bisphosphonate over the course of one year.[11] Merck has received at least 2,400 reports from people who developed the condition after Fosamax® use.[12] More than 1,000 Fosamax® lawsuits, a number including multiple plaintiffs, have been filed against Merck in both federal and state courts. Merck claims, however, that the relationship between ONJ and Fosa-max® is not a causal one, despite the fact that internal Merck documents and email comments made by one of Merck's own scientists, Dr. Donald B. Kimmel, indicate that bisphosphonates cause ONJ.

In 2005, Dr. Kimmel, who was their director of molecular endocrinology, warned that the severe reduction in bone remodeling caused by the bisphosphonate patent medicines is likely to reduce the jaw's natural ability to heal, and that placing too much of a healing demand on patients treated with bisphosphonates can lead to the death of the jaw bone.[13] Merck claims this was just one of "various theories" Kimmel examined when investigating how ONJ might develop.

One data point is uncontestable—ONJ incidence is increasing and occurs most frequently in older women taking bisphosphonates who have undergone dental work.[14] Merck estimates ONJ occurs in 1.6 individuals per 100,000 taking oral bisphosphonates, but a Kaiser Permanente survey found ONJ occurred in roughly 1 in 1,000 respondents who were still or had previously taken these patent medicines.[15] And new reports of ONJ are appearing in the medical journals virtually every month. As of May 10, 2010, more than 1,100 articles discussing bone death related to bisphosphonate use had been published in the peer-reviewed medical literature. These footnotes, in addition to the others in this section, provide just a tiny selection of some of the recent reports.[16] When we started tracking this, we would see one or two reports every few months. Now, we see several every week!

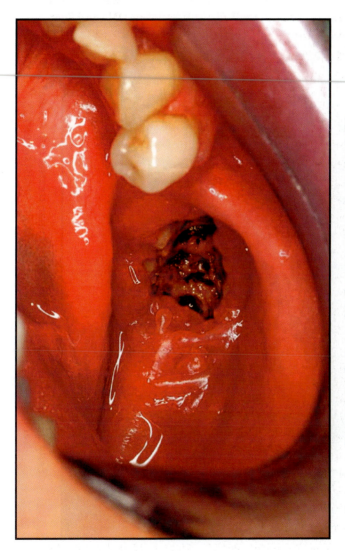

Spontaneous fracture of the lower jaw in woman treated with Aredia® and Zometa® for 24 months (43 years old, breast cancer).

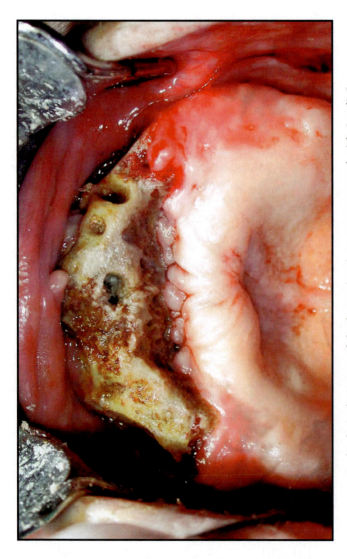

Early clinical picture of the lower jaw in woman treated with Aredia® and Zometa® for 24 months (48 years old, breast cancer)

How Bisphosphonates Cause ONJ

Bisphosphonates accumulate in bones, particularly in the jawbone, and inhibit the bone's natural ability to repair everyday damage by about 90%.[17] The very unpleasant consequences are first apparent in the jaw rather than other bones for several reasons.[18] Bisphosphonates concentrate in the jaw bones because these bones have a greater blood supply than other bones and a faster bone turnover rate, due both to the daily trauma resulting from chewing and the presence of teeth, both of which make daily bone remodeling necessary around the *periodontal ligament*, the ligament that attaches the tooth to its socket in the jawbone.

Many Dentists Will Not Treat Women Taking Bisphosphonates

Even short-term use of oral bisphosphonates significantly increases risk of ONJ following dental work, particularly surgical dental procedures such as root canals or extractions. Sixty percent of all reported cases of ONJ have occurred after dental surgery to treat infections, with the remaining 40% related to infection, denture trauma, or other physical trauma.

In medical circles, Cochrane Reviews are known to be the best single source of scientific evidence about the effects of healthcare interventions. In a Cochrane Review, researchers evaluate the combined results of virtually all the best studies on a topic using rigorous methods carefully designed to prevent bias and errors in interpretation. A Cochrane review of bisphosphonate-related ONJ found that an age of 60 years or older, female sex, and previous invasive dental treatment were the common characteristics of patients taking bisphos-phonates who developed ONJ.[19]

Since the primary target population for bisphos-phonate use is postmenopausal women, many of whom are 60 or older and, as they age, are increas-ingly likely to need some kind of invasive dental pro-cedure, these risk traits for ONJ with bisphosphonate use are far too common for comfort. In fact, they are so common that the American Dental Association has warned dentists to avoid "invasive dental procedures" in patients on IV bisphosphonates and to take a "con-servative" approach to dental procedures for patients taking oral bisphosphonates.

In December 2008, the American Dental Associa-tion updated recommendations for managing patients on oral bisphosphonates by adding a recommendation to dentists to protect themselves by consulting with an attorney to develop an informed consent form for patients taking bisphosphonates that would be certain to satisfy the criteria of the state in which they prac-tice.[20] The American Dental Association's updated rec-ommendations, published November 2011, stress the importance of informing the patient to the fullest extent possible of the risk for ONJ, documenting the discussion and obtaining the patient's written acknowl-edgment of that discussion and consent for the cho-sen course of treatment.[21] Many dentists are becom-ing increasingly reluctant to perform any type of dental work on women taking these patent medicines.[22]

No Cure Exists for ONJ

A key reason for dentists' concern is that bisphos-phonate-related ONJ is extremely difficult to treat.

Affected individuals usually have no symptoms until dying bone becomes infected. Initial symptoms include numbness, heaviness, swelling, pain and infection in the jaw, and loosening of the teeth. Open sores or lesions develop that frequently do not respond to conventional treatments, including debridement (the removal of dead or infected tissue), antibiotics, and hyperbaric oxygen therapy.

Increasing patients' risk of ONJ by prescribing bisphosphonates is far from trivial since, currently, *no definitive cure exists.*[23] Most treatment is only palliative, providing some pain relief without restoring health, and the condition is associated with significant impaired eating ability, pain and disfigurement, resulting in greatly compromised quality of life.[24]

BISPHOSPHONATES PROMOTE CHRONIC ORAL INFECTIONS

Bisphosphonates also contribute to chronic oral infections. Research published in the *Journal of Oral Maxillofacial Surgery* found a direct correlation between bisphosphonate use and the development of *microbial biofilms*, supersized bacterial colonies that cause chronic infections in affected bone.[25]

BISPHOSPHONATES INCREASE RISK FOR ATRIAL FIBRILLATION

A number of recent studies, including a meta-analysis of four studies involving more than 26,000 postmenopausal women, have now reported that bisphosphonates increase risk for "serious atrial fibrillation"— that is, an erratic, irregular heartbeat, by more than

150%.[26] Over the last 20 years, atrial fibrillation has become the most commonly encountered cardiac arrhythmia in clinical practice, accounting for the majority of arrhythmia-related hospital admissions and greatly increasing risk of stroke.[27]

A study published in the *New England Journal of Medicine* in 2007 found Fosamax® increased likelihood of serious atrial fibrillation events by 150%.[28] Data from a more recent study, published in the journal *Menopause* in 2009, show that Fosamax® caused a more than twofold (or 200%) increase in risk for atrial fibrillation.[29] Yet another study, published in the *Archives of Internal Medicine* in 2008, estimates that 3% of *all* atrial fibrillation cases that have occurred since the bisphosphonate patent medicines received FDA approval over 16 years ago may have been due to bisphosphonate [specifically, Fosamax® (alendronate)] therapy, and warns that bisphosphonate use should be closely monitored in populations at high risk of serious adverse effects from atrial fibrillation, which includes patients with heart failure, coronary artery disease, or diabetes.[30]

In other words, those at risk for serious side effects from bisphosphonates include not only women aged 60 and older who might need dental work, but also anyone with heart disease or diabetes—or more than one-third of the entire US adult population.

Bisphosphonates: A Long List of Other Adverse Side Effects

Numerous other adverse effects have also been reported, including:[31]

- **Erosions and ulcerations of the esophagus (throat) and severe damage to the lining of the gastrointestinal tract**

  These are the key reasons for the detailed procedure necessary for taking these patent medicines, which must be consumed with a full 6–8 oz. glass of ordinary (not mineral) water, first thing in the morning after getting out of bed, and at least 30 minutes before ingesting any other food, beverage, or medication, during which time the patient must consume an additional 2 oz. of water and cannot lie down until at least 30 minutes later after food has been consumed.

  The results of the 1-year findings in the Prospective Observational Scientific Study Investigating Bone Loss Experience in the US (POSSIBLE US), published April 2010, showed that 20% of women taking bisphosphonates reported gastrointestinal side effects when they began participating in the study. Side effects frequently became so severe that when the women were questioned again after 6 months, those using bisphosphonates were 139% more likely to have stopped taking the patent medicines.[32]

- **Esophageal Cancer**

  People who take oral bisphosphonates for bone disease for more than five years may be doubling their risk of developing esophageal cancer, according to a study published September 2010 in the *British Medical Journal*.[33] The researchers analyzed data from the UK General Practice Research Database, which includes patient records for around six million people. They focused on men and women aged over 40 years, identifying 2,954 cases of esophageal cancer. Each case was compared with five controls matched for age, sex, general practice, and observation period. People with 10 prescriptions for bisphosphonates—or who had been prescribed bisphosphonates over a period of five years—had nearly double the risk of esophageal cancer compared with people with no bisphosphonate prescriptions.

▪ **Influenza-like illness**

Bisphosphonates may cause a flu-like syndrome, particularly in the early phase of treatment. Onset is sudden, and symptoms commonly include fever, shivering, chills, dry cough, loss of appetite, body aches, and nausea.[34]

▪ **Myalgia (severe muscle pain)**

In clinical trials, approximately 4% of patients treated with Fosamax® (alendronate) developed muscle, bone, or joint pain. The time to onset of severe muscle pain varied from one day to several months after starting treatment. When patients stopped taking alendronate, their myalgia usually—but not always—went away.[35]

▪ **Deterioration of kidney function and kidney failure**

Studies have shown the bisphosphonates, especially zoledronic acid (sold under the trade names of Zometa® and Reclast®), are toxic to the kidneys. The peer-reviewed medical studies show kidney function is harmed in 8.8–15.2% of patients given zoledronic acid.[36]

- **Symptomatic hypocalcemia (too little calcium in the circulation)**

  This can cause seizures, gastric achlorhydria (too little stomach acid to be able to properly digest food), dementia, dangerously low blood pressure, bronchospasm (when the bands of muscle around the airways tighten uncontrollably, as in asthma), and heart failure.

  Reports of symptomatic hypocalcemia are increasing in patients receiving the latest additions to the bisphosphonates, Reclast® and Aclasta®. These patent medicines, which contain zoledronic acid and must be given intravenously, are being promoted as a more "convenient" way to prevent osteoporosis since they are so potent, so poisonous to the normal functioning of osteoclasts, that they are administered only once a year.[37]

- **Bone stress fracture**

  Wait a minute, isn't this what these patent medicines are supposed to prevent? The peer-reviewed research, published in top medical journals on this adverse side effect of bisphosphonates, is discussed next, and proves that bisphosphonates actually *increase* fracture risk.[38]

BISPHOSPHONATES *INCREASE* FRACTURE RISK

Starting in 2005, studies began appearing showing that bisphosphonates' suppression of normal bone remodeling increases fracture risk in as little as 2½ years.

In 2005, in what is called a "case series" in the medical journals, physicians working at the same hospital reported on nine patients who, after 3 to 8 years on Fosamax®, experienced fractures "while performing normal daily activities such as walking, standing, or turning around." In six of these patients, all of whom were told to continue to take Fosamax® after their fracture, healing was delayed, taking from 3 months to *2 years longer* than the time normally expected for healing.[39]

A case report in 2007 alerted physicians that two hospitals had seen 13 women (average age 66.9 years) who suffered thighbone fractures with minimal or no trauma—in other words, during normal daily activities—during a 10-month period (May 2005 to February 2006). Nine of these women had been taking Fosamax®, several for as little as 2½ years.[40]

In another case series, published in 2008, researchers looked at the records of patients admitted to a Level 1 trauma center over a five-year period. They found that low-energy thighbone fractures (i.e., fractures occurring during normal daily activities) with a specific, uncommon *transverse* (crosswise) pattern were associated with Fosamax® use. This is especially concerning since the thighbone is the thickest, strongest bone in the body.

Seventy patients with this type of low-energy thighbone fracture (59 women, 11 men, average age 74.7 years) were identified. Of these, 25 were taking

Fosamax®, and 19 of them suffered a low-energy thighbone fracture with the same unusual pattern. In contrast, only one patient not being treated with Fosamax® had this fracture pattern, which translates to a 98% increased risk for this uncommon type of fracture in patients taking Fosamax®.

While most of the patients experiencing this uncommon type of thigh bone fracture had been taking Fosamax® longer than those who did not have this type of fracture (6.9 years versus 2.5 years, respectively), one patient in this study had been taking Fosamax® for less than 4 years. Thus, although it is clearly true that the longer a woman takes a bisphosphonate, the greater her accumulation of brittle bone and risk of fracture during normal daily activity, in some people, unhealthy bone accumulates much more quickly.

Researchers think that the increased risk of thighbone fracture during normal activity seen with Fosamax® is a result of the accumulation of tiny stress fractures whose healing is prevented by the patent medicine's suppression of osteoclast activity and microdamage repair.[41] In lab animals, Fosamax® increased the number of microcracks by 2- to 7-fold, and a study involving 66 postmenopausal women with osteoporosis found 30% more microdamage in the bones of those taking Fosamax®.[42]

In 2009, physicians at the University Hospitals of Geneva, Switzerland, voiced concerns to the Swiss National Pharmacovigilance Centre about bisphosphonates' long-term harmful effects after admitting a series of eight patients who had been treated with bisphosphonates to their regional hospital for low-energy thighbone fractures. Some of these patients had been on Fosamax® for as little as 16 months; one had been on Boniva® only 4 months.[43]

Numerous papers are now reporting that bisphosphonates' repression of bone turnover actually promotes the accumulation of microcracks and the occurrence of unexpected stress fractures, characteristically at the subtrochanter of the femur (below the trochanter but in the upper part of the body of the thigh bone, see images on pages 30 and 31).[44] In some especially unfortunate individuals, these fragility fractures are occurring in both femurs simultaneously!* [45]

The question researchers are now asking is, "How long can a person take bisphosphonates before these patent medicines *cause* a fragility fracture?" The current estimate is a maximum of five years.[46]

In 2008, the FDA questioned Merck about increasing reports of femur fractures spontaneously occurring in women taking Fosamax® during normal daily activities. It took Merck more than a year to respond, but 16 months later, they very quietly added "low energy femoral shaft and subtrochanteric fractures" to the list of possible side effects in the patent medicine's package insert.

According to ABC News senior health and medical editor, Dr. Richard Besser, neither Merck nor the FDA made any effort to inform doctors or the public that all the bisophosphonates—including not just Fosamax®, but Actonel®, Boniva®, and Reclast®—*cause* fractures.

---

* The numerous endnotes listed in this citation are just a representative sampling, taken from among dozens of papers now appearing in the peer-reviewed medical literature on this highly negative outcome of bisphosphonate use.

Both the FDA and Merck refused a request by ABC News for an interview, although the FDA announced in a drug safety communication issued March 10, 2010, that they would look into whether there is an increased risk of "atypical subtrochanteric femur fractures" in women using bisphosphonates.[47]

Following their review of all available data on bisphosphonate use, on October 13, 2010, FDA issued a bulletin[48] warning patients and health care providers that all the bisphosphonates prescribed for osteoporosis increase risk for atypical thigh bone fractures and announced that the bisphosphonates must change their labeling and include a Medication Guide to ensure physician and patient awareness of this risk. The FDA bulletin includes two recommendations: (1) that health care professionals reevaluate the need for continued bisphosphonate use in patients who have been taking these patent medicines for longer than five years, and (2) that patients taking bisphosphonates report any new thigh or groin pain to their health care provider and be evaluated for a possible femur fracture. Patients and health care professionals are asked to report side effects with bisphosphonate use to the FDA's MedWatch Adverse Event Reporting program at www.fda.gov/MedWatch or by calling 800-332-1088.

Not only do the bisphosphonates increase risk of femur fracture, but they also greatly increase the likelihood that the broken bone will not heal. In June 2009, a study involving 19,731 patients with thighbone fractures was conducted at Harvard Medical School to evaluate the effects of bisphosphonates on bones' ability to heal. Bisphosphonate use more than doubled the risk of "nonunion"—medical jargon

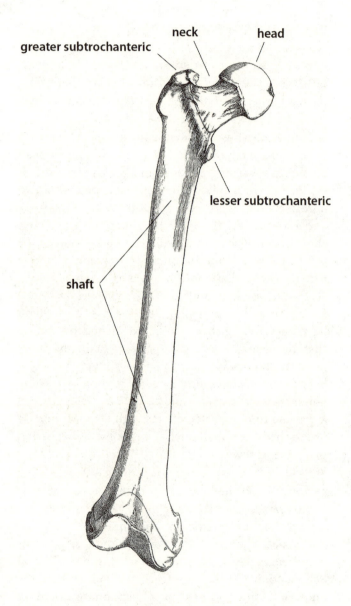

Diagram of femur

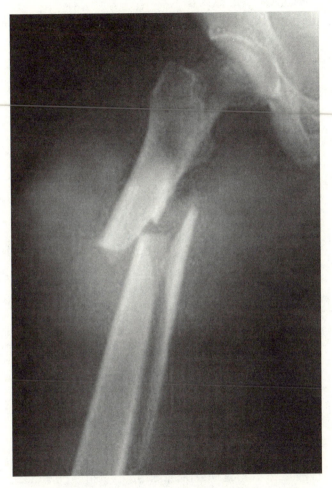

X-ray* showing fracture in the upper half of Dr. Jennifer
Schneider's right femur caused by a subway car jolt
following 7 years of Fosamax® treatment.

---

* Courtesy of Dr. Schneider, from *Stay Young and Sexy with Bio-Identical
Hormone Replacement* (Petaluma, CA: Smart Publications, 2010).

meaning the bone had become incapable of re-joining and could not heal.[49]

What we are now seeing is simply the result of the fact that many women have now been taking bisphosphonates long enough to do very serious damage to their bones. Class action lawsuits brought as a result of bisphosphonate-related osteonecrosis of the jaw are now underway on three continents and are thought to be "a worrying precursor for millions of other consumers who will soon reach the five-year oral half-life of bisphosphonates," which is when the adverse effects of these patent medicines typically begin to become apparent.[50]

Reports of spontaneous fractures will continue to increase until many more class action lawsuits have been brought against the patent medicine companies responsible. Don't wait until the FDA and Merck are forced to acknowledge the harm done to millions of women. If you are taking a bisphosphonate, stop! If your doctor is telling you to start taking any of these patent medicines, refuse—and give him or her a copy of this book, so you can get on a safe bone-building program that works!

BISPHOSPHONATES AND BREAST CANCER

In women with advanced breast cancer that has metastasized to bone, some research suggests that bisphosphonates may be of sufficient benefit to offset their risks *if used short term.*

Cancer cells produce osteoclast-activating factors that play a role in the pathogenesis of bone cancer. Since bisphosphonates poison osteoclasts, these patent medicines may be helpful *in women with advanced breast cancer that has metastasized to bone.*

In some studies, the IV bisphosphonate zoledronate (marketed under the trade names Aclasta®, Reclast®, Zometa®, Zomera®), has been shown to reduce bone pain, help prevent fracture and spinal cord compression, and improve quality of life. However, with the increasing use of bisphosphonates for metastatic bone disease has also come to light the fact that these patent medicines have toxic effects, including ONJ,* that greatly promote morbidity in patients with advanced cancer.[51]

Since even in women without cancer, bisphosphonate therapy, especially with zoledronte (marketed under the trade names Aclasta®, Reclast®, Zometa®, Zomera®) taken for longer than two years, greatly increases risk of ONJ, medical authorities do not recommend the use of bisphosphonates for women with early stage breast cancer.

Oral bisphosphonates have been used to help lessen bone loss in postmenopausal women with estrogen-receptor positive breast cancer who have been prescribed patent medicines called aromatase-inhibitors. *Aromatase* is an enzyme involved in the formation of the most potent form of estrogen, *estradiol*, which can contribute to the progression of hormone positive breast cancer. However, since estrogen plays an important role in preventing excessive bone loss, aromatase-inhibiting patent medicines also promote bone loss, greatly increasing risk of osteoporosis.

Recently, two studies have suggested that bisphosphonates may be linked to a reduction in breast cancer risk. One study using data from the Women's Health Initiative found 32% fewer cases of invasive breast

---

* See previous images on pages 17 and 18.

cancer in women who used bisphosphonates. The second, an Israeli study, found that more than five years of bisphosphonate use was associated with a 29% reduction in risk of postmenopausal breast cancer. Whether these associations are simply coincidence or really indicate that bisphosphonates may help reduce breast cancer risk remains unknown. All the experts agree that more studies are necessary to find out.[52]

But why should women even consider risking the serious side effects clearly associated with all the bisphosphonates when there are completely safe and effective ways to reduce breast cancer risk—and improve overall health—using research-proven diet, supplement, and lifestyle choices with *no* toxic side effects?

Even in women with breast cancer, supplementation with the naturally occurring mineral, strontium, which not only reduces bone resorption but stimulates the formation of healthy new bone (especially when combined with calcium and other nutrients necessary for bone re-mineralization, such as vitamins D and K_2), does a much better job of building healthy bone than bisphosphonates any day! [53]

More Evidence Confirms Bisphosphonates (e.g., Fosamax®, Reclast®, Aclasta®, Actonel®, Boniva®) Are NOT Your Bones' Best Friends

Since the publication of the first edition of *Your Bones* in April 2011, a great deal more evidence has surfaced confirming that your risk of an osteoporotic fracture is not going to be lessened—but, in fact, may be increased, by taking any of the bisphosphonates.

As of April 2012, 630 papers had been published in the peer-reviewed medical literature on PubMed discussing adverse events caused by the bisphosphonates, including 201 review articles. (These are papers that summarize a number of studies in one article.) Here's a quick overview of just a small selection from the important recently published papers that provide many reasons why relying on a bisphosphonate, like Fosamax®, Boniva®, or Reclast®, is more likely to harm you rather than help your bones.

BISPHOSPHONATES NOT HELPFUL, MAY HARM, WOMEN WITH BREAST CANCER

Cancer cells stimulate osteoblasts (the cells that break down old bone), thus increasing the rate at which bone is lost. Plus, when old bone is broken down, bone-derived growth factors are released that nearby cancer cells could possibly co-opt for their own growth. So, it was hypothesized that giving women with early stage breast cancer a bisphosphonate along with chemo might help preserve their bone mass, reduce their likelihood of dying and, if treatment were successful, of having a recurrence of their cancer.

Unfortunately, this hope has not panned out.

Results of a large, randomized trial involving 3,360 women with early stage breast cancer, published in the *New England Journal of Medicine,* October 13, 2011, found that adding zoledronic acid (an IV-delivered bisphosphonate, trade names Reclast®, Aclasta®) to adjuvant chemotherapy in patients with early-stage breast cancer not only does *not* improve rates of recurrence or survival, but can *cause* osteonecrosis of the jaw (ONJ), death of the jawbone.[54]

FOSAMAX® CONTINUES TO SUPPRESS NORMAL BONE REBUILDING IN THE SPINE FOR AT LEAST 1 YEAR AFTER STOPPING TREATMENT

In this study, published in the journal *Osteoporosis International* October 8, 2011, postmenopausal women who had taken Fosamax® for at least three years discontinued treatment and were checked six months and one year later. Bone remodeling in their lumbar spines (lower back) was still suppressed after one year, and their spinal bone mineral density was significantly decreased.

What this means is an increased risk for a spinal fracture. How long will it take before the lumbar spine begins to rebuild in these women? No one knows.

The study authors' conclusion: "Further clinical studies are required to fully evaluate the persistence of BP [bisphosphonate] treatment." Our conclusion: you have to be nuts to take these patent medicines![55]

FDA WARNS DOCTORS: DO NOT USE THE BISPHOSPHONATE, ZOLEDRONIC ACID (RECLAST®, ACLASTA®) IN PERSONS WITH KIDNEY DISEASE

After cases of acute renal failure requiring dialysis or having a fatal outcome (PR-speak for "the patient died") following Reclast® use were reported to the FDA, the agency demanded labeling for this bisphosphonate be revised to state: "Reclast® is contraindicated in patients with creatinine clearance less than 35 mL/min or in patients with evidence of acute renal impairment."[56]

What's creatinine? Creatinine is a breakdown or waste product from creatine phosphate in muscle.

Creatine phosphate is a compound that provides a rapidly accessible source of high-energy phosphates in our muscles and brain, and is usually produced at a fairly constant rate by the body. (The energy currency our cells use, ATP, stands for adenosine triphosphate.) When creatine phosphate is used to produce ATP, creatinine is a resulting byproduct that is excreted from the body via the kidneys.

The creatinine clearance rate is the rate at which a person's kidneys are able to filter out or clear this creatinine from the blood passing through them and is considered an accurate indication of how well the kidneys are able to do their filtering job overall. A creatine clearance rate of less than 35 mL/min indicates that clearance is too slow—in other words, that kidney function is impaired. *Many* patent medicines, including the bisphosphonates, are eliminated through the kidneys.

The revised label also tells healthcare professionals to be sure to screen people before administering Reclast® to ensure they have identified "at-risk patients". So, who is "at risk" of renal failure from Reclast® besides folks with a creatinine clearance less than 35 mL/min? Anyone using potentially kidney-damaging (nephrotoxic) patent medicines at the time Reclast® is given.

Whoa! *Many* commonly taken patent medicines are potentially nephrotoxic, including non-steroidal anti-inflammatory patent medicines (e.g., acetaminophen [Tylenol®], ibuprofen [Advil®, Motrin®], aspirin), and patent medicines taken for high blood pressure (e.g., ACE inhibitors, Angiotensin Receptor Blockers, diuretics). "At risk" folks also include people who are dehydrated either before or after Reclast® is given. Among older individuals (aged 65 and older), the sense of thirst is often diminished, and dehydration is all too common.[57]

BISPHOSPHONATES MAY CAUSE HYPOCALCEMIA

As mentioned on pages 86–92, calcium plays many other vital roles in our bodies in addition to serving as a key component of our bones. Hypocalcemia is the medical term for low blood levels of calcium, which cause electrolyte disturbances and disruption of nervous system functioning. In medical school, doctors-to-be are given the mnemonic "CATS go numb" to help them remember the key presenting symptoms for hypocalcemia. These are convulsions, cardiac arrhythmias (erratic heartbeat), tetany (involuntary muscle contractions, including laryngospasms, which are spasms of the vocal chords that prevent breathing), and numbness/parasthesias in hands, feet, around mouth and lips. Parasthesias, tingling "pins and needles" sensations around the mouth and lips, and in the hands and feet, are often the first symptom of hypocalcemia, which is taken quite seriously since it can cause death.

Bisphosphonates induce hypocalcaemia, both by their poisoning of osteoclasts (thus preventing them from removing old bone, which releases calcium into the bloodstream), and also by increasing the maturation of osteoblasts present, not in normal healthy bone, but in bone cancers. Bisphosphonates increase not only the production of osteoblasts in bone cancers, but their activity in cancerous bone. Thus, doctors are being warned that patients with bone-metastatic prostate cancer may be more susceptible to symptomatic hypocalcaemia following bisphosphonate therapy, and studies are just now being designed to identify risk factors for hypocalcemia in these patients.[58]

ORAL BISPHOSPHONATES INCREASE RISK FOR ESOPHAGEAL CANCER

This adverse effect of the bisphosphonates had been noted earlier, but was strongly denied by the patent medicine companies. The results of this study, published in 2010, are going to be harder to discount.

A study of almost six million people that was conducted in Great Britain involved 2,954 men and women over age 40 with esophageal cancer. Incidence of esophageal cancer was 30% greater in people with one or more previous prescriptions for oral bisphosphonates compared to those with no such prescriptions. In people who had been given 10 or more prescriptions for an oral bisphosphonate, risk for esophageal cancer was increased 93%. Use of an oral bisphosphonate for more than 3 years increased risk an average of 224%. (Note, this was the *average* increase in risk, the range ran from 147% to 343%!)

Risk for esophageal cancer did not differ significantly by bisphosphonate type—all the bisphosphonates increased risk. And risk in those with 10 or more bisphosphonate prescriptions did not vary by age, sex, smoking, alcohol intake, or body mass index; by diagnosis of osteoporosis, fracture, or upper gastrointestinal disease; or by prescription of acid suppressants, non-steroidal anti-inflammatory patent medicines, or corticosteroids. Risk increased in everyone taking any bisphosphonate.[59]

ORAL BISPHOSPHONATES CAUSE CONJUCTIVITIS, UVEITIS AND SCLERITIS— INFLAMMATORY EYE DISEASES

Inflammatory eye diseases, including conjunctivitis, uveitis and scleritis, are now being noted in patients taking oral bisphosphonates and have been conclusively linked to the use of these patent medicines. Conjunctivitis (aka "pink eye") is inflammation of the conjunctiva (the outermost layer of the eye and the inner surface of the eyelid), and produces a gritty, burning sensation in the eye. Its most common causes are viral or bacterial infections, or an allergic reaction. Now we can add bisphosphonates to the list of suspects. While typically not serious, conjunctivitis is extremely unpleasant and may require treatment with antibiotics. When bisphosphonates are the cause, only discontinuation of their use will cure the condition.[60]

Uveitis and scleritis are much more serious. Uveitis, inflammation of the middle layer of the eye, is estimated to be responsible for approximately 10% of the blindness in the United States and requires urgent referral to an ophthalmologist for treatment to control the inflammation. Scleritis, inflammation of the sclera or white of the eye, is a condition for which treatment is less urgent, but is also a serious inflammatory eye disease that typically requires treatment with corticosteroids and may necessitate eye surgery. Severe cases of scleritis can also result in blindness.

In April 2012, a retrospective study was published of British Columbia residents who had visited an ophthalmologist from 2000 to 2007 (934,147 people), and this group included 10,827 first-time users of oral bisphosphonates. Bisphosphonate users had a 45% elevated risk of uveitis and a 51% increased risk for scleritis. The paper concludes with the warning: "Patients taking bisphosphonates must be familiar with the signs and symptoms of these conditions, so that they can immediately seek assessment by an ophthalmologist."[61]

ORAL BISPHOSPHONATES INCREASE RISK FOR MANY INFLAMMATORY JAW DISEASES, NOT JUST ONJ

Danish researchers compared the incidence of inflammatory jaw diseases—osteomyelitis (inflammation of bone marrow inside the jawbone), osteitis (inflammation of the alveolar socket that surrounds the teeth), periostitis (inflammation of the connective tissue surrounding the jawbone), and sequestrum (when a piece of dead bone separates from the remaining normal bone as it is dying)—between Danish patients who had been prescribed oral bisphosphonates to treat osteoporosis (103,562 people) and those who had not used a bisphosphonate (310,683 people) between 1996 and 2006. After adjusting for a variety of factors that might have increased risk for inflammatory jaw disease, such as diabetes and chemotherapy, alendronate (Fosamax®) was found to more than triple risk of inflammatory jaw disease, and etidronate (Didronel®) more than doubled the risk.[62]

BISPHOSPHONATES DO CAUSE "ATYPICAL" FEMUR FRACTURES—NO DOUBT ABOUT IT!

When the first edition of *Your Bones* was published in 2011, Merck was still claiming that bisphosphonates were not the cause of an unusual fracture of the femur that had begun to literally pop up in an increasing number of people who had been taking these patent medicines for several years. Now the papers being published in the medical journals are telling physicians what the x-ray features are of these, not all that infrequently seen, femur fractures.[63]

Here's the description of these "atypical femur fractures" in medical-speak: "A common radiographic pattern has been identified, namely a simple transverse fracture with unicortical beaking occurring through an area of hypertrophic lateral cortex."

Radiologists are being urged to look for this pattern since it has been noted that in patients in whom one femur has suffered an "atypical" femur fracture, compliments of a bisphosphonate, the other femur is highly likely to have also deteriorated and to be at greatly increased risk of breaking. Doctors are now being told to be sure to check the other "contralateral" leg, so if it's getting ready to break, "prophylactic internal fixation," i.e., surgery to install a pin for support, can be performed before it breaks as well. Cessation of "bisphosphonate therapy" is also strongly recommended.[64]

Research published February 2011 in the aptly named journal, *Injury*, comments on the "recent surge in interest on bisphosphonate-related femoral fractures," which prompted National University Hospital in Singapore to look at the records of patients over age 60 admitted for femur fractures between January 2003 and 2007. All of the patients who had taken alendronate (Fosamax®) exhibited the same "atypical" fracture pattern described above, and all had complained of thigh pain three weeks to as long as two years before the fracture. The conclusion of the study reads: "Low-impact femoral shaft fractures in elderly patients on long-term alendronate therapy represent a new entity of insufficiency fractures, with characteristic low-impact modes of injury and fracture patterns on radiograph. Prodromal [literally, precursor or early symptom] thigh pain is a warning sign for impending fracture in this group of patients and should be evaluated closely."[65]

A number of other recent papers are also warning physicians about these "atypical" fractures and recommending patients taking any of the bisphosphonates be told to immediately report thigh pain since this can signal an impending fracture, that fractures can occur with complete absence of any trauma, and that both femurs may break at once![66] This paper by Nieves and Cosman, published in *Current Osteoporosis Reports* in March 2010, is especially disconcerting since, after noting that the bisphosphonates cause thigh bones to break, and outlining the x-ray features that will confirm this has occurred, this article concludes with the following statement: "There is no rationale to withhold bisphosphonate therapy from patients with osteoporosis, although continued use of bisphosphonate therapy beyond a treatment period of 3 to 5 years should be re-evaluated annually." WHAT? The possibility of having both your femurs break during normal daily activities in complete absence of any trauma is insufficient reason to recommend against taking a bisphosphonate?

Too many papers have come out in the last two years reporting the numerous adverse effects of the bisphosphonates (oral and IV) to discuss them all, but here are a few highlights:

- Atypical femur fractures are showing up— not just in women, but also in men given bisphosphonates.[67]

■ Increasing reports of "non-traumatic stress fractures in bilateral femoral shafts." (This is "medspeak" for both thigh bones break at once for no
apparent reason—except bisphosphonate use!)[68]

So many case reports and single studies have told
of adverse events caused by bisphosphonates that
numerous reviews have been published to summarize
many of these papers in one article. A PubMed scan
for reviews discussing bisphosphonate-caused adverse
events produced 201 papers as of April 9, 2012. If you
would like to read some of the papers coming out in
the medical journals, please refer to the endnotes
listed under this paragraph's citation number.[69]

If you look at these review articles and begin with
the earliest ones, then progress to the most recent,
you will notice a clear pattern: first, it is denied that
the bisphosphonates might cause the adverse effect,
then it is said that causality is uncertain but may exist,
then the claim changes to "bisphosphonates cause
this adverse event, but occurrence is rare," and finally,
we are told that bisphosphonates cause this adverse
event, e.g., osteonecrosis of the jaw, atypical femur
fractures, and that doctors should inform patients of
this risk and watch for any of the signs of impending
adverse outcome, e.g., thigh pain, which may indicate
impending femur fracture.

Bisphosphonate-related osteonecrosis of the jaw
(ONJ, also now given the acronym BRONJ in the medical literature) is a good example. First they told us it
didn't exist, then they told us it was extremely rare, now
they are telling us precisely how bisphosphonates cause
it and that our genetic inheritance may increase our risk
by 580%. A recent review of case reports and cohort
studies published in the *Journal of Dental Research* found

bisphosphonate use is strongly associated with ONJ: odds ratios of 299.5 for IV bisphosphonates and 12.2 for oral bisphosphonates. This means with IV bisphosphonate use, you are 229.5 times more likely to develop ONJ, and with oral bisphosphonates, you are 12.2 times more likely to develop ONJ. Even when cancer patients were excluded, bisphosphonate use still produced an odds ratio of 7.2 for producing ONJ. Higher risk of ONJ began within two years of bisphosphonate use and increased four-fold after two years.[70] Again, there are way too many papers coming out now to list them all, but here's a sampling of the recent papers discussing bisphosphonate-caused ONJ:[71]

- Bisphosphonates (alendronate [Fosamax®]; risedronate [Actonel®]) given via weekly injection caused so many adverse effects within three months of the onset of a two year study of 198 postmenopausal women with osteoporosis (T scores ≤ 2.5) in Malaysia that many refused to continue. At the conclusion of the study, 36 participants (20%) had quit therapy, 19 (10.6%) did not come to the clinic follow-up (one would assume this means they also quit), and 53 (26.8%) did not come in even for the bone mineral density scan.[72]

- A Working Group of the European Society on Clinical and Economic Aspects of Osteoporosis and Osteoarthritis and the International Osteoporosis Foundation reviewed the evidence that long-term treatment with bisphosphonates causes subtrochanteric (femur) fractures. Their findings: An estimated one per 1,000 patients on a bisphosphonate will suffer an "atypical subtrochanteric fracture" caused by the bisphosphonate. Physicians are told to "remain vigilant in assessing their patients treated with bisphosphonates for the treatment or prevention of osteoporosis and to advise patients of the potential risks."[73]

■ A nationwide cohort study from Denmark whose results were published in March 2011 compared risk of "atypical femur fracture" in all users of bisphosphonates between 1996 and 2006 (103,562 people) with risk for an "atypical femur fracture" among age-and-sex-matched controls in the general population (310,683 individuals). Adjustments were made for prior fracture, use of systemic hormone therapy, and use of systemic corticosteroids. Alendronate (Fosamax®) was found to have a hazard ratio of 2.41, which means it more than doubled risk of subtrochanteric fractures. Etidronate almost doubled fracture risk (hazard ratio = 1.96), but the hands down winner here was clodronate (marketed as Bonefos®, Loron®, and Clodron®); this bisphosphonate increased risk for "atypical femur fracture" by a factor of 20! (HR = 20.0)[74]

■ Even patients taking bisphosphonates who have *no symptoms* may have "incomplete atypical femoral fractures." In May 2012, researchers at the Department of Radiology, Hospital for Joint Diseases, New York University School of Medicine, published the results of a study in which they examined 200 femur x-rays in 100 patients who had been on bisphosphonates for 3 or more years (93 women and 7 men, ranging in age from 47–94 years). They discovered that two of these asymptomatic patients, who were only 50 and

57 years old, actually had "incomplete" atypical femur fractures. One of the women had "incomplete atypical femur fractures" in both her legs. The researchers note that two out of 100 patients is a much higher incidence rate than has yet been reported in the medical literature. What does this mean? If you are taking a bisphosphonate, even if you have no symptoms, your femurs may actually still be partially broken already, and obviously, on their way to a complete break.[75]

THE LATEST FDA ADVISORY COMMITTEE BULLETIN: LIMIT BISPHOSPHONATE USE TO A MAXIMUM OF 3 YEARS—LONGER USE MAY CAUSE ATYPICAL FEMUR FRACTURES, ONJ, ESOPHAGEAL CANCER

On September 9, 2011, a joint FDA advisory committee meeting of the Advisory Committee for Reproductive Health Patent Medicines, and the Patent Medicine Safety and Risk Management Advisory Committee, was held in response to these increasing reports of adverse events—including "atypical femur fractures, osteonecrosis of the jaw, and esophageal cancer"—caused by the bisphosphonates. The question raised was, should the FDA change the label on all the bisphosphonates to lessen the amount of time for which these patent medicines should be approved for use from five to a maximum of three years?

Current labeling for the bisphosphonates states that clinical data on each patent medicine's safety and effectiveness is of limited duration—one to four years, depending on the product—and no optimal duration of therapy is known. The labeling states that patients' need for therapy should be reevaluated "on a periodic basis." The National Osteoporosis Foundation recommends bisphosphonates be used in osteopenic patients only when their 10-year fracture risk exceeds 3% for the hip or 20% for a major osteoporotic fracture. FDA has stated that bisphosphonates' fracture-prevention efficacy is limited to five years with no additional benefits related to osteoporotic fractures after that time.

The panel heard from women who were taking bisphosphonates to prevent osteoporosis when suddenly, during normal activities, their femurs (thigh bones)—very painfully—broke. One woman was standing on a subway train. When it came to a halt and her weight transferred onto one leg, its femur snapped, and she collapsed. Other women related similar stories—a teacher reaching for something in class, a grandmother taking a big step towards her grandchild, a woman just walking outside her front door to pick up the morning newspaper. In each case, despite the complete absence of any trauma or excessive stress, their femurs just snapped.

The panel was also concerned with bisphosphonates' link to "deterioration of the jawbone." In 2005, the FDA added a warning on bisphosphonates about osteonecrosis of the jaw, a supposedly rare disease. Data presented to the panel, however, indicate that risk for osteonecrosis of the jaw is not so rare and increases significantly after four years or more of bisphosphonate use. Why the jaw is especially susceptible to harm from bisphosphonates is explained in the section "How Bisphosphonates Cause ONJ."*

Other data indicate a link between long-term use of bisphosphonates and esophageal cancer. A study

---

* Page 19.

published in 2009 in the *New England Journal of Medicine* used data from FDA's Adverse Event Reporting System to identify and describe 23 patients taking Fosamax® who were diagnosed with esophageal cancer.

After hearing all this, what do you think the committee did? The majority (17–6) voted to endorse a label change, restricting bisphosphonate use to a maximum of three years.

To quote Sonia Hernandez Diaz, MD, associate professor of epidemiology at Harvard School of Public Health: "What we're talking about today is using these patent medicines for more than three years, and I'm not convinced at all that there are any good data that, even for subgroups of patients, they should be continued [past three years]."[76]

Another member of the panel, Kathleen Horner, clinical pharmacy specialist in ambulatory care at the University of Iowa Hospitals and Clinics, suggested that a so-called patent medicine holiday of two to five years may be an option for patients who have taken a bisphosphonate for at least two years with good adherence to the regimen, have not suffered a fracture, and whose bone mineral density is in the osteopenic or normal range. "There's not really data out there to support or not support this idea of a patent medicine holiday. But I think it's reasonable to try," said Horner. The advisory committee discussed patent medicine holidays but concluded that there is insufficient evidence about whether the strategy is beneficial or harmful. Doesn't this "no real data, but reasonable to try" FDA approach to experimenting with our lives concern you?

Translation—at best—when you take a bisphosphonate, even FDA now admits that you are placed at increased risk of ONJ, atypical femur fracture, esophageal cancer, musculoskeletal pain, and kidney toxicity—and they forgot to mention a few other items appearing in the research such as atrial fibrillation (erratic heartbeat, which significantly boosts risk of heart attack), scleritis and uveitis (eye inflammatory diseases that can cause blindness). If you escape all this—and whether you will is truly a crap shoot—what have the bisphosphonates done for you? They have poisoned your osteoclasts, preventing normal bone remodeling and left you with increasingly brittle, fracture-prone bones. And after a maximum of five years, you can expect no further "benefit."

MAJORITY OF PATIENTS ARE NOT BEING INFORMED OF THE REAL RISKS ASSOCIATED WITH THE BISPHOSPHONATES

In 2003, the first case reports appeared describing bisphosphonate-induced osteonecrosis of the jaw (BRONJ). So the patent medicine companies profiting from the bisphosphonates have been aware of this highly adverse effect for at least 10 years; however, don't expect them to help get the word out about the risks associated with these (or any) patent medicine any time soon. Unfortunately, many physicians rely on information provided by the patent medicine reps whose job it is to get them to prescribe more patent medicines, e.g., bisphosphonates, so they may not be as aware as we would wish of information meriting a warning to their patients.

In a recent study, 62% of patients received most of their knowledge about their prescribed bisphosphonate from the package insert. Despite knowing that the patient was being given a bisphosphonate, 80% of dental treatments were continued without modifications. Only 32% of patients who received intravenous bisphosphonate treatment were aware of their possible risks of developing ONJ, even though the IV versions of the bisphosphonates have a much worse risk profile for causing ONJ than the oral forms. (As noted above, the odds ratio for IV bisphosphonates causing ONJ is a whopping 299.5 versus the much lower, although still not inconsequential, odds ratio of 12.2 for the oral forms.)[77] We wrote *Your Bones* so that YOU would not be among the uninformed.

COMBINATION OF MICRONUTRIENTS FOR BONE (COMB) STUDY PROVES NATURAL APPROACH BETTER THAN PATENT MEDICINES

In February 2012, right after the annual meeting of the American Academy of Orthopaedic Surgeons officially warned doctors that the bisphosphonates increase risk for "atypical femur fractures," the results of the one-year long Combination of Micronutrients for Bone (COMB) Study were published in the prestigious *Journal of Environmental and Public Health*.[78] The COMB study unequivocally demonstrated that providing our bones with the nutrients they need along with regular weight-bearing exercise is as or more effective than any of the bisphosphonates or strontium ranelate,* and a lot less expensive!

---

* Strontium ranelate is the unnatural patent medicine version of natural strontium. The many reasons you do not want to take strontium ranelate, but should consider including a natural form of strontium (e.g., strontium citrate) in your bone-building program, are discussed on pages 248–256.

What was the protocol utilized in the COMB Study? Daily vitamin D_3 (2,000 IU), DHA (250 mg), K_2 (in the form of MK-7,100 mcg), strontium citrate (680 mg), magnesium (25 mg), and dietary calcium. In addition, daily impact exercise was encouraged. (All are discussed in detail in *Your Bones*.)

As one of the lead researchers, Dr. Stephen Genuis, noted, not only was this combination of nutrients that bones require "at least as effective as bisphosphonates or strontium ranelate* in raising BMD levels in hip, spine, and femoral neck sites," but the nutrient supplement regimen was also effective "in individuals where bisphosphonate therapy was previously unsuccessful in maintaining or raising BMD."

What a concept—by providing our bodies with the nutrients our bones require and enjoying a little weight-bearing exercise, we can build strong bones for life, safely, effectively—naturally!

Next up: why the new osteoporosis patent medicines—denosumab (Prolia®) and teriparatide (Forteo®) may be *even worse* than the bisphosphonates!

Denosumab (aka Prolia®, Xgeva®)— Even Worse than the Bisphosphonates

Like the bisphosphonates, denosumab (trade names Prolia®, Xgeva®[79]) also prevents osteoclasts from removing old, damaged or worn out bone. It just does so via a different action than the bisphosphonates— an action that may turn out to have even more harmful side effects. Instead of poisoning already mature osteoclasts (which is what the bisphosphonates do), denosumab prevents the precursor cells for osteo-clasts from ever developing into osteoclasts.

MECHANISM OF ACTION— HOW DENOSUMAB WORKS

Denosumab (Prolia®, Xgeva®) does this by binding to and thus blocking off the RANK ligand (RANKL). RANKL is a protein whose job is to bind to a cell receptor called RANK that is found on several differ-ent cell types, just *one* of which is osteoclast precur-sor cells. RANK (an acronym that stands for "recep-tor activator of nuclear factor-kappa B") is activated by the RANK-Ligand (RANKL). RANK is produced by osteoblasts (yes, *osteoblasts*—these bone-build-ing cells work in concert with osteoclasts to continu-ously replace old or damaged bone with new bone). When RANKL activates the RANK receptor on the precursor cells for osteoclasts, this signals these osteoclast-wannabes to develop into mature osteo-clasts ready to remove worn out bone. By prevent-ing RANKL from doing its job, denosumab (Prolia®, Xgeva®) prevents osteoclasts from ever maturing and doing theirs.

DENOSUMAB—WHAT PROBLEMS MIGHT ARISE?

Since denosumab, like the bisphosphonates, prevents normal bone remodeling, one would expect the deno-sumab twins, Prolia® and Xgeva®, to produce simi-lar adverse effects, and they do.[80] Far fewer studies tracking outcomes are available in comparison to the bisphosphonates because denosumab just got FDA approval as Prolia® in June 2010, and as Xgeva® in November 2010. But, already denosumab has been found to cause osteonecrosis of the jaw.[81] Given the hundreds of studies which have now confirmed that, by preventing normal bone remodeling, the bisphosphonates cause not only ONJ, but "atypical" femur fractures, one wonders why the pharmaceutical companies are now attempting to sell us yet another patent medicine that prevents osteoclast function.

Denosumab's most common side effects, noted to date, include infections of the urinary and respiratory tract, cataract, constipation, rashes, and joint pain. A small study has also already found slightly increased risk of cancer and severe infections. Other trials have shown significantly increased rates of eczema and skin infections so severe they required hospitalization.

Why might denosumab increase risk of ONJ, other severe infections or cancer? Well, guess what else must bind to RANKL in order to develop—T and B cells, key cells of our immune system! In the case of ONJ specifically, both the bisphosphonates and denosumab increase susceptibility to infections in the oral cavity and impair mucosal healing. Removing any surface areas of infected bone—the job of osteoclasts—is an important defense against infection on bone surfaces that is blocked by both the bisphosphonates and denosumab, and, in addition, denosumab may interfere with monocyte and macrophage function.[82] Obviously, the potential adverse ramifications related to these facts of human physiology were somehow overlooked when FDA gave denosumab its stamp of approval.

Osteoclasts and Our Immune System— Tight Buddies

Recent papers have begun to discuss "the tight relationship between osteoclasts and the immune system." A new interdisciplinary research field called "osteoimmunology" is just beginning to look at the interplay between our bones and immune system. Already, however, a substantial body of evidence is showing that our bones and immune system are connected by two-way regulatory mechanisms that bring them into much closer association to each other "than one could ever predict"—to quote a review paper published January 2012.[83] Well, we are predicting that by causing osteoclast genocide, denosumab is going to produce some extremely unhappy, "unexpected" (but should have been!) results.

Osteoclasts are strongly linked to our immune system because they belong to the monocyte/macrophage family (these are the white blood cells of our innate immune system), have tight relationships with B and T cells (the adaptive immune system's fighter squadrons), and differentiate (develop into mature osteoclasts) in response to RANKL, which is also produced by lymphocytes and—here's the real stinger—RANKL regulates lymphopoiesis!

What's Lymphopoiesis, and Why Should I Care?

Lymphopoiesis is the generation of a broad class of immune cells called lymphocytes, which include natural killer cells, T cells and B cells. And we (all of us, including the pharmaceutical companies) should care because lymphopoiesis is *absolutely necessary for life*.

Mature lymphocytes are cells that are a critical part of our immune system, and (except for memory B and

T cells which are slightly longer-lived), our immune defender cells have very short lives (just days or weeks) and must be continuously generated. Were this generation to stop, the body would be largely undefended from infection. And how are these immune cells generated? *By RANKL's binding to cell receptors on their precursor cells.* And what does denosumab do? It binds to and uses up all available RANKL.

Both pre-osteoclasts and immune cell precursors share the requirement of activation by RANKL, which allows them to develop into mature, active cells. Because osteoclasts share this need for RANKL activation with our immune cells, it has recently been hypothesized that *osteoclasts are actually immune cells themselves.*

Back in 2009, before its FDA approval, a red flag was raised about denosumab's across-the-board shut down of RANKL in an editorial in the *New England Journal of Medicine*: "Perhaps the major concern about long-term use of denosumab relates to its possible effects on the immune system, since RANKL is expressed not just on bone cells but also on immune cells."[84]

DENOSUMAB'S ALREADY RECOGNIZED ADVERSE EFFECTS

It seems we don't have to wait "long term." After just a few years since denosumab's FDA approval, side effects are already being seen that certainly suggest its effects on immunity are an issue! Compared to placebo, denosumab has produced significant increases in rates of eczema and hospitalizations for cellulitis, which is inflammation of connective tissue either localized or spread throughout the body along with severe inflammation of the dermis (the layer of the skin immediately below the skin's surface or epidermis) and its subcutaneous layers (which consist of connective tissue). In a study involving 314 postmenopausal women with low bone mineral density who were treated with denosumab, neoplasms (cancers) developed in 6 patients and serious infections in 3, whereas none of the 46 patients in the placebo group had such complications.[85]

At the May 2012 Annual Meeting of the Society for Investigative Dermatology, one of the presentations, entitled "Denosumab is associated with dermatologic toxicity in the FDA-Adverse Events Reporting System (AERS) database," discussed reports of "cutaneous [skin] adverse events" (CAE) reported to the FDA's AERS, from June 1, 2011 to June 30, 2012. Of the 33 reports of denosumab-associated CAE, 29 were women, ranging in age from 54 to 86 years, 21 of whom had been given Prolia®. These women experienced hair changes, stomatitis (inflammation of the mucous lining of any part of the mouth, e.g, cheeks, lips, tongue, gums), dry skin, and skin rash, which included exfoliative dermatitis (skin inflammation so severe the skin peels). "Serious CAE" requiring hospitalization occurred in 81.8% of these people; two women died. The comment made by the researchers, "Denosumab-associated dermatologic toxicity warrants further close monitoring." Our comment: Don't let the makers of Prolia® experiment on YOU![86]

As Amgen, the patent medicine company that developed and holds the patent on denosumab, has noted, the patent medicine produces the same adverse effects as the bisphosphonates.[87] "Overall rates of adverse events and serious adverse events were generally similar between the two patent medicines." Here Amgen is referring to denosumab (Prolia®/Xgeva®) and zoledronic acid (this is the bisphosphonate marketed under the trade names Zometa®, Reclast®, and Aclasta®). Common side effects for zoledronic acid (and denosumab) include osteonecrosis of the jaw, back pain, pain in the extremities, musculoskeletal pain, high cholesterol levels, and urinary bladder infections.

Of major concern is that far fewer studies have been done using denosumab than the bisphosphonates. As mentioned above, denosumab was only approved by the FDA for use in postmenopausal women with risk of osteoporosis under the trade name Prolia® in June 2010, and for prevention of "skeletal-related events" in patients with bone metastases from solid tumors under the trade name Xgeva® in November 2010. The point being that we only have short-term results as of yet. Denosumab, however, may have much nastier outcomes in store for us than the bisphosphonates because, by binding to RANKL, this patent medicine interferes with our production of immune cells.

A recent review (Bridgeman, et al.) of what research has been done on Prolia® for reduction of bone loss in postmenopausal osteoporosis (from 1995–2011) summarizes a long list of adverse effects associated with the patent medicine:[88]

- After 24 months, compared with placebo, denosumab was associated with significantly greater prevalences of urinary tract infection and hypertension.
- After 12, 24, and 48 months, the most commonly reported adverse effects with denosumab

use included upper respiratory tract infection, arthralgias, back pain, and nasopharyngitis.

- Infections requiring hospitalization were reported in denosumab-treated patients [10/314 (3.2%)] but not in patients given alendronate (Fosamax®) or placebo.

- Prevalence of malignant neoplasms (cancer) were higher in the denosumab than in the Fosamax® (alendronate) or placebo groups (4.8%, 4.3%, and 4.3%, respectively), as was the overall prevalence of serious adverse events after 48 months of treatment (17.8% for denosumab, 17.4% for Fosamax®, and 10.9% for placebo).

- A greater number of patients developed infections that required hospitalization in the denosumab group compared with placebo (8 vs 1). For some reason, for which no justification or explanation is given, "Infections were not considered to be related to denosumab." The types of infections included pneumonia, urinary tract infection, pyelonephritis, diverticulitis, appendicitis, sepsis, and cellulitis.

- Four patients in the denosumab group were reported to have neoplasms compared with one patient in the placebo group, but for some reason for which, again, no explanation is given, the higher incidence of cancer in those given denosumab is said to not be related to the patent medicine.

- Other adverse events reported at significantly greater rates with denosumab compared with placebo included constipation (11.0% vs 4.8%), sore throat (9.1% vs 3.0%), and rash (8.5% vs 3.0%)

If all this weren't sufficient cause for concern, Bridgeman, et al., go on to also warn that patent medicine/patent medicine interactions may be a serious problem with denosumab:

> Studies of the potential for denosumab to affect the metabolism of other pharmacologic agents were not identified in the literature search. (Translation—no studies looking into this have been conducted.) However, based on reports of serious infections associated with the use of denosumab, the concurrent use of immunosuppressants, including corticosteroids, chemotherapeutic agents, and immune modulators, may increase the risk for infection.*

Elsewhere we are simply told that data regarding interactions between denosumab and other patent medicines are "missing." (Translation—they haven't looked into this.) But we are assured such interactions are "rare," so "it is unlikely that denosumab exhibits any clinically relevant interactions."

(Translation—we haven't seen this yet, so we are not going to worry about it until enough people have been harmed that a class action suit is brought.)[89]

The following quote from the concluding section of Bridgeman, et al.'s review of the research on denosumab use in postmenopausal women at risk of osteoporosis summarizes the adverse events already seen:

---

* Many patent medicines fall under these classifications including patent medicines prescribed for allergies, asthma, depression, epilepsy, and insomnia. "Bone-Busting Patent Medicines," pages 124–139, discusses a number of these patent medicines, which are also known to promote osteoporosis.

Adverse events reported with the use of denosumab have included back pain (34.7%); pain in the extremities (11.7%); general musculoskeletal pain (7.6%); elevated cholesterol (7.2%); inflammation of the bladder (5.9%); and dermatologic conditions including dermatitis, eczema, and rashes (combined prevalence, 10.8%). Serious adverse events have included hypocalcemia (1.7%), pancreatitis (0.2%), and severe infection (0.2%). Several cases of osteonecrosis of the jaw have also been reported.

Shockingly, the next sentence, the concluding statement of this review, is:

Based on the data from the available literature, denosumab is an efficacious and well-tolerated treatment for postmenopausal osteoporosis.

This was such a non-sequitur to me, I read the paragraph several times trying to make sense of it—I couldn't.

NO FREEDOM FROM SEVERE ADVERSE EVENTS WITH DENOSUMAB

FREEDOM (Fracture Reduction Evaluation of Denosumab in Osteoporosis) was an international multicenter, randomized, double-blind, placebo-controlled study of postmenopausal women with osteoporosis, who were randomly assigned to receive placebo (a group of 3,906 women) or denosumab (60 mg) every 6 months (3,902 women).

Papers discussing the results of FREEDOM[90] note that serious adverse events of infections involving the gastrointestinal system, kidneys and urinary tract, ear, and heart (endocarditis, inflammation of the inner layer of the heart) occurred significantly more in the denosumab group compared with placebo, but, as usual, we are told, just a few women were affected.

Serious adverse events of skin infections (erysipelas and cellulitis) were also more frequent in denosumab-treated subjects. Erysipelas, from the Greek for "red skin," and also called "St. Anthony's fire" is an acute streptococcus bacterial infection of the top layer of the skin and the superficial lymph nodes. Key risk factor for erysipelas: immune deficiency. Cellulitis, as mentioned above, is inflammation of connective tissue and is also caused by bacteria entering the skin, usually by way of a cut, abrasion, or break in the skin that can be so small it is not visible. Group A Streptococcus and Staphylococcus are the most common of these bacteria. Both are part of normal skin flora and would normally cause no infection. But give someone denosumab, and "normal" immunity may be compromised.

The researchers propose that denosumab's inhibition of RANKL in keratinocytes (the cells that make up 95% of the outer layer of our skin) may decrease the number of regulatory T cells (whose job it is to suppress excessive immune responses), leading to an increased inflammatory response in the skin. So, the appearance of skin lesions suggests a more severe inflammatory response in subjects receiving denosumab, which (1) resulted in their needing to be hospitalized, and (2) is just what we want to avoid to build bone! Remember, chronic inflammation activates osteoclasts.

Bottom line—taking denosumab resulted in "significantly more serious adverse events of infections that were associated with hospitalization" than taking placebo. Given this, what's planned for denosumab's use in postmenopausal women at risk of osteoporosis: "The benefit/risk profile of denosumab continues to be evaluated in ongoing clinical trials, including an open-label extension of the phase 3 pivotal fracture trial that is planned to follow up subjects for up to 10 years." Wanna bet denosumab causes some very nasty "adverse events" to occur in some of these "subjects"?

DENOSUMAB HAS LITTLE BENEFIT, NASTY SIDE EFFECTS IN MEN WITH PROSTATE CANCER

Most recently, Amgen has attempted to have denosumab, as Xgeva®, also approved to increase bone mass in men with non-metastatic prostate cancer who are at high risk for fracture because they are being given "androgen deprivation therapy" (patent medicines that shut off men's production of testosterone). Remember, in men, a little testosterone is converted into estrogen, which plays a very important role in building men's bones. Patent medicines that prevent a man from producing testosterone therefore also cause him to lose bone.

Amgen approached FDA for approval using data from its study of 1,432 men with non-metastatic, castration-resistant prostate cancer. These men were randomly assigned to receive calcium and vitamin D supplements plus either 120 mg subcutaneous denosumab every four weeks or placebo. (Dosing for denosumab is a 60 mg subcutaneous injection every six months for postmenopausal osteoporosis and 120 mg every 4 weeks for patients with solid tumors.)

Men in this study who were given denosumab did have, on average, about four months longer before developing bone metastases compared to those in the placebo group (29.5 months versus 25.2 months), *but the men's overall survival and cancer progression-free survival were not any better in the denosumab group versus placebo. Nor did denosumab lessen the men's pain or improve their health-related quality of life compared to placebo.*

As expected from prior studies, denosumab did, however, cause a number of adverse effects in these men, including more hypocalcemia (1.7% versus 0.3% with placebo) as well as a 5% rate of osteonecrosis of the jaw, which didn't occur at all in the control group. Just think about this—it's bad enough having prostate cancer and suffering the effects of having your testosterone wiped out, but to also have to endure a rotting jaw is completely unacceptable!

FDA REVIEWERS CONCERNED ABOUT "UNRESOLVED SAFETY ISSUE": MIGHT DENOSUMAB CAUSE CANCER?

FDA reviewers were also concerned about an "unresolved safety issue": whether denosumab might *cause* cancer to spread to non-bony sites. Why is the FDA concerned? Remember denosumab works by shutting down RANKL, which is required for the activation of our T and B immune cells. In just living our lives, normal bodily metabolism and environmental exposures result in each of us experiencing insults to our cells' DNA that produce hundreds of *potentially* cancerous cells every day; our immune system, if not overloaded and not prevented from functioning properly, destroys them.

Amgen argued that denosumab should be approved for the added indication anyway "because no other therapy has been shown to prevent the development of bone metastases in patients with non-metastatic castrate-resistant prostate cancer." Am I missing something in the logic chain here? Denosumab should be approved—not because it has been shown to help prevent bone cancer in men with non-metastatic prostate cancer or extend their lives or even improve the quality of whatever time they have—but because no other patent medicine has been shown to do so?[91]

DENOSUMAB—ANOTHER PHARMACEUTICAL COMPANY EXPERIMENT—ON US!

Even for its use only to prevent excessive bone loss in individuals with osteoporosis, denosumab only received approval by the FDA as of 2010. As two recent papers in leading medical journals focusing on osteoporosis clearly warn, bone remodeling continues throughout the human lifetime, so any treatment used to prevent excessive bone loss must be safe *over many years*—for which reason, "the collection of long-term efficacy and safety data [on denosumab] is warranted."[92] "Denosumab has been introduced recently, and its extra-skeletal effects still have to be assessed."[93]

Despite these concerns voiced in leading medical journals and by the FDA, the fact that denosumab has already been found to produce adverse effects, and its far less than stellar results in men with non-metastatic castrate-resistant prostate cancer, a *Wall Street Journal* post entitled, "Analysts React to FDA Panel: 'It Wasn't a Perfect Day for Amgen,'" noted that annual worldwide sales of denosumab are still projected to reach $5 billion by the year 2015.[94] Well, at least Amgen should have plenty of money available for the lawsuits sure to come when denosumab's impact on bone and immune health has resulted in serious harm to sufficient people. Don't be one of them!

Haven't the atypical fractures and osteonecrosis of the jaw caused by the bisphosphonates provided a clear enough warning? Why would we want to expose ourselves to yet another patent medicine that shuts off osteoclasts and prevents the normal levels of bone remodeling essential for healthy bones? And denosumab's undesirable long-term effects could be much, much worse because this patent medicine not only prevents osteoclasts from developing, but does so by locking up RankL, which key cells of our immune system, our T and B cells, also require in order to develop.

Why You Should Forego Forteo®

Forteo® (teriparatide) is a portion of human parathyroid hormone—a fragment that includes the amino acid sequence 1-34. The full molecule of parathyroid hormone (PTH) contains 84 amino acids. PTH regulates calcium and phosphate metabolism in our bones and kidneys. If chronically elevated, PTH depletes bone because, when your blood levels of calcium are too low, PTH increases osteoclast activity, so calcium will be liberated from bone to increase calcium levels in the blood. However, if PTH is elevated intermittently—which is what once daily injections of teriparatide are supposed to do (this patent medicine must be taken as an injection)—osteoblasts get activated more than osteoclasts, so the net effect is increased bone mineral density.

Sounds good at first blush, right? Unfortunately, however, like all the other patent medicines, "teriparatide" *is not produced by your body,* it's literally a foreign molecule, and as such, much more likely to cause problems, just like all the other patent medicines intended to prevent or treat osteoporosis. Forteo® has a number of side effects including not only nausea, leg cramps and dizziness, but an increased risk of bone tumors and osteosarcoma (bone cancer)—as the following quote from "Present at the beginning: a personal reminiscence on the history of teriparatide," an article published in *Osteoporosis International,* March 2011, clearly states. Written by Dr. Marcus, one of the researchers involved with the development of teriparatide, this paper is an up-close-and-personal recounting of teriparatide's development.[95]

Here's a quote from Marcus' history of teriparatide:

> The ability of parathyroid glandular extracts to stimulate bone acquisition in rodents was established in the 1920s, but interest in this action lay dormant for almost 50 years until application of contemporary laboratory methods permitted the large-scale production of an amino-terminal fragment of PTH, (1–34) hPTH (teriparatide), which was capable of carrying out all known actions of the full-length (1–84) PTH molecule. In the 1970s, largely stimulated by the efforts of a British pharmacologist, Dr. John Parsons, the scientific community began to revisit these anabolic actions and showed that single daily injections of teriparatide dramatically increased bone mass in several

mammalian species and restored bone in oöphorectomized rats [female rats whose ovaries have been removed to simulate menopause]. Shortly thereafter, human studies confirmed a striking increase in trabecular bone mass and showed also that an important part of teriparatide's action is to increase cortical bone. Eli Lilly and Company conducted a formal registration trial in postmenopausal women with osteoporosis.

The unexpected occurrence of osteosarcomas in Fisher 344 rats treated long term with teriparatide provoked an abrupt cessation of that trial, but ambiguity concerning the relevance of this rat finding to human disease, combined with significant antifracture efficacy, led to FDA approval of teriparatide for men and postmenopausal women with osteoporosis 'at high risk for fracture' in 2002. Subsequently, teriparatide has been approved also for treatment of patients with glucocorticoid-associated osteoporosis, and papers indicating utility of this agent for dental and orthopedic applications have begun to appear.

Our takeaway from this is that even though teriparatide long term caused osteosarcoma in rats—almost 45% of the rats treated with this patent medicine at the highest-tested dose level developed this aggressive form of bone cancer—FDA approved it anyway, saying whether it would do so in humans was unknown. Since our bones are remodeling throughout our lives, any bone-building regimen must be followed long term, which means For-teo® must be taken long term for meaningful benefit. Treatment with teriparatide is approved by the FDA for a limited duration of 18–24 months; in many European countries approval is limited to 18 months.

Also, prior radiation exposure, another potential promoter of osteosarcoma, is considered a big red flag. If you have had prior radiation exposure (x-rays, radiation therapy for cancer), teriparatide is contraindicated for you. [96]

It is important to not only recall that in the animal studies, long-term treatment with teriparatide caused bone cancer in almost half the animals, but also to know that the studies run on humans to date have been short term, a maximum of 36 months. There are two problems with the latter: First, no one has any idea whether the people who have been given Forteo®, even short term, will later develop bone cancer as a result. Secondly, as we keep repeating, bone remodeling is *not* short term! It is a life-long process.

As the following quote from an article in *Arthritis and Rheumatism* makes clear, researchers are concerned about the long-term consequences of Forteo's use, even when restricted to short-term use in patients on glucocorticoid-mimicking patent medicines. This is an experiment that is far from risk free:

> In some recent studies, the period of treatment with teriparatide was prolonged to 24–30 months. It has been reported that a longer treatment period may have a role in the development of various pathologies in animals, one of which is osteosarcoma. Although this has not been observed in

humans to date, longer-term use of teriparatide, especially in the young population that makes up a great proportion of patients with glucocorticoid-induced osteoporosis, may cause risks. Because the exact relationship between the occurrence of osteosarcoma and the duration of treatment has not been clearly elucidated, it is difficult to determine an exact duration of treatment after which risk might develop. The most significant problem that patients will experience is not patent medicine tolerance, but malignancy.

In the study by Saag, et al., published in the November 2009 issue of *Arthritis & Rheumatism*, teriparatide was used for up to 36 months in a patient population with a short duration of osteoporosis, which carries more prominent risks. We believe this prolonged treatment may have increased the risk of osteosarcoma occurrence. Although it has been reported that the teriparatide-related risk of osteosarcoma development is low, there are still no clear scientific data, and the general recommendation about this treatment is to closely follow up patients who have risk factors. Therefore, we have the following questions about the study by Saag, et al.: How was the treatment duration planned? Were the patients evaluated for risk of osteosarcoma development before the study? Did the authors experience difficulties with the ethical approval process? And how will the study patients be

followed up prospectively in terms of osteosarcoma risk?[97]

Good questions.

Teriparatide's use in men with glucocorticoid-induced
osteoporosis, where short-term use might make sense
and should be associated with less long-term risks, is
easier to comprehend. But Forteo® is being recommended for treatment of postmenopausal osteoporosis
as well. And, as we write this, Columbia University is
running a trial in which they are giving Forteo® to premenopausal women with "idiopathic" osteoporosis for
24 months. "Idiopathic" simply means they don't know
why these younger, premenopausal women have lost so
much bone. I, Lara, was just such a young woman well
on my way to osteoporosis with "idiopathic osteopenia"
in my late 40s. The key cause of my "idiopathic osteopenia"? Insufficient vitamin D.

In the study eligibility section, we are told that
"Women with levels of 20–30 ng/mL will be eligible
after treatment with vitamin D has resulted in levels
>30 ng/mL."[98] Has anyone considered that once these
women have achieved vitamin D levels of >30 ng/mL—
which is at the lowest end of the "normal" range (optimal is 60–80 ng/mL), they may not need intervention
with a patent medicine to build bone? That giving them
sufficient vitamin D to get their blood levels of 25(OH)D
into the low 60s ng/mL, along with vitamin K_2, calcium,
magnesium, and boron, some weight-bearing exercise,
and a healthful diet might more than do the trick? Actually, they already tried this in the COMB study, and it
worked, very well.*

---

* See pages 76–79.

We have a few other suggestions for these researchers interested in treating "idiopathic osteopenia/osteoporosis": all of Part 3 of this book, pages 83–164, which discusses many factors, any one of which can give you osteoporosis, and all of which are treatable, naturally, safely, inexpensively, and very effectively—without patent medicines! I don't know how you feel about being part of an experiment to see how many humans develop bone cancer from taking this patent medicine, but I, Lara, would be unwilling to participate! Especially when we can have healthy bones for life naturally—as I have learned through personal experience and which has now been demonstrated in the COMB study (discussed below, page 76) in which the key nutrients recommended in *Your Bones* outperformed the bisphosphonates and strontium ranelate, safely building bone—even in women whose BMD had not been helped by these patent medicines.

Review articles (which summarize the results on a number of studies in the peer-reviewed medical literature) back in 2008 were already warning of adverse effects caused by teriparatide, including hypercalcemia (abnormally high blood levels of calcium), hypercalciuria (abnormally high levels of calcium in the urine, which can damage kidneys and result in kidney stones), and hyperuricemia (abnormally high levels of uric acid in the blood, which predisposes to gout).[99]

WHAT ARE THEY SEEING IN THE MOST RECENT STUDIES BEING PUBLISHED ON EARLY OUTCOMES USING FORTEO®?

In a clinical study of older people (aged 52 to 69) who had one or more collapsed spines, no underlying diseases and no history of bone tumor, hyperparathyroid, hypercalcemia, "common unwanted effects were:"

- **Hypercalcemia**: excessively high blood levels of calcium, a serious condition whose most common cause is abnormal parathyroid gland function.*

- **Hyperuricemia**: high levels of uric acid in the blood, which as noted above, is a key symptom of gout and if very high, can cause kidney failure.

- **Hypomagnesia**: low blood levels of magnesium—also serious. Hypomagnesia is not the equivalent of magnesium deficiency and can be present without it, although hypomagnesia often indicates systemic magnesium insufficiency. Symptoms include: weakness, muscle cramps, cardiac arrhythmia, increased irritability of the nervous system with tremors, athetosis (involuntary convoluted, writhing movements of the fingers, arms, legs, and neck), jerking, nystagmus (involuntary eye movement that can result in reduced or limited vision), and an extensor plantar reflex (often a sign of B_{12} deficiency). In addition, there may be confusion, disorientation, hallucinations, depression, epileptic fits, hypertension, tachycardia (very rapid heartbeat), and tetany (involuntary muscle contractions).

---

* See pages 114–117.

These highly undesirable effects were seen within the first month of "therapy" with Forteo® in 5.5% (hypercalcemia), 54.56% (hyperuricemia) and 43% (hypomagnesia) of subjects. By the end of the 6th month, they occurred 1.38%, 8.77% and 5.5% respectively—not as alarming, but still much too frequent to pass off as unlikely.[100] Case reports are now beginning to appear warning physicians, and we quote, "although teriparatide seems quite effective in the treatment of osteoporosis, it may cause life-threatening hypercalcemia. Therefore, patients should be closely monitored if symptoms of hypercalcemia are present during teriparatide treatment."[101]

Most recently, teriparatide has been found to increase blood and urine levels of the stress hormone, cortisol when given to postmenopausal women with osteoporosis. The women's cortisol levels had increased above baseline after just 6 months of teriparatide treatment (20 micrograms self-administered by injection daily). After 12 months, the increase in cortisol levels was significant.[102] This is not surprising since teriparatide causes a spike in parathyroid hormone levels, and parathyroid hormone increases the adrenal glands' secretion of cortisol.

Why Might Elevated Cortisol Levels Be a Problem for Your Bones?

Cortisol is the body's own premier natural glucocorticoid. As discussed in the "Bone-Busting Patent Medicines" section,* chronic exposure to high levels of glucocorticoids kills osteocytes (the kind of cells that osteoblasts become once they begin building the bone matrix). Even

---

* Pages 124–139.

"subclinical" elevations in cortisol levels (an increase in cortisol levels small enough to cause no noticeable symptoms) is associated with increased occurrence of osteoporosis and vertebral fractures—and high blood pressure, type 2 diabetes, high cholesterol, and central obesity, the unhealthiest type of obesity in which fat deposits are concentrated around the abdominal organs.[103]

And you'll really love this—researchers have no idea if stopping treatment with teriparatide will restore cortisol levels back to normal. They think cortisol levels will probably drop back down and suggest, you guessed it, running more studies "to observe if the cortisol values continue to increase and if the effect of teriparatide is reversible."[104]

If all these risks are not enough to cause you to think twice about using Forteo®, let me add another reason I would be hesitant to abnormally boost my PTH every day: above normal levels of PTH have also been associated with cognitive decline and dementia (Alzheimer's). The connection is that sustained elevated levels of PTH in the brain increase risk of calcium overloading, which leads to impaired blood flow and brain degeneration.*[105]

Interestingly, when PTH activity is excessive, the human body attempts to inhibit PTH production in two ways: by increasing blood levels of calcium and decreasing blood levels of magnesium. Both are being seen in response to teriparatide. Wouldn't this suggest the body is sending a clear, "No thanks" message in response to treatment with this patent medicine?

Don't be part of the tereparatide experiment!

---

* Parathyroid hormone's effect on bone is discussed in more detail on pages 114–117.

Latest Research Proves You Can Restore the Health of Your Bones— Safely and Effectively—Naturally

Why participate in yet another pharmaceutical company experiment and expose yourself to these risks when the latest research proves you can maintain and restore the health of your bones—safely and effectively—naturally?

As we mentioned earlier in relation to the bisphosphonates,* in February 2012, right after the annual meeting of the American Academy of Orthopedic Surgeons officially warned doctors that the bisphosphonates increase risk for "atypical femur fractures," [106] the results of the one-year long Combination of Micronutrients for Bone (COMB) Study were published in the prestigious *Journal of Environmental and Public Health*. The COMB study unequivocally demonstrated that providing our bones with the nutrients they need along with regular weight-bearing exercise is as or *more effective* than any of the bisphosphonates or strontium ranelate (the unnatural patent medicine version of strontium). And a lot less expensive!

What was the protocol utilized in the COMB Study? Daily vitamin D_3 (2,000 IU), DHA (250 mg), K_2 (in the form of MK-7,100 mcg), strontium citrate (680 mg), magnesium (25 mg), and dietary calcium. In addition, daily weight-bearing exercise was encouraged.[107]

As one of the lead researchers, Dr. Stephen Genuis, noted, not only was this combination of nutrients

---

* Pages 26–32.

that bones require "at least as effective as bisphosphonates or strontium ranelate in raising BMD levels in hip, spine, and femoral neck sites," but the nutrient supplement regimen was also effective "in individuals where bisphosphonate therapy was previously unsuccessful in maintaining or raising BMD."

What a concept—by providing our bodies with the nutrients our bones require and enjoying a little weight-bearing exercise, we can build strong bones for life, safely, effectively—naturally!

Also in February 2012, positive results were seen after just six months in another bone-building nutrient-combination study. This research, conducted at the Osteoporosis Research Center, Creighton University Medical Center, in Omaha, Nebraska, was published in the *European Journal of Nutrition*.[108] This was a double-blind study involving 70 postmenopausal women who ranged in age from 52 to 57 years, and who were just one to three years post menopause. In other words, these were women who had very recently gone through menopause and were still within the span of years during which bone loss is at its peak level.

The researchers examined the effects on bone mineral density of taking a daily supplement providing either calcium (500 mg calcium carbonate) by itself or along with a bone-nutrient support blend called geniVida®, which contained an isoflavone found in soyfoods called genistein (30 mg), vitamin D_3 (800 IU), vitamin K_1 (150 micrograms), and omega-3 essential fatty acids (1 gram total, 2/3 of which was eicosapentaenoic acid [EPA] and 1/3 of which was docosahexaenooic acid [DHA]).

In regards to the calcium dosage, when added to the women's consumption of calcium from their diet, their total calcium intake was at least 1,200 mg per day. Also, it is important to note that the 30 mg dose of genistein is the amount typically consumed in Japan by Japanese following a traditional diet, and is lower than the doses of 80, 100, and 200 mg/day of supplemental isoflavones that have been used with mixed results in other studies. It appears that isoflavones, and specifically genistein, stimulate bone formation at lower concentrations, but may inhibit it at higher concentrations.

As mentioned, this was a double-blind study. Half the women were given a capsule containing geniVida® plus a second capsule containing 500 mg of calcium carbonate, while the remaining women received a placebo capsule without geniVida® and a second capsule providing 500 mg of calcium carbonate. The researchers did not know which women were in either group.

After the BMD results were collected and the code was broken, it was revealed that women in the placebo group *lost* an average of 1.2% and 1.1% BMD at the femoral neck and Ward's triangle (the section of the femur used to evaluate BMD on DXA scans), respectively. In contrast, women in the geniVida® group *gained* 0.1% and 2.3% at these sites, respectively. Bone-specific alkaline phosphatase, a marker of osteoblast activity and bone formation, significantly increased, and N-telopeptide, a marker of bone resorption, significantly decreased, only in the geniVida® plus calcium group, indicating a significant boost in healthy bone remodeling activity in these women. No significant adverse events were reported in either the placebo or geniVida® groups; in fact, more symptoms, none serious, were reported by those taking placebo.

The "take home" message from the latest studies: our medical paradigm is changing from one that pretends a "silver bullet" (usually a patent medicine, but sometimes one or maybe two nutrients, like calcium plus vitamin D) can fix our disintegrating bones to a much more intelligent comprehensive paradigm that prescribes a healthy dose of all the nutrients our bones require plus regular weight-bearing exercise.* Follow this prescription and you'll have strong, healthy bones for life—naturally.

GET YOUR BONES OFF PATENT MEDICINES!

Just in case you are not already convinced, we'll let Rizzoli and Reginster, physicians working in the Division of Bone Diseases, Department of Medical Specialties, Geneva University Hospitals and Faculty of Medicine, Geneva, Switzerland, sum it up in this quote from their recent paper [109] entitled, "Adverse Patent Medicine Reactions to Osteoporosis Treatments":

> The bisphosphonates are associated with gastrointestinal effects, acute phase reactions, and musculoskeletal pain, and, more rarely, cases of atrial fibrillation, subtrochanteric fracture, osteonecrosis of the jaw, cutaneous hypersensitivity reactions and renal impairment. It is too soon for pharmacovigilance data on denosumab, but it has been associated with cutaneous effects and possibly osteonecrosis of the jaw (to date, only in metastatic cancer). The selective estrogen receptor modulators may induce hot flushes and leg cramps, and—more rarely—venous thromboembolism and stroke. Strontium

* Discussed in Chapter 7, page 167.

ranelate is associated with headache, nausea, and diarrhea, and, more rarely, cutaneous hypersensitivity reactions and venous thromboembolism, while teriparatide and parathyroid hormone are associated with headache, nausea, dizziness and limb pain. The management of osteoporosis should entail weighing the probability of adverse reactions against the benefits of therapy—that is, reduction of fracture risk.

Personally, we cannot see why anyone would take any of the osteoporosis patent medicines the pharmaceutical companies are pushing—whether the bisphosphonates, denosumab or teriparitide, since the latest studies (discussed above) are now proving combinations of bone-building nutrients will enable you to restore the health of your bones safely and effectively—naturally. We suggest you take FDA's bisphosphonate holiday recommendation* a big step further for womankind (and mankind) and go on a permanent patent medicine holiday!

SAY BYE-BYE TO THE BISPHOSPHONATES, DENOSUMAB, AND TERIPARATIDE!

Since bone is constantly remodeling throughout our lives, any therapy used to promote bone health in aging women must be one a woman can rely upon for the rest of her life. Obviously, it makes little sense to take a patent medicine that, at best, only conserves old, worn-out bone, and may, in the case of the bisphosphonates and denosumab, increase fracture risk within as little as four months!

---

* See page 49.

Even a quick look at the many serious risks associated with taking any of these patent medicines, especially when combined with the fact that the bisphosphonates and denosumab actually increase your likelihood of developing bones so brittle they break during normal daily activities, provides sufficient reason to question the advisability of relying on any of them to prevent osteoporosis!

A substantial amount of top quality, peer-reviewed research shows that the balance between osteoclasts' demolition of old, worn-out bone and osteoblasts' reconstruction of healthy, new bone can be restored safely without recourse to dangerous and expensive patent medicines.

What we need to do is identify and control the factors that are causing our osteoclasts to become hyperactive, so they remove too much bone, and to be sure we are providing our osteoblasts with an adequate supply of all the materials they need to build new bone. Once this is accomplished, our bodies will happily set about doing what they are born already programmed to do—provide us with strong bones for life, naturally.

PART 3

What Increases Your Risk for Osteoporosis?

CHAPTER 3

What You Don't Know Can Give You Osteoporosis

I N THE FOLLOWING CHAPTERS, we look at the key factors affecting bone remodeling and the nutrients our bodies need to build healthy bones. You'll find it easy to identify which of these factors applies to YOU, and which nutrients your bones need that your current diet and supplement program is not adequately supplying.

Once you have recognized what YOU—not some imaginary "average" person—need, you can take the steps necessary to protect and enhance the health of your bones. Safeguard and nourish your bones, and they will repay you by beautifully supporting you throughout a long and vibrant life.

Are You Sure You're Getting Enough Calcium?

As we get older, we normally lose a tiny amount of bone each year. Not getting enough daily calcium can greatly accelerate our rate of bone loss.

Although most of us think we get plenty of calcium, surprisingly, a review of data from the most recent NHANES (National Health and Nutrition Examination Survey) found that 60% of Americans are not getting enough calcium, even when including both food and supplements, to meet current recommendations for adequate calcium intake.[110]

Recommendations for adequate intake (AI) of calcium were issued by the Institute of Medicine at the National Academy of Sciences in 1998. For those most at risk for osteoporosis—women approaching or currently experiencing their transition through menopause—these recommendations are:

- 31–50 years: 1,000 mg
- 51+ years: 1,200 mg
- Postmenopausal women not taking hormone replacement therapy: 1,500 mg

To determine whether you are, in fact, consuming enough calcium to maintain your bones' health, you'll want to take a look at your typical diet and, if you are taking supplements, the amount of calcium they contain.

On the next page is a list of foods rich in calcium, and the amount of calcium a typical serving of each provides. You can easily check whether you are getting enough calcium. For 5 to 7 days, keep a food and supplement diary each day, then look to see how much calcium you're really getting.

FOODS RICH IN CALCIUM

FOOD	SERVING SIZE	CALCIUM
Cow's milk,* 2% fat	1 cup	297 mg
Yogurt, low-fat	1 cup	447 mg
Cottage cheese, 1% fat	1 cup	100 mg
Mozarella cheese, part-skim	1 ounce	183 mg
Swiss cheese	1 ounce	265 mg
Goat milk	1 cup	326 mg
Salmon, canned	4 ounces	300 mg
Sardines, canned with bones	2 ounces	240 mg
Spinach, steamed	1 cup	245 mg
Collard greens, steamed	1 cup	226 mg
Kale, steamed	1 cup	94 mg
Romaine lettuce	2 cups	40 mg
Broccoli, steamed	1 cup	75 mg
Green beans	1 cup	57 mg
Cabbage, shredded, steamed	1 cup	46 mg
Sesame seeds	1/4 cup	351 mg
Tofu	4 ounces	100 mg
Orange	1 raw	52 mg
Almonds	1 ounce (about 20 nuts)	70 mg

* However, don't rely on cow's milk as your primary source of calcium. The nearly 78,000 woman *Harvard Nurses Study* determined that osteoporosis risk actually increased with increased use of milk and dairy products.

I NEED MORE THAN CALCIUM TO PREVENT OSTEOPOROSIS?

Yes, most definitely! Normal bone metabolism is an intricate interplay among more than two dozen nutrients, including, in addition to calcium, the vitamins D, K, B_6, B_{12}, and folate, and the minerals boron, magnesium, zinc, copper, manganese, molybdenum, selenium, silicon, and phosphorous. What you need to know about each one of these nutrients to build and maintain healthy bone is laid out in the sections "Strong Bones for Life, Naturally"* and Appenix B "Vitamin and Mineral Essentials for Healthy Bones."† Our agenda here is to convince you that your bones need a good deal more than calcium to stay strong.

As mentioned earlier, our hormones play key roles in maintaining healthy bone. In women, estrogen regulates osteoclasts, keeping them under control, so they only remove dead demineralized bone, and progesterone helps activate osteoblasts, which build new bone. Levels of both hormones begin to decline several years before menopause, during the time in a woman's life called *perimenopause* ("peri" = around).

While the average age at which perimenopause begins is 47.5 years in the Western world, for some women this transition to menopause begins in their early 40s. Average length of time during perimenopause is about four years, with menopause most often occurring around the age of 51 (or 49 in women who smoke).[111]

In men, hormones also play a key role in maintaining bone mass. Testosterone's importance in maintaining

* See page 167
† See page 339.

bone mass in men is not as well recognized as the roles played by estrogen and progesterone in women, but the androgens (male hormones) are known to be involved in the development of osteoblasts, and some testosterone is metabolized into estradiol, the most potent form of estrogen, which also plays an important role in men's healthy bone remodeling.[112]

As men age, their testosterone levels decline, although not as early or as abruptly as women's levels of estrogen and progesterone do. However, by age 60, virtually all men have experienced a drop in their levels of male hormones or androgens, which increases the rate at which men lose bone. Androgen deprivation therapy, which is commonly used in the treatment of prostate cancer, results in a 3% to 5% yearly loss in bone mineral density and is well known to promote osteoporosis in men.[113]

In addition to the nutrients noted above and our sex hormones, a variety of genetic and lifestyle factors affect our body's ability to maintain a healthy balance between bone resorption and formation. Let's take a look at the most important of these next.

I NEED STOMACH ACID TO ABSORB CALCIUM?

Yes! Despite the fact that TV commercials tell us that heartburn and indigestion are caused by too much stomach acid, *too little* stomach acid not only results in the same symptoms (heartburn or reflux from half-digested food backing up the throat, bloating, belching, and gas), but promotes osteoporosis because, without sufficient stomach acid, we cannot absorb calcium.

In order for calcium to be absorbed in the intestines, it must first be made soluble (able to be dissolved) and ionized (made to have fewer electrons) by stomach acid. Studies have found that almost 40% of postmenopausal women are severely deficient in stomach acid![114]

Not surprisingly, decreased stomach acid is common in both women and men who frequently take antacids to relieve heartburn or indigestion. Over-the-counter antacids, such as Maalox®, Tums®, or Rolaids®, neutralize acid already present in the stomach, while the acid-blocking patent medicines, including the H2 blockers (e.g., Pepcid®, Tagament®, Axid®) and the proton pump inhibitors (e.g., Prilosec®, Nexium®, Prevacid®), suppress the stomach's ability to produce acid. Among the acid-blocking patent medicines, H2 blockers are less harmful to bone than the proton pump inhibitors because H2 blockers only decrease the amount of stomach acid produced, while proton pump inhibitors completely shut down the stomach's ability to produce stomach acid.

Relying on these patent medicines instead of taking a look at the diet and lifestyle habits that are the *cause* of our upset stomachs is like turning off the fire alarm and going back to bed while the house continues to burn down. Not only do all the antacid patent medicines fail to address the reasons for our indigestion problems, but they promote other ones, including osteoporosis.

When we turn to supplements to ensure we are getting enough calcium, having enough stomach acid can be especially important. Calcium carbonate, the least expensive and therefore the most commonly used form of calcium in nutritional supplements, is neither soluble nor ionized. Individuals who produce little stomach acid only absorb about 4% of an oral dose of calcium carbonate, and even persons who produce normal amounts of stomach acid absorb only 22% of an oral dose of this form of supplemental calcium.[115]

Fortunately, even patients with low stomach acid will absorb much more—about 45%—of the calcium from supplements providing calcium in the form of *calcium citrate*.[116] In a number of studies involving healthy women, women with low stomach acid production, and women who had undergone gastric bypass surgery (gastric bypass restricts food intake, thus lowering the amount of *all* vitamins and minerals, including calcium, available to be absorbed from the digestive tract), calcium citrate has been shown to be a much more effective means of delivering calcium into the bloodstream than calcium carbonate.[117]

Regardless of whether you suspect your production of stomach acid is low or you have no problems digesting your food (and therefore are producing enough stomach acid to do so), if you are taking a supplement containing calcium carbonate, be sure to take it with a meal to maximize your production of stomach acid and your ability to absorb its calcium.[118] If you're uncertain, why not just switch from calcium carbonate to calcium citrate?

IS YOUR DIET LEACHING CALCIUM FROM YOUR BONES?

A slightly alkaline body chemistry, which is what is seen in individuals whose diet includes lots of plant foods (vegetables, fruits, beans, whole grains, nuts and seeds, etc.), is required for good bone health. A diet high in animal protein results in an acidic body chemistry, which our bodies attempt to buffer by withdrawing alkaline minerals, i.e., calcium, from our bones.

Research has very clearly shown that a diet too high in protein greatly increases the amount of calcium released from our bones and excreted in the urine. In a study that looked at the effects of diets containing varying amounts of protein on the bones of women with osteoporosis, raising their daily protein intake from 47 to 142 grams *doubled* the amount of calcium lost in their urine.[119] This is one reason why vegetarian diets (both those that include dairy products and eggs as well as vegan diets) are associated with a lower risk of developing osteoporosis.[120]

How Much Protein Do YOU Need?

Three steps are necessary to figure this out, each of which is explained below. Here is what you will be doing: first, you'll determine your ideal weight. Then you'll convert your ideal weight from pounds to kilograms. And lastly, you'll multiply your ideal weight in kilograms by 0.8 to determine the number of grams of protein *your* body needs each day. If you do not want to bother with this, the chart below will give you a reasonable estimate of how many grams of protein you need each day.

STEP ONE: DETERMINING YOUR IDEAL WEIGHT

Your daily protein requirements are based on your *ideal* weight, not your current weight. Ideal weight for a woman 5 feet (60 inches) tall is 100 pounds. If you are taller than 5 feet, add 5 pounds for each additional inch in your height over 60 inches. So, for example, if you are 5 feet 6 inches tall, your ideal weight would be

5 feet (100 pounds) plus 6 inches (5 pounds x 6 inches = 30 pounds) for a total of 130 pounds.

DAILY PROTEIN REQUIREMENTS BY WEIGHT

HEIGHT	IDEAL WT. IN LBS.	IDEAL WT. IN KGS.	GRAMS OF PROTEIN NEEDED
5'2"	110.00	49.5	39.6
5'3"	115.00	51.75	41.4
5'4"	120.00	54	43.2
5'5"	125.00	56.25	45
5'6"	130.00	58.5	46.8
5'7"	135.00	60.75	48.6
5'8"	140.00	63	50.4
5'9"	145.00	65.25	52.2

STEP TWO: CONVERT YOUR IDEAL WEIGHT IN POUNDS TO KILOGRAMS

One pound = 0.45 kilograms, so to convert your weight in pounds to kilograms multiply your weight in pounds by 0.45. For example, 130 pounds multiplied by 0.45 = 58.5 kilograms.

STEP THREE: MULTIPLY YOUR WEIGHT IN KILOGRAMS BY 0.8

The US Recommended Daily Allowance (RDA) for protein intake is 0.8 grams of protein per kilogram of ideal body weight each day. To find the number of grams of protein you need daily, multiply your weight in kilograms by 0.8. Thus, for the 5 foot 6 inch woman in our example, whose ideal weight is 130 pounds or 58.5 kilograms, the calculation is 58.5 x 0.8 = 46.8 grams.

Unfortunately, diets containing significantly more protein than is needed are quite common in the United States. Analysis of NHANES (National Health and Nutrition Examination Survey) data show that daily protein intakes ranging from 91 to 113 grams are typical in the majority of adults (19 and older), and decrease to amounts that still remain quite a bit higher than needed—around 66 to 83 grams per day—in many elders 71 years or older.[121]

On the other hand, somewhere between 15 to 38% of adult men and 27 to 41% of adult women have dietary protein intakes *below* the RDA.[122] A diet too low in protein has been associated with reduced absorption of calcium from the intestines, which researchers are concerned may also increase bone loss.[123]

To determine *your* typical protein intake, keep a food diary for three to five days (if you kept a food diary to check that you were getting enough calcium, you can use that here as well), then use the list of protein-rich foods listed in the following table to check and see if you are supplying your body with sufficient protein to meet your needs—but not overdoing it.

FOODS RICH IN PROTEIN

FOOD	SERVING SIZE	PROTEIN
Cod, baked/broiled	4 ounces	26 grams
Tuna, yellowfin, baked/broiled	4 ounces	34 grams
Snapper, baked/broiled	4 ounces	30 grams
Halibut, baked/broiled	4 ounces	30 grams
Scallops, baked/broiled	4 ounces	23 grams
Shrimp, steamed/ boiled	4 ounces	24 grams

FOOD	SERVING SIZE	PROTEIN
Sardines, canned	1 can, 3.75 ounces	23 grams
Salmon, baked/broiled	4 ounces	29 grams
Chicken breast, roasted	4 ounces	33 grams
Turkey breast, roasted	4 ounces	33 grams
Beef tenderloin, lean, broiled	4 ounces	32 grams
Lamb loin, roasted	4 ounces	30 grams
Calf's liver, braised	4 ounces	25 grams
Egg, whole, boiled	1	6 grams
Tofu	4 ounces	10 grams
Tempeh, cooked	4 ounces	21 grams
Soybeans, cooked	1 cup	29 grams
Split peas, cooked	1 cup	16 grams
Kidney beans, cooked	1 cup	15 grams
Lima beans, cooked	1 cup	15 grams
Black beans, cooked	1 cup	15 grams
Navy beans, cooked	1 cup	15 grams
Pinto beans, cooked	1 cup	14 grams
Garbanzo beans, cooked	1 cup	15 grams
Lentils, cooked	1 cup	18 grams
Peanuts	1/4 cup	10 grams
Pumpkin seeds	1/4 cup	9 grams
Cow's milk	1 cup	8 grams
Yogurt, low-fat	1 cup	13 grams
Cottage cheese	3 ounces	14 grams
Mozzarella cheese, part skim	1 ounce	7 grams
Cheddar	1 ounce	8 grams
Cheddar, low fat	1 ounce	10 grams
Feta	1 ounce	5 grams
Parmesan	1 ounce	8 grams

FOOD	SERVING SIZE	PROTEIN
Oats, whole grain, cooked	1 cup	6 grams
Bread, whole wheat	1 slice	3 grams
Bread, white	1 slice	2.5 grams
Pasta, whole wheat, boiled	3 ounces	9 grams
Pasta, refined flour, boiled	3 ounces	7 grams
Rice, brown	7 ounces	5 grams
Rice, white	7 ounces	5 grams
Asparagus	3.5 ounces	3 grams
Broccoli	3.5 ounces	3 grams
Cauliflower	3.5 ounces	3 grams
Spinach	3.5 ounces	2 grams
Tomato	3.5 ounces	2 grams
Yam	3.5 ounces	2 grams
Beet	3.5 ounces	2 grams
Onion	3.5 ounces	2 grams
Sweet corn	3.5 ounces	2.5 grams
Mushrooms	3.5 ounces	2 grams

Refined Sugars Make Your Belly Fat but Your Bones Skinny

Consumption of refined sugars, such as the high fructose corn syrup now added to virtually every processed packaged food and beverage, promotes acidic body chemistry. Similar to what happens when you eat too much animal protein, when your diet is loaded with refined sugars, your urinary excretion of calcium increases.

The average American consumes 125 grams of sucrose (table sugar) and 50 grams of corn syrup each day in processed foods, which also contain other refined simple sugars (e.g., dextrose). (Since neither of your authors consumes any sucrose or corn syrup at all, there are at least one or two people who must be consuming 250 grams [almost 9 ounces] of sucrose and 100 grams [approximately 3½ ounces] of corn syrup daily, for a grand total of over three-quarters of a pound of just these two simple sugars daily!) And that doesn't even count carbonated beverages (sodas) high in both refined sugars and phosphates, both of which promote bone loss.[124] Our genes, which have changed only about 0.01% since the Paleolithic era when the only refined sugar humans encountered was a very occasional bit of honey, are not equipped to handle this sugar tsunami.

While 99.9% of our genetic profile is still Paleolithic, 70% of the average caloric intake of Americans comes from food products that did not even exist for our Paleolithic ancestors, for example, cookies, French fries, corn chips, or soft drinks. Somehow, our ancestors not only survived but evolved. Humans today may not be faring as well. Research published in the *New England Journal of Medicine* indicates that the current generation of children in the US is likely to live shorter lives than their parents, largely because the rapid rise in obesity, if unchecked, will shorten life spans by as much as five years.[125]

Soft Drinks Are Hard on Bones

Soft drinks hit your bones with a double whammy since they dose you not only with refined sugars, but large amounts of phosphates, and no calcium. When phosphate levels are high, and calcium levels are low, calcium is—you guessed it—once again pulled out of your bones to restore balance. The "average" American consumes 15 ounces of soda pop every day.[126] Even if you drink "diet soda," your bones are still being assaulted by phosphates.

Greens Give the Go-Ahead for Great Bones; Their Absence Slams the Brakes on Bone-Building

Green leafy vegetables are packed with all the vitamins and minerals necessary for bone health, including calcium, vitamin K, boron, and magnesium. Unfortunately, very few Americans are eating leafy greens.

According to research conducted by the Center for Disease Control and Prevention, adults in the US average, at best, no more than 3.4 servings per day of fruits and vegetables *combined*.[127] Data collected by the second National Health and Nutrition Examination Survey showed that only 27% of Americans were eating at least three servings of vegetables daily (and this included potatoes, of which the vast majority were consumed in the form of French fries or potato chips).[128]

Since a serving of vegetables is just one-half cup (the equivalent of five broccoli florets, ten baby carrots, or half a baked sweet potato) or one cup of leafy greens (such as lettuce, spinach, kale, collards, or Swiss chard), these statistics go a long way towards explaining why osteoporosis is so common. Our bodies simply cannot build bone unless we provide them with the necessary ingredients to do so. It's like asking someone to whip up an omelet with no eggs.

"Bs" for Better Bones

The B vitamins—vitamin B_6, vitamin B_{12}, folate, and riboflavin—are involved in a cellular process called *methylation*, which jump starts and stops many vital processes in the body. Methylation is so important to so many of the biochemical processes that support our life that it occurs throughout the body billions of times every second!

At one of the steps in the methylation cycle, the amino acid *methionine* must be converted into another amino acid called *cysteine*, and this conversion requires vitamin B_{12} and the activated forms of vitamin B_6 and folate. The activated forms of vitamin B_6 and folate are produced by an enzyme called *flavin adenine dinucleotide* or *FAD*, which requires riboflavin (vitamin B_2) as a necessary component (co-factor).

Why do you need to know about all of this? If any of these B vitamins are not available throughout the body in adequate amounts, the methylation cycle stops midway at the point where an intermediate product called *homocysteine* gets produced. And homocysteine is a very nasty, very inflammatory compound—the molecular equivalent of a terrorist with an acid-spray gun.

When levels of homocysteine get too high within our cells, it leaks into the bloodstream and wreaks all kinds of havoc throughout the body. In addition to promoting osteoporosis,[129] high levels of homocysteine are strongly linked to cardiovascular diseases including atherosclerosis, peripheral artery disease, heart attack, and stroke;[130] neuropsychiatric diseases such as Alzheimer's dementia, Parkinson's disease, schizophrenia, and depression;[131] kidney disease;[132]

rheumatoid arthritis;[133] and worsening the vascular complications associated with type 2 diabetes.[134]

Homocysteine harms bone, specifically, because concentrations of homocysteine—which, by the way, typically increase during and after menopause—interfere with collagen cross-linking, and this results in the production of a defective bone matrix.[135] In other words, the internal structure of bone built when homocysteine levels are high is defective.

The impact of high homocysteine levels on bone health can be quite significant. In one study involving 1,002 men and women whose average age was 75, those with high levels of homocysteine (>14 micromol/liter) had a 70% higher risk of hip fracture.[136]

B vitamin deficiencies are quite common in the US, and they typically increase with age. Even during childbearing years, women are at increased risk of B vitamin deficiency due to the widespread use of oral contraceptives, which lower blood levels of vitamins B_6 and B_{12}, putting premenopausal women at increased risk of cardiovascular disease.[137]

Among individuals 65 and older, the most recent NHANES data indicates that only 38% have adequate blood levels of folate.[138] A study involving one hundred and fifty-two consecutive outpatients, ages 65 to 99, found that 14.5% were deficient in B_{12}.[139] Large surveys in the US have repeatedly found that at least 6% of those aged 60 or older are vitamin B_{12} deficient and that the likelihood of deficiency increases with age, so that closer to 20% of Americans have marginal B_{12} levels in later life.[140] Incidence of deficiency is even higher in individuals with type 2 diabetes, due in part to the fact that metformin (a patent medicine that lowers blood sugar levels and is prescribed for people with type 2 diabetes) inhibits B_{12} absorption. A recent study of individuals with type 2 diabetes revealed that 22% were B_{12} deficient.[141]

DO YOU HAVE ENOUGH OF THESE "Bs" ON BOARD?

Use the 5-to-7-day food diary you kept to estimate your calcium and protein intake to get an estimate of how much B_6, B_{12}, folate, and riboflavin your typical diet is giving you each day. If you are taking a multiple vitamin and mineral supplement, be sure to add in the B vitamins it supplies when you check to see if you are meeting your bones' needs for B vitamins.

Recommended daily intake of B vitamins for bone health:

- B_6: 50 milligrams
- B_{12}: 500 micrograms
- Folate: 2,000 micrograms
- Riboflavin: 25 milligrams

As the tables on the following pages show, simply enjoying one meal that includes a large tossed salad (leafy greens plus some favorite vegetables, such as carrots, celery, bell pepper, broccoli, cauliflower, beets, or green beans), along with 4 ounces of fish or a cup of beans, and snacking on a handful of peanuts, sunflower seeds, and/or an orange, a banana, or some papaya, can help meet your bones' vitamin B needs.

BEST FOOD SOURCES OF VITAMIN B$_6$:

FOOD	SERVING SIZE	AMOUNT OF B$_6$
Tuna, yellowfin, baked or broiled	4 ounces	1.18 mg
Cod, baked or broiled	4 ounces	0.52 mg
Snapper, baked or broiled	4 ounces	0.52 mg
Salmon, baked or broiled	4 ounces	0.52 mg
Halibut	4 ounces	0.45 mg
Chicken breast, roasted	4 ounces	0.64 mg
Turkey breast, roasted	4 ounces	0.54 mg
Spinach, raw	1 cup	0.44 mg
Banana	1	0.68 mg
Potato, baked with skin	1 cup	0.42 mg
Avocado slices	1 cup	0.41 mg
Green peas, boiled	1 cup	0.35 mg

BEST FOOD SOURCES OF VITAMIN B$_{12}$:

FOOD	SERVING SIZE	AMOUNT OF B$_{12}$
Calves' liver, braised	4 ounces	41.39 mcg
Snapper, baked or broiled	4 ounces	3.97 mcg
Salmon, baked or broiled	4 ounces	3.25 mcg
Beef tenderloin, lean, broiled	4 ounces	2.92 mcg
Lamb loin, roasted	4 ounces	2.45 mcg
Halibut	4 ounces	1.55 mcg
Cod, baked or broiled	4 ounces	1.18 mcg
Yogurt, low-fat	1 cup	1.38 mcg

FOOD	SERVING SIZE	AMOUNT OF B_{12}
Cow's milk, 2%	1 cup	0.89 mcg
Egg, whole, boiled	1	0.49 mcg

BEST FOOD SOURCES OF RIBOFLAVIN:

FOOD	SERVING SIZE	AMOUNT OF RIBOFLAVIN
Cow's milk, nonfat	8 ounces	0.6 mg
Cheese, Danish blue	1 ounce	0.6 mg
Cheese, Parmesan	1/3rd ounce	0.5 mg
Cheese, Cheddar	1 ounce	0.5 mg
Yogurt	6 ounces	0.2 mg
Beef sirloin	3 ounces	0.3 mg
Corn flakes, enriched	1 ounce	1.3 mg
Chicken liver	4 ounces	1.7 mg
Egg, boiled	1 large	0.5 mg
Almonds	10 nuts	0.9 mg
Cashews	10 nuts	0.2 mg
Walnuts	5 nuts	0.1 mg
Salmon, baked or broiled	3 ounces	0.2 mg
Sardines	3 ounces	0.3 mg
Crab	3 ounces	0.2 mg
Chicken	3 ounces	0.2mg
Mushrooms	3 ounces	0.4 mg
Broccoli	3 ounces	0.2 mg
Spinach, raw	1 cup	0.42 mg
Bread, whole wheat	1 slice	0.06 mg
Prunes	8	0.2 mg
Apricots, dried	1 ounce	0.2 mg
Avocado	1/2	0.1 mg

BEST FOOD SOURCES OF FOLATE:

FOOD	SERVING SIZE	AMOUNT OF FOLATE
Calves' liver, braised	4 ounces	860.70 mcg
Lentils, cooked	1 cup	357.98 mcg
Spinach, boiled 1 minute	1 cup	262.80 mcg
Asparagus, boiled 1 minute	1 cup	262.80 mcg
Navy beans, cooked	1 cup	254.80 mcg
Pinto beans, cooked		294.12 mcg
Chickpeas (garbanzos), cooked	1 cup	282.08 mcg
Black beans, cooked	1 cup	255.94 mcg
Collard greens, steamed	1 cup	176.70 mcg
Turnip greens, cooked	1 cup	170.50 mcg
Lima beans, cooked	1 cup	156.23 mcg
Romaine lettuce	2 cups	151.98 mcg
Beets, cooked	1 cup	136.00 mcg
Split peas, cooked	1 cup	127.20 mcg
Papaya	1	115.52 mcg
Brussels sprouts, steamed	1 cup	93.60 mcg
Avocado slices	1 cup	90.37 mcg
Peanuts	1/4 cup	87.53 mcg
Sunflower seeds	1/4 cup	81.86 mcg
Winter squash, baked	1 cup	57.40 mcg
Cauliflower, steamed	1 cup	54.56 mcg
Green beans, steamed	1 cup	41.63 mcg
Oranges	1	39.69 mcg
Summer squash, cooked slices	1 cup	36.18 mcg
Celery, raw	1 cup	33.6 mcg

FOOD	SERVING SIZE	AMOUNT OF FOLATE
Bell pepper, raw slices	1 cup	20.24 mcg
Carrots, raw	1 cup	17.08 mcg

"C" Your Way to Stronger Bones

Vitamin C stimulates the activity of akaline phosphatase, an enzyme that is a marker for the formation of the bone-building osteoblasts; is necessary for the formation and secretion of osteoid, a cartilage-like material into which the osteoblasts deposit calcium; and is also required for the cross-linking of collagen fibrils in bone, which helps to form a strong bone matrix. Not getting enough vitamin C means not enough bone-building cells or docking stations for calcium inside your bones.[142]

A number of recent studies have confirmed vitamin C's importance for bone health. Researchers analyzing seventeen years of follow up data from the Framingham Osteoporosis Study noted that study participants whose diets provided the most vitamin C had significantly fewer hip and other fractures compared to those whose diets provided the lowest amounts of vitamin C.[143] A study carried out at the Hospital of Jaén, in Spain, confirmed this. This study involved 167 people aged 65 or older who had had a fragility fracture (a fracture that occurs during normal daily activities as a result of having weak, thin bones) plus 167 healthy controls of comparable age and sex. When study participants' diet was assessed for vitamin C intake, and their blood levels of vitamin C were measured, those whose diets provided the most vitamin C (and thus those whose blood levels of vitamin C were highest) were found to have a 69% lower risk of fracture![144]

In another recent study, this one conducted in Australia, researchers randomly selected 533 nonsmoking women and checked their blood levels of a key biochemical marker of bone breakdown called C-telopeptide (CTx). Not only was CTx much lower in women taking supplemental vitamin C, but the longer the women had been taking vitamin C, the lower their CTx level.[145]

Many Americans are consuming far too little vitamin C to maintain healthy bones. In the third National Health and Nutrition Examination Survey (NHANES III, 1988–1994), approximately 13% of the US population was vitamin C deficient (blood levels lower than 11.4 micromols per liter). The most recent NHANES (2003–2004) showed some improvement, finding frank vitamin C deficiency in 7.1% of Americans.

However, there is a big difference between outright vitamin C deficiency—we're talking so little vitamin C that these folks were at risk for scurvy—and having

FOODS RICH IN VITAMIN C

FOOD	SERVING SIZE	AMOUNT OF VITAMIN C
Papaya	1	187.87 mg
Bell pepper, red, raw, slices	1 cup	174.8 mg
Broccoli, steamed	1 cup	123.40 mg
Brussels sprouts	1 cup	96.72 mg
Strawberries	1 cup	81.65 mg
Oranges	1	69.69 mg
Cantaloupe	1 cup	67.52 mg
Kiwifruit	1	57.00 mg

enough of this nutrient available in your body to promote strong, healthy bones![146] Although the RDA for vitamin C was recently increased to 75 mg per day in women and 90 mg per day in men, this recommendation is still based on how much vitamin C is needed to prevent frank deficiency (think scurvy), not how much is needed to promote optimal health. In the medical research, intakes of vitamin C much higher than the RDAs have been related to better bone health. In postmenopausal women, greater bone mineral density was reported as vitamin C intake from supplements increased from 0 to 500 to 1,000 mg per day.[147]

In addition, vitamin C plays many vital roles in our white (immune) blood cells and is therefore rapidly depleted when we are ill, when we consume foods or beverages high in sugar, or when we are exposed to cigarette smoke.[148] Vitamin C levels are one-third lower in smokers compared to nonsmokers.[149] All these circumstances greatly increase our needs for vitamin C.

Pull out your trusty food diary and see how much vitamin C your diet is giving YOU each day.

CHAPTER 4

What Else Increases My Risk for Osteoporosis?

Osteoporosis, a Family Affair?

THE LEVEL OF PEAK bone mineral density or bone mass, which our bodies attain between 20 and 30 years of age, is greatly influenced by genetic factors.[150] Some studies suggest that up to 80% of how much peak bone mass each of us achieves is related to genetic factors! Young daughters of women with osteoporotic fractures have lower bone mass compared with other children their age, and *first-degree relatives* (the parents, brothers, sisters, or children) of women with osteoporosis tend to have lower bone mass than do first-degree relatives of women who do not have a family history of osteoporosis.[151]

The rate at which we lose bone after menopause is also impacted by our genetic inheritance. Although the genetic impact on the rate at which bone is lost with aging is less dramatic than our genes' effects on how much peak bone mass we achieve, our genes may still account for up to 56% of the variation in the rate at which bone loss occurs among different individuals.[152]

SO, WHAT DOES THIS MEAN FOR YOU?

Just as some people can smoke for 50 years and never develop lung cancer or COPD (chronic obstructive pulmonary disease), some people have an inborn ability to build and keep very strong, dense bones. If your mother, aunt, and/or grandmother experienced a broken hip or other fragility fracture, however, chances are that you are not one of them!

This does *not* mean you are doomed to develop osteoporosis. You absolutely can be the first woman in your family in generations to go through your entire life with the beautiful, erect posture that comes from strong, healthy bones. But you will need to make the diet, lifestyle, and supplement choices outlined in this book that optimize bone health. Your bones need all the help you can provide.

Gastric Bypass: Free Pass? Not for Your Bones

Gastric bypass (or small-bowel resection) reduces the amount of absorptive surface area in the intestines, and by doing so lessens the body's ability to absorb not just fat and calories, but also all the nutrients needed to maintain and form healthy bone.

The gastric bypass (the medical term for it is the Roux-en-Y procedure) is the leading surgery to treat morbid obesity performed in the United States. Since this operation causes the primary sites where calcium absorption occurs to be bypassed, patients become deficient in calcium and vitamin D. In response to these deficiencies, the body up-regulates the secretion and activity of parathyroid hormone. Parathyroid hormone has two bone-related effects: it causes an increase in the production of the most active form of vitamin D (1,25-dihydroxyvitamin D), which helps us absorb more calcium from food, but it also causes increased bone resorption (bone breakdown) to liberate more calcium for calcium's many other uses in the body.[153]

Calcium wears a lot of "hats" in the body, playing vital roles in a number of critical physiological processes not related to its use in bone. These include helping blood to clot, so we don't bleed to death when cut; helping nerves to send impulses and muscles to contract (in the case of the heart muscle, contraction = heartbeat); and regulating our cell membranes, so our cells can allow entry of what they need and send out what they don't.

Because these activities are essential to life, the body tightly controls the amount of calcium in the blood to ensure that sufficient calcium is available for them. Our bones, where approximately 99% of the calcium in our bodies is stashed, serve as a calcium "bank" from which withdrawals can be made to maintain normal blood concentrations whenever the need arises—which it surely will after gastric bypass (or if we fail to consume calcium-rich foods and/or supplemental calcium sufficient to meet our body's needs).

Gastric banding, another surgical procedure for morbid obesity, is a safer, potentially reversible, and effective alternative to the Roux-en-Y gastric bypass that has not been shown to produce as much bone loss as the Roux-en-Y procedure. In gastric banding, an inflatable silicone device is placed around the top portion of the stomach to create a small pouch at the top of the stomach that holds about 3.5 to 6.5 ounces of food. When a person eats, the pouch quickly fills with food, and the band slows its passage from the pouch to the lower part of the stomach. As soon as the upper part of the stomach registers as full, the brain is sent a message that the entire stomach is full, which helps the person eat smaller portions, eat less often, and lose weight over time. Within six to eight years, weight loss from gastric banding is comparable to that achieved by gastric bypass; however, many physicians and patients choose gastric bypass because it results in faster weight loss and resolution of diabetes.[154] The fact that some of the weight lost comes from the patient's bones is somehow overlooked.

WHAT DOES THIS MEAN FOR YOU?

Either of these surgeries will lessen your body's ability to absorb calcium and the other nutrients necessary for bone health. If you have had or are considering either of these surgical interventions for morbid obesity, please discuss the potential adverse effects on your bones with your physician. Medical journal articles alerting physicians to these concerns are just beginning to appear, and many doctors remain unaware of these issues.[155]

Although increasing calcium or vitamin D intake does not suppress parathyroid hormone or prevent the acceleration in bone resorption caused by gastric bypass, it is possible that highly absorbable supplements may help lessen the damage.[156] Anyone who has had either of these surgeries should be using calcium supplements providing calcium citrate and not calcium carbonate.*

The Liver–Kidney Connection to Bone

You've probably heard something about how important vitamin D is for bone health. Here's why: vitamin D stimulates the absorption of calcium from the intestines and also calcium's resorption from the kidneys, greatly improving the likelihood that adequate calcium will be present in the bloodstream for all the body's calcium needs.

However, these effects of vitamin D do not occur until *after* vitamin D has been converted into its most active form in the body. This conversion occurs in two stages, the first of which takes place in the liver, and the second in the kidneys. For this reason, dysfunction in either the liver or the kidneys can compromise vitamin D activation, calcium absorption, and bone health.

Approximately 23% of patients with chronic liver disease have osteoporosis. You may be thinking that this couldn't possibly concern you, that liver disease is uncommon and caused only by alcoholism or hepatitis. You'd be wrong.

Today, the most rapidly increasing liver disease is nonalcoholic fatty liver disease or NAFLD, and it is caused by insulin resistance and type 2 diabetes. Following menopause, risk for NAFLD goes up significantly. In a surprising 55% of women over age 60, liver function is compromised by NAFLD.[157] High blood

---

* See page 206.

pressure and diabetes also increase risk for chronic kidney disease, which is estimated to affect 11.5% of adults aged 20 or older in the US.[158]

WHAT DOES THIS MEAN FOR YOU?

NAFLD and other liver diseases often produce no noticeable symptoms and may therefore go undiagnosed. Particularly if you have been diagnosed with MetS (metabolic syndrome) or type 2 diabetes, be sure your annual physical includes the standard lab tests that check liver function.[159]

Symptoms of worsening kidney function are also unspecific and may go unnoticed. Symptoms include feeling generally unwell and loss of appetite. Check to be sure that the lab tests run for your annual physical include *creatinine*. Higher levels of creatinine indicate a decrease in kidney function and the ability to excrete waste products.

Anyone suffering from chronic liver or kidney disease is at significantly increased risk for vitamin D deficiency and osteoporosis. Supplemental vitamin D has been found to help lessen bone loss associated with liver and/or kidney disease.[160]

What's Hyperparathyroidism and Why Should My Bones Care?

Hyperparathyroidism is overactivity of the parathyroid glands (hyper = excessive, above normal), resulting in excessive production of parathyroid hormone. Hyperparathyroidism is divided into "primary" and "secondary" types.

"Primary" hyperparathyroidism is relatively rare. It's a disease of the parathyroid glands themselves, usually of unknown origin, and is almost always the more severe form. Sometimes surgery is required as part of treatment.

"Secondary" hyperparathyroidism is almost always milder, and not always diagnosed as such. Secondary hyperparathyroidism is not a disease (as the primary form is) but a protective response by the body to increase blood levels of calcium from unhealthy low levels caused by inadequate calcium intake or the many other causes listed below.

But, although parathyroid hormone causes an increase in the body's production of the most active form of vitamin D (1,25-dihydroxyvitamin D), which helps us absorb more calcium from our intestines, parathyroid hormone also causes increased osteoclast activity and bone resorption (bone breakdown) in order to liberate calcium from bone for calcium's many other immediate uses in the body.

Blood levels of calcium low enough to cause secondary hyperparathyroidism are typically due to not getting enough daily calcium, vitamin D deficiency, chronic kidney disease, chronic liver disease, low levels of stomach acid (hypochlorhydria, relatively common after age 50), malabsorption of calcium (and other minerals, most often caused by "hidden" gluten sensitivity), or gastric bypass surgery. Obesity has also been shown to increase parathyroid hormone levels, which, in addition, tend to increase with age in both men and women.

Above normal levels of parathyroid hormone have recently been associated not only with osteoporosis, but also with cognitive decline and senile dementia (Alzheimer's disease). The connection is most likely explained by the fact that sustained high levels of parathyroid hormone in the brain increase risk of calcium overloading, which leads to impaired blood flow and brain degeneration.[161]

Fortunately, a recent study involving 37 institutionalized women, ranging in age from their late 70s to late 80s, has shown that consumption of a fortified dairy product, containing only about 17–25% of the recommended daily intakes for calcium and vitamin D, lowered levels of parathyroid hormone and increased levels of both vitamin D and markers of bone formation in just one month.[162]

WHAT DOES THIS MEAN FOR YOU?

Especially if you are taking teriparatide (Forteo®*) the lab tests ordered at your annual physical should include blood levels of parathyroid hormone. Normal values range from 10–55 picograms per milliliter (ng/mL); however, recent research suggests values higher than 30 may indicate suboptimal intake of calcium and vitamin D.[163]

Higher than normal levels of parathyroid hormone indicate that you are not meeting your body's needs for calcium and vitamin D, and that you are at increased risk not only for osteoporosis but cognitive decline and Alzheimer's disease. Work with your doctor to increase your consumption of calcium and vitamin D, and recheck your levels of parathyroid hormone after a month to two months on your new and improved bone health promotion program.

---

* See page 66. See also pages 314–316.

IS YOUR THYROID ON OVERDRIVE?

Hyperthyroidism (a "hyperactive" thyroid) is a well-known risk factor for osteoporosis, regardless of sex or age. The hormones produced and secreted by the thyroid gland regulate the body's metabolic rate. When thyroid hormone levels are too high, regardless of whether we are pre- or post-menopausal, female or male, it's like putting the body into overdrive, accelerating all its metabolic activities, including the rate at which bones are remodeled, all the time.

Each bone remodeling cycle involves 3–5 weeks of bone breakdown by osteoclasts followed by about 3 months during which osteoblasts lay down new bone to replace the bone that was removed. The result of the fast-forward bone metabolism seen in hyperthyroidism is increased bone resorption that leads to a loss of approximately 10% of bone mass per remodeling cycle. Not surprisingly, this can quickly result in lowered bone mineral density and increased risk of fracture.[164] Fortunately, hyperthyroidism is relatively uncommon.

Do Your Favorite Activities All Involve Sitting?

If you want to keep your bones, get moving! Exercise helps build and maintain bone mass by stimulating osteoblasts. It's true that younger individuals get more bone-building bang-for-their-exercise-buck—a 2–5% increase in bone mineral density (BMD) per year—but us older folks can still expect regular exercise to deliver a net gain in BMD of 1–3% per year.[165]

In contrast, if most of your day involves sitting, your sedentary lifestyle is rapidly and dramatically accelerating the loss of your bones. Numerous studies have confirmed this.[166] In one of the most recent, researchers studied 59 postmenopausal women with osteoporosis or osteopenia, 30 of whom followed a weight resistance exercise program for one year while the remaining 29 did not exercise. At the end of the study, the exercising women showed a 1.17% *increase* in BMD in the lumbar spine. The sedentary women *lost* 2.26% in their lumbar spine BMD.[167]

Aerobics, weight bearing, and resistance exercises have all been shown to be effective in increasing the bone mineral density of the spine in postmenopausal women, and walking is especially effective for building bone in the hips.[168]

Just walking briskly for 15 to 20 minutes a day can be the deciding factor in whether you lose or gain bone mass. In another recent study involving 37 sedentary women, 20 women remained sedentary while 17 took up brisk walking for an average of just 16.9 minutes each day. In the same study, in a second group of 31 women, 15 women who had been walking regularly for 1 year returned to their former sedentary lifestyle, while the remaining 16 women continued their brisk walking for a second year. These 16 women walked an average of 20.8 minutes daily—an amount of time you could clock in during your lunch hour. By the end of the study, BMD, measured in the *calcaneus* (anklebone) had decreased significantly (by 2.7%) in the women who stopped walking and returned to a sedentary lifestyle, but increased significantly (7.4%) in the women who had been sedentary but changed their lifestyle to include a daily brisk walk.[169]

Even if you already have been diagnosed with osteopenia or osteoporosis, exercise can be a huge help in restoring the health of your bones. In another recent study, researchers looked at the effects of a group exercise program on BMD, pain, and quality of life in postmenopausal women with osteoporosis (16 women, average age 55.2 years) and osteopenia (17 women, average age 55.4 years). Each group followed the same group exercise program. For one hour three times a week for 21 weeks, all the women did a series of breathing, warm-up, stretching, strengthening, balance, stabilization, and cooling exercises. After the 21-week program, both groups showed significant improvements in their DXA-score ("Dual-Energy X-ray Absorptiometry" is the gold standard x-ray procedure used to evaluate bone density. This was previously shortened to "DEXA," but is now called "DXA."*), pain score, BMD, and all the parameters of the Quality of Life Questionnaire of the European Foundation for Osteoporosis. Following the exercise program, 43.8% of the osteoporotic women had a DXA-score that now showed only osteopenia, and 23.5% of the osteopenic women had a DXA-score falling within the normal range![170]

Getting Any . . . Sunshine?

Are your bones getting their daily dose of sunshine vitamin? Sunshine begins your body's bone-building process. Sunlight on exposed, *sunscreen-free* skin changes a compound in the skin called 7-dehydrocholesterol into vitamin D_3 (cholecalciferol). (Sunscreen SPF 8 reduces sunlight's ability to trigger the conversion of 7-dehydrocholesterol into vitamin D_3 by 95%.)

---

* See page 158.

This is the first of the three steps through which your body activates vitamin D into the form in which it is able to stimulate the absorption of calcium.

You don't have to spend hours being unprotected from the sun's skin-wrinkling rays or possibly increasing your risk for skin cancer. In the summer, all you need is 20–30 minutes of sun exposure, during which time, as much as 10,000 IU of vitamin D can be produced in our skin.

Once awakened by the kiss of sunlight on your skin, cholecalciferol is transported to the liver and converted into 25-hydroxycholecalciferol [25(OH)D$_3$], a compound five times as potent as cholecalciferol. 25-hydroxycholecalciferol is then sent to the kidneys where it is converted into 1,25-dihydroxycholecalciferol [1,25(OH)D$_3$], which is 10 times as potent as cholecalciferol and the most active form of vitamin D in the body.*

If you live north of 35° latitude (i.e., in any of the states north of North Carolina, Tennessee, Arkansas, Oklahoma, New Mexico, or Arizona, or in the northern part of California, or in Oregon or Washington state), you are at increased risk for vitamin D deficiency. Why? Because the wavelength in sunlight needed to produce vitamin D in the skin (UVB radiation of 290 to 320 nm) is not available in these areas during the winter months and possibly for even more of the year.

In addition to people living in northern latitudes, individuals whose sun exposure is limited are at significant risk for vitamin D deficiency.[171] This would include those who are homebound or work in occupations that

---

* You can see why liver or kidney problems can cause bone loss. For more on this, see page 113.

keep them indoors, preventing exposure to sunlight; wear clothing that completely covers the body (we knew wearing a burqa would not only keep us off the Best Dressed List, but is physically bad for us);[172] or always use sunscreen.

Even if you live in a sunny climate, sun exposure alone may not produce blood levels of vitamin D adequate for bone (and overall) health. Your vitamin D levels (as measured by the serum 25-hydroxyvitamin D test) should be at the very least 30 nanograms per milliliter (ng/mL) or 75 nanomoles per liter (nmol/L, an alternate measurement that is often used). Many physicians now recommend that 25-hydroxyvitamin D levels be between 60 and 100 ng/mL, the so-called "tropical optimum." But even in Hawaii, one recent 3-month study found that only half of the healthy and racially diverse young adult participants, whose average sun exposure was 29 hours each week, achieved blood levels of vitamin D of 30 ng/mL (75 nmol/L).[173]

If you are deficient in vitamin D, you will not absorb calcium effectively. Without adequate vitamin D, the intestine absorbs only 10–15% of the dietary or supplemental calcium you consume.[174]

Many studies have documented the key role vitamin D plays in bone health. Most of the research has been done using both calcium and vitamin D, but even a study using vitamin D_3 alone found that supplementation with 700 IU/day reduced the rate of hip fracture in elderly women (average age 84) by nearly 60%—from 1.3% to 0.5%.[175]

In another study of 3,270 healthy women, whose average age was again 84, for 18 months, half the women were given 800 mg of vitamin D along with 1,200 mg of calcium daily, while the other half received a placebo.

Among those treated with vitamin D and calcium, the number of hip fractures was 43% lower and the number of nonvertebral fractures was 32% lower compared to those given the placebo. BMD in the femur (thigh bone) increased 2.7% in the women taking vitamin D and calcium, while decreasing 4.6% in the placebo group.[176]

Other large studies have confirmed these results, including a 2-year, multicenter study involving 583 institutionalized women whose average age was 85 years. In the women given vitamin D_3 (800 mg) along with calcium (1,200 mg) daily, parathyroid hormone levels returned to normal within 6 months (one of the effects of too little vitamin D is increased levels of parathyroid hormone, which causes increased osteoclast activity and bone breakdown*). In the women receiving vitamin D and calcium, BMD remained stable, while decreasing 2.36% in the women receiving the placebo.[177]

The bone-health bottom line here is: you should consider a vitamin D_3 supplement. In healthy adults who regularly avoid sunlight exposure or always use sunscreen (like most of us wrinkle-avoiding women), a review of the research by the Vitamin D Council (www.vitamindcouncil.org), a nonprofit organization whose directors are among the world's leading experts on vitamin D, indicates a necessity to supplement with 2,000 to 5,000 IU of vitamin D daily. [178]

According to the Vitamin D Council, you can ensure your vitamin D levels are adequate for bone health by:

- Regularly getting outside to enjoy a half hour of midday sun exposure in the late spring, summer, and early fall, exposing as much of your skin as

---

* See page 114.

possible (but being careful not to get a sunburn). Then you can apply sunscreen and don a hat.

- Taking 5,000 IU of vitamin D_3 per day for 2–3 months, then getting a blood test run to check your levels of 25-hydroxyvitamin D_3. Work with your doctor to adjust your dosage of supplemental vitamin D so your blood levels are *at least* 30 ng/mL (75 nmol/L). A number of medical experts involved in vitamin D research now feel that optimal blood levels of vitamin D should run between 50–80 ng/mL (or 125–200 nmol/L) year-round.

Gloria Vanderbilt Once Said, "A Woman Can't Be Too Rich or Too Thin." She Was Half-Wrong.

Anorexia nervosa, an eating disorder characterized by intense fear of gaining weight and becoming fat, despite being underweight (weighing less than 85% of the weight considered normal or healthy for one's height and build), causes bone loss, particularly in the spine and hip.[179] This is not surprising since bones cannot be built without a whole team of nutrients and also respond by strengthening when stressed by weight—which is why resistance exercises help build bone.

Heavier women put some stress on their bones just by walking around; thin women don't. But this is not a recommendation to become obese. Being overweight promotes inflammation and is much more harmful than helpful to your bones. Stress your bones by exercising, and not only will you build bone, you'll fit into your skinny jeans.

Avoiding food, self-induced vomiting, use of laxatives, diuretics, and/or appetite suppressants is a sure-fire recipe for bone starvation. Lack of sufficient nourishment not only causes a premenopausal woman to stop menstruating and lose bone, but also causes her to lose muscle and turn into a Skeletor cartoon character look-alike.

The stress that muscles put on bone when they contract is a key "time to build more bone" signal. Women are already at a bone-building disadvantage compared to men because our muscles are smaller. Cannibalize your muscles, and you thin your bones. The complete loss of menstrual periods, *amenorrhea*, occurs largely because the body is no longer willing to use the energy needed to produce estrogen, which as mentioned earlier,* regulates osteoclasts, preventing them from removing too much bone. Maybe you should stop reading now and go get a healthy, calcium-rich snack?

Bone-Busting Patent Medicines

Many commonly prescribed patent medicines *cause* osteoporosis. These include patent medicines prescribed to treat epilepsy, anxiety, insomnia, depression, schizophrenia, restless leg syndrome, type 2 diabetes, chronic pain, allergies, asthma, and autoimmune diseases.

ANTICONVULSANT PATENT MEDICINES USED TO MANAGE EPILEPSY

Since the first edition of *Your Bones* was published, I (Lara) have learned a great deal more about this,

---

* See page 6.

inspired by Julie, who wrote me that, although only age 50, she has severe osteoporosis. Her doctors say her bones are "like twigs." In the last 2½ years, she has suffered fractures of both her hip and leg. When I wrote back in hopes of helping her figure out why her bones have become so brittle at such a young age, she replied she already knew why:

> I have had epilepsy since I was six months old. All epilepsy drugs cause a deficiency in calcium and vitamin D. This is a known fact, and I should have had regular blood tests throughout my life to monitor this, and, hopefully prevent the osteoporosis. This, of course, was never done, and even now they don't do it, so I have given up asking for it to be done. They only did a test to check bone density a few years ago. By that time, I already had the condition, and it was just a matter of time before I had the first fracture, a couple of years later.

Needless to say, I was very distressed that her doctors did not monitor the effects on her bones of the patent medicines they prescribed to manage her epilepsy. Her osteoporosis could have been prevented!

If you must take anticonvulsants, I want you to know that out-of-control bone loss does not need to be in your future! If you have epilepsy, there is much you can do to safely, effectively and naturally protect your bones—and, should you have already developed osteoporosis, to restore your bones' health.

How Anticonvulsant Patent Medicines Cause Bone Loss

In the first edition of *Your Bones*, I wrote (p. 106) about the fact that anticonvulsant patent medicines used to manage epilepsy (e.g, phenytoin [trade name, Dilantin®]; primidone, phenobarbital [trade name, Luminal®], valproic acid [trade name, Depacon®]) greatly increase risk for osteoporosis. These patent medicines all interfere with vitamin D absorption and metabolism, may cause deficiency of folate and/or vitamin B6, and reduce blood levels of vitamin K—all of which play important roles in bone health.*

Julie lives in Europe, where the latest position statement issued by the European Menopause and Andropause Society (EMAS), January 11, 2012, notes that 50–70% of all Europeans are deficient in vitamin D. Since her needs for this nutrient critical for bone health are increased by the anticonvulsants required to manage her epilepsy, it's highly likely that Julie—and anyone else requiring chronic treatment with anticonvulsants—needs even more than the 4,000 IU/day of vitamin D now recommended by the lead author of the EMAS position paper, Dr. Pérez-López, for postmenopausal women with any of the following risk factors for vitamin D insufficiency: obesity, dark skin, intestinal malabsorption, or residing close to the North or South poles.[180]

---

* As discussed beginning on page 168 for vitamin D, page 199 for folate/B6, and page 172 for vitamin K.

BENZODIAZEPINE PATENT MEDICINES USED TO MANAGE ANXIETY, DEPRESSION, SCHIZOPHRENIA, AND RESTLESS LEG SYNDROME CAUSE BONE LOSS

The benzodiazepines, (e.g., Valium®, Xanax®, Librium®, Halcion®—and many others),[181] another class of patent medicines frequently prescribed to treat not just epilepsy, but also anxiety, insomnia, depression, schizophrenia, and restless leg syndrome, also cause significant bone loss. Many recent studies confirm this.

One study conducted in Spain, for which results were published in 2008, assessed risk factors for osteoporosis and fractures in a large sample of women—4,960 postmenopausal women aged 50 to 65 years, who were being seen at 96 different primary care facilities across the country. The two top risk factors identified for osteoporosis were low intake of calcium and benzodiazepine use.[182]

How Benzodiazepine Patent Medicines Cause Bone Loss

The latest medical journal review articles (reviews are papers that summarize the results of many studies) are now warning physicians that the entire class of benzodiazepines (and as noted above there are numerous patent medications in this group[183]) cause chronic elevation of the hormone, prolactin. These patent medicines bind to and block off dopamine receptors in the hypothalamus. (The hypothalamus is an area in the brain containing small clusters of neurons that link the nervous system to the endocrine system via the pituitary gland.) By this action, the benzodiazepines prevent dopamine, another important neurotransmitter, from being secreted. Unfortunately, shutting down the secretion of dopamine causes prolactin levels to rise because dopamine is what turns off the pituitary gland's secretion of prolactin.

How Does Having Chronically High Levels of Prolactin Cause Bone Loss?

High prolactin levels (a condition referred to in the medical literature as "hyperprolactinaemia"), suppress the activity of the hypothalamic-pituitary-gonadal axis. This triad of endocrine glands interacts and secretes a number of hormones involved with reproduction. The hypothalamus produces gonadotropin-releasing hormone (GnRH). The anterior portion of the pituitary gland produces luteinizing hormone (LH) and follicle-stimulating hormone (FSH), and the gonads (ovaries in women, testes in men) produce estrogen and testosterone, respectively.

More accurately, the pituitary's secretion of FSH and LH are what signal the gonads to produce estrogen, progesterone, and testosterone. Since estrogen and progesterone play very important roles in maintaining healthy bones in women, inhibiting their production, by inhibiting that of FSH and LH, causes bone loss. Estrogen prevents excessive activation of osteoclasts (the specialized cells that break down old bone), while progesterone activates osteoblasts (specialized cells involved in building new bone). This is why the drop off in the production of these hormones that occurs with menopause contributes to bone loss. Even in men, estrogen is essential for bone health. Men convert a small, but very necessary amount, of testosterone into estrogen, which plays a critical role in maintaining men's bones. This is why the aromatase inhibitor patent medicines used to treat prostate cancer, which shut down testosterone (and therefore estrogen) production, cause rapid bone loss in men.

SSRIS AND TRANQUILIZERS COMMONLY USED TO MANAGE ANXIETY AND DEPRESSION CAUSE BONE LOSS

A study, published February 2011, which involved more than 27,000 postmenopausal women in Canada, found that selective serotonin reuptake inhibitors (SSRIs, e.g., Prozac®, Paxil®, Zoloft® and many others)[184] increased risk for osteoporosis by 46%, atypical antipsychotics (tranquilizers, also called 2nd generation antipsychotics, e.g., trade names Zyprexa®, Risperdal®, Seroquel®, Geodon®, Zeldox®, Ablify®[185]) increased risk by 55%, and benzodiazepines (e.g., Diazepam®, Xanax®, Paxil®, Librium®, Valium®, and many others; SSRIs are among the benzodiazepines) increased risk by 17%.[186]

Another very large study conducted in Spain—this one included more than 63,000 subjects—found SSRIs to be associated with the highest adjusted odds of osteoporotic fractures—a 45% increased risk. Monoamine oxidase inhibitor antidepressants (MAOIs are less frequently prescribed these days; the most commonly used MAOI is Emsam®, a transdermal patch of the MAOI, selegiline) increased risk for osteoporosis 15%, and benzodiazepines increased risk by 10%. A dose-effect relationship was seen with SSRIs and benzodiazepines—the longer any of these patent medicines was used, the greater the increase in risk for osteoporosis. In contrast, lithium, which is prescribed to manage bipolar disorder, was associated with a 37% lower risk for fracture.[187]

SSRIs are very commonly prescribed antidepressants—e.g., Prozac®, Valium®. These patent medicines are supposed to just increase brain levels of the neurotransmitter, serotonin, by preventing its reuptake by the neurons that secrete it. However, it has recently been revealed that SSRIs also inhibit dopamine production and neurotransmission[188]—which, as explained above, causes high prolactin levels, endocrine dysfunction, and bone loss.

Researchers have now reported very high rates of osteoporosis and osteopenia in people taking long-term psychoactive patent medicines (e.g., anticonvulsants, benzodiazepines), and the higher the dose and longer the patent medicines were taken, the greater the bone loss.

Young Caucasian women have been found to be especially vulnerable to developing high prolactin levels (hyperprolactinaemia), with the resulting inhibition of estrogen and progesterone production, and bone loss. Younger women taking any of these patent medicines and experiencing menstrual problems (an indication that the patent medicine is disrupting normal function of the hypothalamic-pituitary-gonadal axis) should immediately alert their doctors and request tests to evaluate their prolactin levels and BMD.

Ideally, work with a physician knowledgeable about integrative, holistic, and/or naturopathic medicine, who can help you identify the underlying causes of your health issues and help you restore your health using effective and safe, natural means.*

---

* To find these physicians in your area, please see "Where Can I Find an 'Integrative' Doctor Who will Help Me Build and Keep My Bones Strong, Naturally," in the "Resources" section, page 353.

You do *not* want a prescription for yet another patent medication, like a bisphosphonate (e.g., Fosamax®, Boniva®, Reclast®), or one of the other patent medicines that are now being advocated since women are aware of the bisphosphonates' adverse effects and are refusing to take them. The two latest patent medicines the pharmaceutical companies are telling doctors to prescribe are denosumab (trade names, Prolia®, Xgeva®) and teriparatide (trade name, Forteo®*), neither of which will help you restore normal bone rebuilding, and both of which can have significant adverse side effects.

If you must take a psychoactive medication, please discuss which patent medicine might be least harmful to your bones with your doctor. Some of these patent medicines have a lesser antagonizing effect on dopamine receptors in the brain. Others are potent dopamine receptor antagonists, and remember, it is by antagonizing dopamine receptors that antipsychotic patent medicines cause hyperprolactinaemia—and thus osteoporosis. Conventional psychoactive patent medicines all cause hyperprolactinemia, but a few of the so-called "atypical" psychoactive patent medicines, supposedly, do not. We've provided references[189] for the latest studies discussing this in the peer-reviewed medical literature. Share these with your doctor and ask for help finding the psychoactive patent medicine with the lowest prolactin-raising profile.

If you are taking one of these patent medicines because you suffer from depression, once again, working with a physician who can help you understand and naturally correct the underlying causes of your depression is

---

* Discussed on pages 66–76.

your best option. If you feel you must take a patent medicine, you might ask your physician about switching to a tricyclic antidepressant. (Also, once again, there are way too many of these patent medicines to list here. This endnote provides a link to the full listing online.[190]) Tricyclic antidepressants do not appear to promote bone loss and, in one study, were associated with 43% lower risk for osteoporosis.[191]

PATENT MEDICINES COMMONLY PRESCRIBED FOR TYPE 2 DIABETES CAUSE BONE LOSS

Use of the diabetes patent medicines Avandia® or Actos® for more than a year doubles to triples your risk of hip fractures. These patent medicines, members of a class of insulin-sensitizing medications called thiazolidinediones, have now been shown to also increase risk of fractures of the arm, wrist, hand, spine and foot, as well as the hip—in both men and women, even women younger than age 50 (and thus likely to be premenopausal)—by 43%. Furthermore, fracture risk increases with duration of "therapy"; four or more years of exposure to these patent medicines doubles risk of fracture.[192]

The thiazolidinediones (also known as glitazones and given the acronym TZDs) account for approximately 21% of the oral blood sugar-lowering patent medicines used in the US. Although their main therapeutic effects occur in fat tissue, muscles, and the liver, studies have conclusively shown they negatively affect bone as well. They do so by triggering mesenchymal stem cells, which can become any one of several different types of cells, including osteoblasts, chondrocytes (cells that produce cartilage) or adipocytes (fat cells), into choosing to become adipocytes. When you take these patent medications, your body makes more fat and less bone.

New research has also revealed that the TZDs initially increase osteoblast production from mesenchymal stem cells (which seems like a good thing), but then immediately cause such great disruption of normal energy production in the cells' mitochondria (the organelles in our cells responsible for producing the energy they need) that a dramatic increase occurs in reactive oxygen species (ROS, one of the two key forms free radicals). This surge in ROS triggers the osteoblasts to commit apoptosis (suicide).[193]

OPIOID PATENT MEDICINES COMMONLY USED TO MANAGE CHRONIC PAIN CAUSE BONE LOSS

Used in the management of chronic pain, opioid patent medicines (e.g., morphine, codeine, hydrocodone, oxycodone, methadone, tramadol) greatly impact the production of a number of hormones, including several with significant effects on bone in women: prolactin, estrogen, and thyroid stimulating hormone (TSH). A study of 47 women, aged 30 to 75, who were using oral or transdermal opioids for control of non-malignant pain found estradiol levels were 57% lower than in control subjects! [194]

Opioid patent medicines disrupt normal regulation of hormone production in the hypothalamic-pituitary axis. They increase production of prolactin (discussed above in relation to the benzodiazepines under "How Does Having Chronically High Levels of Prolactin Cause

Bone Loss?"*); inhibit estrogen production so effectively that among premenopausal women, menstruation typically ceases soon after initiating opioid therapy; decrease production of DHEA, and also increase production of thyroid stimulating hormone (TSH), which directly suppresses bone remodeling. The combined effect of suppressing estrogen and DHEA production while increasing that of prolactin and TSH is greatly increased risk of osteoporosis.[195] Women needing opioids for relief of chronic pain should discuss bioidentical hormone replacement with their physicians.[196]

Men's bones are also negatively affected by the use of opioids to manage chronic pain. Chronic opioid use causes secondary hypogonadism (abnormally low function of the hypothalamic-pituitary-gonadal-axis and thus lowered production of testosterone [and therefore estrogen] required for the maintenance of healthy bone in men), and promotes bone loss in the estimated 5 million men in the US and Canada treated with opioids for chronic non-cancer pain. [197]

SO-CALLED "GLUCOCORTICOID" PATENT MEDICINES, COMMONLY USED TO MANAGE ALLERGIES, ASTHMA, AND AUTOIMMUNE DISEASES, CAUSE BONE LOSS

This class of patent medicines, the so-called "glucocorticoid" patent medicines, are often mistakenly referred to as "cortisone." Our natural glucocorticoids are a class of steroid hormones whose role within our immune system is to tune down an excessive immune response that is producing too much inflammation.

---

* See page 128.

The so-called glucocorticoid patent medicines, which exert far stronger immune suppression than is normally produced by our own glucocorticoids, include Prednisone®, Prednisolone®, Kenalog®, Dexamethasone®, and nearly anything else ending with -one, (all of which are much more accurately described as "pseudo-glucocorticoids" or "glucocorticoid mimicking patent medicines") along with the non-patentable Cortef®, which is bio-identical cortisol, but as a prescription is often used in excess of normal body levels.

These patent medicines kill *osteocytes* (which is what osteoblasts turn into after they begin secreting the bone matrix). Thus, the glucocorticoid patent medications cause a rapid weakening of bone architecture (within 6 months of initiating treatment) even at very low doses. In addition, these patent medicines deplete the body of vitamin D_3, interfering with normal calcium metabolism and absorption. One reason smoking is so harmful to bone is that nicotine causes the body to produce excess cortisol.[198]

Pseudo-glucocorticoid therapy is the leading "iatrogenic" (a term that means "caused by a medical treatment," in this case, patent medicine-induced) cause of osteoporosis. Several large case-control studies have confirmed strong associations between pseudo-glucocorticoids and greatly increased risk of fractures.[199]

Often, the first indication of a problem is a fracture—typically in the lumbar spine or femur—and these fractures occur in 30 to 50% of patients receiving long-term pseudo-glucocorticoid therapy. In patients with pseudo-glucocorticoid-induced osteoporosis, bone mineral density drops rapidly (a 6 to 12% loss within the first year and approximately 3% loss yearly thereafter). However, risk of fracture escalates by as much as 75% within the first three months after beginning to take a pseudo-glucococorticoid, well before a substantial drop in BMD occurs, which indicates that the pseudo-glucocorticoids have other adverse effects on bone beyond their effects on BMD.[200]

An increase in the risk of vertebral and hip fractures occurs rapidly after the start of treatment with pseudo-glucocorticoids and has been reported to occur with doses as small as 2.5 to 7.5 mg of prednisolone per day (equivalent to 3.1 to 9.3 mg of prednisone per day). In a study of two groups of patients 18 to 64 years of age, one group receiving 10 mg of prednisone per day for more than 90 days and a second group not given pseudo-glucocorticoids, receiving pseudo-gluococorticoids was associated with an increase in hip fractures by a factor of 7 and an increase in vertebral fractures by a factor of 17.7! Inhaled pseudo-glucocorticoids, as well as alternate-day and intermittent oral regimens have also been shown to significantly increase fracture risk.[201]

ANTACIDS, HISTAMINE H2-RECEPTOR BLOCKERS, AND PROTON-PUMP INHIBITORS COMMONLY USED TO TREAT INDIGESTION, HEARTBURN, AND GERD, CAUSE BONE LOSS

For calcium to be absorbed, it must first be made soluble and ionized by stomach acid. These patent medicines inhibit or even totally shut down your body's ability to produce stomach acid.[202]*

---

* For a full discussion please see pages 89–91, "I Need Stomach Acid to Absorb Calcium?"

Antacids do not shut off the production of stomach acid; they neutralize it after it has been produced. The effect on calcium absorption, however, is the same—its absorption is inhibited. Commonly available antacids include: Duracid®, Tempo®, Maalox®, Mylanta®, Gelusil®, Gaviscon®, Amphojel®, Riopan®, Mi-Acid® Gelcaps, Mylanta® Gelcaps, Rolaids®, Tums®, Milk of Magnesia®, Alka Seltzer®, and Bromo Seltzer®.

H2-blockers block the action of the histamine-producing cells in the lining of the stomach. When normally activated, these histamine-producing cells signal the acid-producing cells in the stomach to secrete HCl (stomach acid). When prevented from turning on by H2-blockers, the histamine cells send no message, so no stomach acid is produced. H2-blockers include: Cimetidine (Tagamet®), Ranitidine (Zantac®), Famotidine (Pepcid®), Nitazidine (Axid®).

Proton pump inhibitors block the action of a mechanism—called the proton pump—which is inside the cells in the stomach lining that produce and secrete stomach acid. PPIs are the most potent of the acid blockers; just one pill can reduce stomach acid secretion by 90–95% for almost an entire day. These powerful patent medicines produce a variety of adverse effects. In addition to promoting osteoporosis, PPIs commonly cause diarrhea, skin reactions, headache, and less frequently, impotence, breast enlargement in men, and gout. Long-term use has been shown to cause severe symptomatic hypomagnesia (levels of magnesium low enough to cause potentially fatal electrolyte disturbances and cardiac arrhythmia).[203] PPIs include: omeprazole (Prilosec®), lansoprazole (Prevacid®), rabeprazole (AcipHex®), esomeprazole (Nexium®), and pantoprazole (Protonix®).

THE GOOD NEWS: YOU CAN HALT AND EVEN REVERSE PATENT MEDICINE-CAUSED BONE LOSS—NATURALLY

The good news for anyone with one of the above conditions being treated with one of these bone-busting patent medications is that even if you must continue to take these patent medicines, you absolutely can combat their side effects on your bones' health, naturally. Findings in the research studies show that "active management" of bone loss in those with patent medicine-associated osteopenia/osteoporosis "can halt or even reverse this process."[204]

Obviously, intelligent "active management" does not mean taking yet another patent medicine, like a bisphosphonate, with even more bone- and health-destroying side effects! Intelligent "active management" means supplying your bones with all the nutrients they require to remodel, rebuild, and maintain healthful structure and function. It also means correcting or avoiding, when at all possible, the many other factors in our modern lifestyle that promote bone loss (which are discussed in "Part 3: What Increases Your Risk for Osteoporosis?").

An ounce of prevention—in the form of an intelligent, natural bone-building program—can help prevent much needless misery from these bone-busting patent medicines.

If, like Julie, you are having difficulty getting your doctor to monitor the effects on your bones of the medications you are being prescribed to manage your epilepsy, depression, anxiety, insomnia, chronic pain, allergies, or asthma, please share this information with your doctor. The footnotes provided cite the most recent papers in the peer-reviewed medical journals. Educate your doctor, so you can get the health care you deserve. If your doctor refuses to become educated, find another, more competent physician.

Are Your Bones Going up in Smoke?

Smokers lose bone more rapidly, have lower bone mass (a full one-third of a standard deviation less at the hip and a one-tenth standard deviation less for all sites combined), and a higher fracture rate. In addition, women who smoke reach menopause, when estrogen levels plummet causing bone loss, up to two years earlier than their nonsmoking peers.[205]

Approximately 19% of the hip fractures occurring in a study that pooled data from three population studies involving a total of 13,393 women and 17,379 men were attributable to smoking.[206] In other research, smoking increased risk of spinal osteoporosis in men by 230%![207]

WHY IS SMOKING SO HARMFUL TO YOUR BONES? TWO KEY REASONS: CADMIUM AND NICOTINE

Cadmium

Cadmium, a toxic metal that is present in the environment both naturally and as a pollutant from industrial and agricultural sources, stimulates the formation and activity of osteoclasts, the cells that break down bone.[208] Cadmium also inhibits the normal inactivation of cortisol. While cortisol is an essential-to-life hormone, excess amounts of cortisol are known to contribute to osteoporosis and hypertension, as well as other problems. The two main sources of exposure to cadmium in the general population are tobacco smoking and food grown in areas in which the soil or coastline waters are contaminated with high levels of cadmium.

Cigarettes are loaded with cadmium. About 10% of the cadmium they contain is inhaled through smoking, and since cadmium is much more effectively absorbed through the lungs than the gut, as much as 50% of the cadmium inhaled via cigarette smoke may be absorbed. Smokers typically have 4–5 times higher blood concentrations and 2–3 times higher kidney concentrations of cadmium.[209]

Cadmium gets into the food supply in foods harvested from cadmium-polluted areas, including shellfish (oysters, mussels, etc.[210]); vegetable, grain, and fruit crops; and meat and dairy products derived from animals pastured in areas with high levels of cadmium in the soils.[211] In general, cadmium concentrations in urban areas tend to be higher than in rural areas of the United States.[212] In areas with high soil levels of cadmium, house dust can also be an important route of exposure.[213]

The use of cadmium to stabilize plastic, as a red and yellow pigment, and in corrosion-resistant coating for steel and copper alloys has declined, but this toxic metal is still widely used in batteries, predominantly rechargeable nickel-cadmium (Ni-Cd) batteries, and in cadmium telluride solar panels. Cadmium may also be present in children's jewelry imported from China. In 2010, a US Consumer Product Safety Commission investigation found 12% of the 103 such items tested from New York, Ohio, Texas, and California contained at least 10% cadmium; one of the items tested contained 91% cadmium.[214]

Classified as a carcinogen, cadmium accumulates in the human body, has a half-life for elimination ranging from 20 to 40 *years*, and is mainly stored in the liver and kidneys. Cadmium causes kidney dysfunction, kidney stone formation, osteomalacia (bone pain), and osteoporosis.[215] (As noted in our discussion of how vitamin D is activated in the liver and kidneys into the form in which it helps the body absorb calcium,* cadmium can really mess this up.)

Analysis of NHANES (National Health and Nutrition Examination Survey) data indicates that women 50 years of age or older with urinary cadmium levels between 0.50 and 1.00 microgram/gram creatinine[†] had a 43% greater risk for hip-BMD-defined osteoporosis, compared to women with urinary cadmium levels less than 0.50 microg/g. [216]

You can minimize your exposure to cadmium by not smoking or hanging out with people who do; avoiding consumption of oysters, scallops, and shellfish from coastal areas along the New England states and Great Lakes with high cadmium levels; dusting regularly and using a HEPA air filter to improve the air quality in your home and office.

---

* Page 113.

† Creatinine is used as a marker since it is excreted at basically the same rate by everyone, while the amount of urine we produce can vary greatly from person to person. For this reason, the amount of creatinine present in a urine sample is used as a means of standardizing kidney output of other compounds in the urine, such as, in this case, cadmium. Seventy-three percent of US women aged 50 or older are estimated to have cadmium body burdens of greater than 0.50 micrograms/gram creatinine. These results suggest that 31% of the osteoporosis prevalence among American women at least 50 years old may be attributable to cadmium!

Nicotine

Nicotine, even in low concentrations, depresses osteoblast activity. Levels of osteocalcin—a protein secreted
by osteoblasts that plays a key role in depositing calcium in bone—are much lower in smokers.[217] If you
smoke to keep your weight down, you'll be interested
to know that osteocalcin also plays important roles in
promoting insulin secretion and insulin sensitivity.
Insulin is the hormone that gets sugars inside your
cells where they can be burned for energy instead of
stored as fat. Lack of sensitivity to insulin promotes
weight gain and is a key factor in metabolic syndrome,
type 2 diabetes, and obesity. Thus, smoking thins your
bones while expanding your waistline.[218]

In concentrations typically seen in heavy smokers,
nicotine is toxic to osteoblasts.[219] Nicotine also increases
the rate at which the liver clears estrogen from the body,
and thus, in postmenopausal women, can completely
cancel out the benefits of estrogen replacement, not
only on bone health, but on hot flashes, vaginal thinning and dryness, and cholesterol.[220]

Data from the Third National Health and Nutrition
Examination Survey, which included 14,060 subjects,
found that blood levels of cotinine, a metabolite of
nicotine and marker for exposure to cigarette smoke
(whether active or passive), were inversely related to
BMD in both men and women. More nicotine exposure = less bone.[221]

The good news for smokers: if you quit, you will
quickly regain your ability to build bone. When postmenopausal women who smoked at least ten cigarettes a day were randomly assigned to a 4-month
smoking cessation program, and were then followed

for an additional year, the women who quit smoking quickly began rebuilding bone and gained 2.9% in BMD in their femoral trochanter (top of the thigh bone) and 1.52% in their hips.[222]

More than Two Drinks of Liquor Makes Bone Loss Much Quicker

Alcohol has a dose-dependent toxic effect on osteoblast activity. One to two drinks a day appears to be beneficial. More than two drinks a day prevents bone repair and renewal, and significantly increases fracture risk.[223]

Using data from the Third National Health and Nutrition Examination Survey, researchers found that moderate drinkers (less than 29 drinks per month) actually had higher BMD than abstainers. Moderate consumption of alcohol translated to 2.1% higher BMD in men and 3.8% higher BMD in postmenopausal women.[224] Another large study, this one involving 11,032 women and 5,939 men, found no increase in fracture risk when two ounces or less of alcohol was consumed daily, but drinking more than this increased risk of any osteoporotic fracture by 38% and hip fracture by 68%.[225]

Your choice of which alcoholic beverage to consume can also affect the health of your bones. Several recent studies suggest moderate intake (no more than two servings a day) of beer and/or wine may have beneficial effects on bone. (One serving of beer = 8 ounces; one serving of wine = 4 ounces.) A study of 1,697 healthy women, of whom 710 were premenopausal, 176 were perimenopausal, and 811 were postmenopausal, found that beer drinkers had slightly higher bone mass.[226]

A second large study involving 1,182 men, 1,289 postmenopausal woman, and 248 premenopausal women found bone mineral density was 3.0–4.5% greater in men consuming 2 daily drinks of alcohol or beer, and 5.0–8.3 greater in postmenopausal women consuming 1–2 drinks of alcohol or wine daily. More than 2 drinks a day, however, was associated with significantly lower (3.0–5.2% lower) bone mineral density in the hip and spine in men.

Beer's beneficial effects on bone are thought to be due to its silicon content. One can of beer contains around 7 milligrams of silicon; a 4-ounce glass of wine provides around 1 milligram of silicon. (For comparison, a half cup of cooked spinach contains around 5 milligrams of silicon.)

Wine's bone benefits may be linked to its content of phytochemicals, especially the resveratrol present in red wine, which has been shown to have estrogenic effects and might therefore help protect against bone loss in postmenopausal women in whom estrogen levels are low. In rat studies, resveratrol has been shown to have an estrogenic effect and to promote increased BMD in ovariectomized rats (rats whose ovaries have been removed to simulate menopause).[227]

Fluoride: Could Your Tap Water or Toothpaste Be Destroying Your Bones?

Fluoride is present in the environment—everywhere. Fluorine is a common element in the earth's crust, so fluorides are naturally present in the soil, rocks, and water throughout the world. Plus fluorides are widely used in many industrial processes, e.g., coal burning, oil refining, steel production, brick-making, and the production of phosphate fertilizers. However, our main sources of exposure to fluoride are diet (food and water) and fluoride-containing dental products (e.g., toothpaste). Fluoride is found in higher concentrations in soft, alkaline, and calcium-deficient waters, and since the fluoride compounds that occur naturally in drinking water are almost totally bioavailable (90%), they are virtually all absorbed from the gastrointestinal tract. [228]

Although fluoridation of community drinking water to prevent dental caries has been hailed by some as one of the ten most important "public health achievements of the 20th century," along with the claimed decline in tooth cavities has come an increase in dental fluorosis, a disturbance of the production of dental enamel caused by exposure to high concentrations of fluoride between the ages of 3 months and 8 years when teeth are developing. (To be precise, the substance used in water "fluoridation" is flurosiliic acid, an "industrial waste".) In its mild, and surprisingly common, forms, fluorosis shows up as tiny white streaks or specks in the tooth enamel. In its most severe form, the teeth are marred by pitting and brown discolorations, spots and stains that are permanent and can darken over time. Dental fluorosis is highly prevalent worldwide. As of 2005, 23% of persons in the United States aged 6 to 39 years had mild or greater dental fluorosis.[229]

HOW DOES FLUORIDE AFFECT OUR BONES?

Fluoride can act on osteoblasts and osteoclasts. While fluoride may increase bone mass, the newly formed bone lacks normal structure and strength. Under a microscope, the "crystallization pattern" of bone from

FLUORIDE CONTENT OF COMMONLY CONSUMED FOODS AND BEVERAGES

FOOD	MICROGRAMS OF FLUORIDE IN 100 GRAMS (3 OZ)
Wine, red	105
Wine, white	202
Carbonated water, fruit flavored	105
Coffee	91
Fruit juice drink, apple	104
Grape juice blend (apple & grape) Juicy Juice®	102
Grape juice, white	204
Tea, brewed, microwave	322
Tea, instant, powder, prepared with tap water	335
Tea, brewed, decaffeinated	269
Water, tap (Midwest), municipal	99
Water, tap (Midwest) well	53
Water, tap (Northeast), municipal	74
Water, tap (Northeast), well	9
Water, tap (South), municipal	93
Water, tap (South), well	10
Water, tap (West), municipal	51
Water, tap (West), well	24
Oatmeal, cooked	72
French fries, McDonald's®	115
Crab canned	210
Shrimp, canned	201
Shrimp, fried	166
Fish sticks, baked	134
Raisins	234
Potato chips, baked	106

deliberately fluoride-treated animals and humans can be seen to be abnormal. In trabecular bone, fluoride results in an increase in bone volume and thickness without a concomitant increase in connectivity, and this lack of trabecular connectivity reduces bone quality despite the increase in bone mass.

What's Trabecular Bone?

Also called cancellous or spongy bone, trabecular bone is one of two types of tissue that form our bones. It typically occurs at the ends of long bones, like our femurs (thigh bones), right next to joints and also the insides of our vertebrae. Trabecular bone is composed of tiny, lattice-shaped structures, contains lots of tiny blood vessels, and is where our red bone marrow produces blood cells. It's also where calcium ions are exchanged—either added to or withdrawn from bone.

The other kind of bone tissue is called cortical or compact bone. As its name suggests, cortical bone forms the cortex, or outer shell, of most bones. Much denser, stronger, and stiffer than trabecular bone, cortical bone contributes about 80% of the weight of a human skeleton.

If your bones were M&M candies, cortical bone would be the outer candy shell and trabecular bone the chocolate inside. We have way more trabecular than compact bone, but trabecular bone is less dense, less stiff, softer, and weaker. Now, the key point: in osteoporosis, trabecular bone is more severely affected than cortical bone.

How Does Fluoride Cause Bone Loss?

At very low and localized concentrations in dental implants, fluoride encourages osteoblast production and new bone formation, but at higher concentrations, new bone formation is blocked. High systemic (whole body) fluoride exposures can cause skeletal fluorosis, a condition in which bones have become too hard and brittle, ligaments calcify, and bone pain and loss result.

After ingestion, fluorine goes to the stomach where it reacts with stomach acid to form hydrogen fluoride. Hydrogen fluoride is absorbed from the gastrointestinal tract and sent into the portal vein, which delivers it to the liver. The liver is like our body's border control system; it's where everything goes to get checked and cleared before its allowed entry into the bloodstream. Harmful compounds are usually transformed in the liver into something we can excrete and sent out of the body via urine or bile. We do this biotransformation with the help of a variety of liver enzymes that first oxidize the harmful compound and then bind it to a carrier that takes it out. Fluorine, however, is itself such a strong oxidizer—the strongest oxidizer currently known—that it simply scoffs at the liver's comparatively feeble attempts to oxidize it. It is not removed, but instead passes into the bloodstream and gets distributed to all our tissues, including our bones.[230]

Once inside bones, fluorine nukes them through a variety of mechanisms:

- Fluorine wipes out bone cells' ability to produce their most important antioxidant defender, called glutathione, and then wreaks havoc, shutting down osteoblasts and causing inflammation that increases osteoclast production and activity.[231]

- As fluorine accumulates in bone, it shuts down alkaline phosphatase, an enzyme in bone that is involved in the production of osteoblasts. Researchers speculate that after a long period of fluoride exposure, the structure of the alkaline phosphatase enzyme changes because fluoride binds to this enzyme. Fluorine exposure may also reduce the content of copper, zinc, manganese and other trace minerals that other enzymes involved in building bone require for their activity. The end result here is osteoblast production stops.[232]

- Our bones are largely composed of calcium compounds, up to 50% of which are hydroxyapatite.* Fluorine can convert hydroxyapatite to fluorapatite, which changes bones' crystalline structure, delays further mineralization with calcium, and causes a reduction in bones' mechanical strength properties.[233]

- Hydrogen fluoride reacts with calcium to form an insoluble salt, CaF_2. This salt has to be cleared by the body, and as it goes, takes out some calcium from the bone matrix.[234]

- Fluoride induces the secretion of parathyroid hormone.† Parathyroid hormone sets off the production of osteoclasts. It's kind of a convoluted process, but one worth summarizing for you here since it shows how our body's bone-maintaining system is delicately balanced, and sheds some light on why patent

---

* Discussed on page 209.

† Discussed on pages 114-117.

medicines like denosumab and teriparatide, which disrupt normal functioning, can produce very unpleasant results.

What happens is that parathyroid hormone tells osteoblast cells (the cells that produce new bone) to secrete a signaling molecule called RANKL.* RANKL plays a role in initiating the process through which osteoclasts (the cells that break down bone) are made. For this reason, when our parathyroid hormone levels are chronically elevated, so is our production of osteoclasts—and we lose bone.

■ Increased fluoride intake has been repeatedly shown to increase levels of parathyroid hormone circulating in the bloodstream and to cause hyperparathyroidism.[235] Remember that the patent medicine teriparatide (trade name, Forteo®, discussed on pages 66–76), works by causing parathyroid hormone production to spike. And the patent medicine denosumab, (trade names, Prolia®, Xgeva®, discussed on pages 52–66), works by blocking RANKL, which at first may sound like a good idea, but RANKL activity is required to produce the osteoclasts we need to clear out old brittle bone, and RANKL is also necessary for the activation of our B cells and T cells, key players in our immune system.

Bottom line here: Messing with Nature's well laid plans for the ways in which our bones constantly rebuild and maintain themselves (which is what all the patent medicines do) is not a good idea! Providing our bones

---

* Discussed on page 53.

with the nutrients they require to do this job by themselves is much safer—and as the COMB study* demonstrates—more effective.

FLUORIDE IS, LITERALLY, IN OUR WATER. WHAT CAN YOU DO TO PROTECT YOURSELF?

Be sure to include calcium-rich foods in your diet! The
bioavailability of fluoride is generally reduced in humans
when consumed with milk or a calcium-rich diet.[236]

Don't use toothpaste containing fluoride. Check the
ingredient list. Fluoride can appear as sodium fluoride
(NaF), stannous fluoride (SnF2), olaflur (an organic
salt of fluoride), or sodium monofluorophosphate
(Na2PO3F). Most the toothpaste sold in the United
States contains 1,000 to 1,100 parts per million fluo-
ride. In the UK, the fluoride content is often higher; a
NaF of 0.32% (1,450 ppm fluoride) is not uncommon.

In 1997, the Institute of Medicine said fluoride
intakes of 0.01 mg/day for infants through 6 months,
0.05 mg/kg/day beyond 6 months of age, and 3 mg/
day and 4 mg/day for adult women and men (respectively), are adequate to prevent dental caries. IOM
set upper limits (UL) for fluoride at 0.10 mg/kg/day
in children less than 8 years and 10 mg/day for those
older than 8 years.

We feel there is no reason to consume even the lowest amount of fluoride recommended by the IOM. In
the May 2012 issue of *Nutrition & Healing*, Dr. Wright
summarizes more than 30 years of research showing that xylitol, a natural sugar our bodies produce
in tiny amounts, which is also found, again in very

---

* Discussed on pages 51–52.

tiny amounts, in berries and vegetables, not only prevents plaque formation and cavities, but has even been shown to reverse developing cavities and restore healthy tooth enamel—safely.[237]

Studies demonstrate that 4 to 12 grams of xylitol per day is effective, and this is most easily delivered in xylitol-containing chewing gums, which keep the xylitol they contain in contact with teeth far longer than toothpaste or mouthwash. Read product labels; if a piece of gum contains 1 gram of xylitol, then chew 4 pieces throughout the day—or more. Dr. Wright's clinical experience suggests chewing a piece of gum five times a day is ideal.

The preceding table* lists the foods and beverages consumed in the US with the highest fluoride content. Take a look and estimate how much fluoride YOU are ingesting each day. The full listing of 400 foods across 23 food groups can be accessed on-line at the National Fluoride Database.

---

* Table adapted from the National Fluoride Database, a comprehensive, nationally representative database of the fluoride concentration in foods and beverages consumed in the United States that are major fluoride contributors. http://www.nal.usda.gov/fnic/foodcomp/Data/Fluoride/fluoride.pdf .

CHAPTER 5

What Men Don't Know Can Increase Their Risk for Osteoporosis

THE SAME FACTORS THAT affect bone health in women also affect men's bones, although in men, peak bone mass is greater and the decline in male hormones (androgens) occurs somewhat later and is not as rapid. Despite these protective factors, approximately 25% of men will have an osteoporotic fracture during their lifetime, and men account for 30% of hip and 20% of vertebral fragility fractures.

More men will experience an osteoporotic fracture than will have a heart attack or stroke, or will develop Alzheimer's disease, prostate cancer, or lung cancer. The incidence of osteoporosis-related fracture in men exceeds that of lung and prostate cancer combined![238]

What Are the Key Risk Factors for Osteoporosis in Men?

- *Bone-busting patent medicines* (see Chapter 2, beginning on page 11).

- *Vitamin D deficiency*: A number of recent surveys indicate less than 1/3 of white males and less than 1/10 of black males have optimal vitamin D status.[239] One of the latest, the MrOS study, recently found 72% of men were deficient in vitamin D.[240]

- *Hyperthyroidism* (see page 114).

- *Increased parathyroid hormone levels* (see pages 114 and 314–316.).

- *Excessive alcohol consumption* (see page 143) for men, it's "more than 2 drinks of liquor, and bone loss is quicker."

- *Smoking* (see page 139).

- *Gastrointestinal disease*: not only do the pro-inflammatory compounds produced by the body in conditions such as Irritable Bowel Syndrome and Crohn's Disease promote disturbances in bone and mineral metabolism,[241] but the patent medicines used to suppress symptoms (e.g., corticosteroids, stomach acid blockers) prevent healthy bone remodeling.[242]

- *Osteoarthritis*: inflammation activates osteoclasts and promotes bone lss.[243]

- *Andropause*: lack of testosterone results in insufficient production of estrogen to maintain bone (see page 89).[244]

- *Sarcopenia* (loss of muscle mass with aging): the drop in male hormones that occurs with aging reduces not only muscle mass but bone mass, and is associated with an increase in fat mass. More than one-third of people over age 65 years fall annually, and approximately 5% of falls lead to fracture.[245]

- *Prostate cancer*—androgen deprivation therapy (same reasoning as Andropause; see page 89).[246]

- *Malabsorption of calcium and other minerals secondary to hypochlorhydria* (low stomach acid) is more common in older men, especially those over 60.

- *Malabsorption of calcium, other minerals, amino acids, and other nutrients secondary to "hidden" (no symptoms or minimal symptoms) gluten sensitivity.* Osteoporosis or osteopenia (beginning bone loss) in men under 50 is frequently due to "hidden" gluten sensitivity, which is most accurately detected by testing for secretory IgA gluten antibodies in a stool specimen (see Appendix A).

CHAPTER 6

Chances Are, You Are Already Losing Bone

I F YOU ARE CONSUMING the standard American diet, not getting regular exercise, wear sunscreen all the time and/or get little sun exposure, you have lots of company. You are following the normal lifestyle of people living in the United States—and you are losing bone.

Americans' nutrient-poor diet, combined with pandemic vitamin D insufficiency and a couch-potato lifestyle is the perfect recipe for osteoporosis. Plus, because, initially, bone loss causes no symptoms, most people live under the illusion that even women don't lose much bone before menopause—an assumption that could not be further from the truth!

The only way to find out how your bones are doing is by N-telopeptide and DXA Testing, So let's talk about this next.

How Can I Tell if I'm Losing Bone?

You're losing bone. The real question is how much, how quickly? Even in adults, normal healthy bone is dynamic, living tissue that is constantly being broken down (or *resorbed*) and rebuilt. In fact, up to 10% of all your bone mass is likely to be undergoing remodeling at any point in time. Normally, it's a balanced process in which bone rebuilding keeps pace with bone breakdown. In osteoporosis, however, bone resorption outpaces bone formation.

Actually, after age 40, it's normal for bone mass to decline up to 1.5% to 2% per year in men as well as in women, a small loss that should not seriously compromise bone strength. Women, however, are at high risk of losing a good deal more bone mass than men and developing osteoporosis because of their smaller size (smaller muscles, smaller bones) and the drop in female hormones, estrogen and progesterone, that occurs with menopause.

What Tests Are Used to Check for Bone Loss? What Qualifies as Osteoporosis?

DXA AND N-TELOPEPTIDE TESTS

The DXA and N-telopeptide tests are the most widely used tests to evaluate bone mineral density and the rate at which bone is being lost.

In women, the World Health Organization defines *osteopenia* (bone thinning) as a bone mineral density between 1 and 2.5 *standard deviations** and osteoporosis as a bone mineral density 2.5 standard deviations below peak bone mass (the amount of bone mass that is normally seen in a 20 year old healthy female) as measured by *DXA*.[247]

The *DXA*—which stands for "dual energy x-ray absorptiometry"—is the most widely used and most thoroughly studied bone density measurement test. During a DXA, two x-ray beams with differing energy levels are aimed at the patient's bones. The amount of the beams absorbed by soft tissue is subtracted, and the individual's BMD is then determined from the amount of the beams her bones have absorbed.)

The *N-telopeptide* test measures the rate of bone loss. Also written as NTx, this is a urine test, which measures the breakdown products of bone, such as the compound from which it gets its name: cross-linked N-telopeptide of type I collagen. By measuring the amount of this compound excreted in the urine, the NTx measures how quickly bone is breaking down. (Pyrilinks-D is a similar test for bone loss, but much less often used at present. The recently developed serum C-terminal telopeptide [CTx] test may be even more accurate than the NTx.[†])

The DXA test is best used to measure bone density, while NTx urinary bone resorption and CTx serum assessments are used to measure the rate of bone loss and are thus helpful for monitoring the success (or failure) of therapy. The NTx and CTx tests provide much

---

* Standard deviation is a statistical measurement that, in this case, shows how much the bone mass of a specific woman differs from that of the "average" healthy 20 year old woman, which is the time in a woman's life when her bone mass is highest.

† See page 307, Appendix A.

quicker feedback than the DXA, which can take up to two years to detect a therapeutic response. Unfortunately, even though the NTx, CTx (and Pyrilinks-D) tests measure the bone loss side of the everyday, this is only one side of the dynamic "bone building/bone loss" equation. At present, there is no widely available test for the degree of everyday bone-building.

Additional tests may be used to determine potential causes of bone loss. These include gastric acid levels, serum calcium, 24-hour urinary calcium, parathyroid hormone, thyroid stimulating hormone, free thyroxine (the T3 thyroid hormone) levels, serum albumin and serum alkaline phosphatase (which checks on liver function), and vitamin D levels (see Appenix A).

FRAX®—A NEW TOOL FOR ESTIMATING FRACTURE RISK

FRAX® (Fracture Risk Assessment Tool) was developed by the World Health Organization to predict a person's 10-year probability of having a hip fracture or of having any major osteoporotic fracture (spine, hip, forearm, shoulder).

The FRAX® models were developed by gathering data on population-based cohorts (groups of people with various risks for fracture) from Europe, North America, Asia, and Australia and then finding the correlations among risks to determine a subject's absolute risk for fracture.

FRAX® is also called 10-year fracture risk model and 10-year fracture probability. This algorithm estimates the likelihood of a person to break a bone due to low bone mass or osteoporosis over a period of 10 years. The FRAX® output is the 10-year probability of hip fracture and the 10-year probability of a major osteoporotic fracture (clinical spine, forearm, hip or shoulder fracture).

FRAX® is country-specific since the data showed that the risk of osteoporotic fractures varies by as much as 10-fold from one nation to another. FRAX® can calculate osteoporotic fracture risk for people living in Argentina, Australia, Austria, Belgium Canada, China, Colombia, Czech Republic, Denmark, Finland, France, Germany, Hungary, Italy, Japan, Jordan, Lebanon, Malta, Mexico, Netherlands, New Zealand, Philippines, Poland, Romania, Singapore, South Korea, Spain, Sweden, Switzerland, Taiwan, Tunisia, Turkey, the United Kingdom, and the United States.

To calculate your FRAX® score, you will need to provide some information about yourself, including the results from your most recent DXA, specifically the BMD of the neck of your femur, which will be given in grams per centimeter squared or "g/cm2" on your DXA report.

The FRAX® tool is a computer-driven algorithm and is available at http://www.shef.ac.uk/FRAX. Enter this URL into your browser to go to this website page. Click on "Calculation Tool," which appears on the banner that runs across the top of the page. Then click on the area of the world in which you live. You will be given a list of countries in that area. Click on the country in which you live. You will then be asked to click on your ethnicity. Then the "Calculation Tool" page will appear with the information you provided already inserted.

The Calculation Tool page contains a short questionnaire—just twelve questions:

1.   Your age or date of birth: The model accepts ages between 40 and 90 years. If ages below or above

are entered, the program will compute probabilities at 40 and 90 years, respectively.

2. Sex: male or female.

3. Weight: in kilograms.

4. Height: in centimeters.

5. Previous fracture (no or yes): specifically, a previous fracture in adult life occurring spontaneously, or arising from trauma which, in a healthy individual, would not have resulted in a fracture.

6. Parent fractured hip (no or yes): if your mother or father fractured a hip.

7. Current smoking (no or yes).

8. Glucocorticoids (no or yes): Enter yes if currently taking oral glucocorticoids or if you have ever taken oral glucocorticoids for more than 3 months at a dose of prednisolone of 5mg daily or more (or equivalent doses of other glucocorticoids).

9. Rheumatoid arthritis (no or yes): do you have a confirmed diagnosis of rheumatoid arthritis?

10. Secondary osteoporosis (no or yes): enter yes if you have a disorder strongly associated with osteoporosis. These include type I (insulin dependent) diabetes, osteogenesis imperfecta in adults, untreated long-standing hyperthyroidism, hypogonadism or premature menopause (onset earlier than 45 years of age), chronic malnutrition, or malabsorption, and chronic liver disease.

11. Alcohol (no or yes): do you drink more than 3 units of alcohol per day? A unit of alcohol is equivalent to a standard glass of beer (285ml),

a single measure of spirits (30ml), a medium-sized glass of wine (120ml), or 1 measure of an aperitif (60ml).

12. Femoral neck BMD (g/cm2): for this you will need your most recent DXA report. This information will be in your DXA Results Summary and will be listed as "Neck."

Lastly, you will need to know what type of DXA machine was used. Options are GE-Lunar, Hologic, Norland, T-Score, or DMS/Medlink. The type of machine used should appear on every page of your report, most likely on the bottom right corner of each page.

After entering your information, click "Calculate" and your 10-year fracture risks will appear.

You are considered at risk if you have Low bone mass (T-score between -1.0 and -2.5 at the femoral neck or spine) AND a 10-year probability of a hip fracture ≥ 3% OR a 10-year probability of a major osteoporosis-related fracture ≥ 20% based on the US-adapted FRAX algorithm.

What to Expect If You Don't Take Steps to Actively Prevent Bone Loss: What Are the Signs and Symptoms of Osteoporosis?

Initially, as bone thins, its loss rarely produces any symptoms—for which reason, osteoporosis has been called "the silent disease," but this is part of the problem! For many, the first symptom is a broken bone or an alarming DXA test.

As the disease progresses, if symptoms occur, they can include:

- Backache
- Neck pain
- Muscle pain
- Bone tenderness

Late symptoms include:

- Severe backache in either the upper or lower regions of the back
- Loss of height
- Sudden back pain with a cracking sound indicating vertebral (spinal bone) fracture
- Fractures, especially of the hip, arm, or wrist, occurring during normal daily activity or with minor injury, such as slipping and falling
- Spinal deformities—a stooped posture or hunchback, resulting from loss of bone mass and/or from multiple vertebral compression fractures

PART 4

How to Have Strong Bones for Life

CHAPTER 7

Strong Bones for Life, Naturally

What Your Bones Really Need to Stay Strong

As **YOU NOW KNOW,** bone is dynamic, living tissue that is constantly being broken down and rebuilt, regardless of one's age or sex. Until recently, not getting enough calcium and women's postmenopausal drop in estrogen were singled out as the only issues. Today, vitamin D's importance for bone health is once again being recognized.

It's true that calcium, vitamin D, and estrogen play key roles in preventing osteoporosis, but maintaining healthy bones throughout life requires a good deal more than simply calcium, estrogen, and vitamin D. Normal bone metabolism is a complex dance among over two dozen nutrients including the vitamins K (especially K_2), B_6, B_{12}, and folate as well as vitamin D, and the minerals boron, magnesium, phosphorous, zinc, manganese, copper, silicon, molybdenum, selenium—and possibly strontium—as well as calcium.

Also, while estrogen regulates the action of osteoclasts, specialized bone cells that remove dead portions of demineralized bone, progesterone is required by the osteoblasts, the bone-forming cells that pull calcium, magnesium, and phosphorous from the blood to build new bone mass.

What you need to know about each of these factors essential for building and maintaining healthy bones is discussed below and in Appendix B.

Bone-Building Vitamins

VITAMIN D

What it Does

Vitamin D is essential for calcium's absorption from the intestines, and for its re-absorption from the kidneys (so it is not excreted in the urine), and therefore increases calcium's availability, while also stimulating its use in bone. Vitamin D deficiency leads not only to muscle weakness, which increases the risk of falling, but to osteopenia and osteoporosis—all three increase your risk of fracture.

In addition to its roles in calcium absorption, vitamin D is now known to affect genetic transcription—the process that directs our cells' DNA to turn on certain genes, which then send out messenger RNA to make certain proteins, while turning off other genes and preventing the production of other proteins. It's complicated, but what it boils down to is that not having enough vitamin D on board can result in a wide array of harmful outcomes, including not only osteoporosis, but also depression, many common cancers, autoimmune diseases like multiple sclerosis, susceptibility to infectious diseases, and cardiovascular diseases. Your entire body, not just your bones, needs vitamin D!

How Much Do I Need?

Most Americans are not getting anywhere near enough vitamin D. Current official recommendations for women aged 50 or older are only 600 IU per day, but leading vitamin D researchers and the majority of experts believe we need *at least* 1,000 IU per day. Many vitamin D experts are now recommending somewhere between 2,000 IU and 5,000 IU, or even as much as 10,000 IU, per day. Americans' average daily intake of vitamin D, which is found in small amounts in fortified milk and in fatty fish such as salmon and sardines, is only 200 IU![248]

To determine if you are vitamin D deficient—or more likely, how serious a vitamin D deficiency you have—it's best to have a blood test run to check your levels of 25-hydroxyvitamin D_3 [you may also see this written as $25(OH)D_3$ or $25(OH)D$].

If your blood levels of vitamin D are not *at least* 30 ng/mL (or if the "nmol/L" measure is used, your blood levels should be at least 75 nmol/L), work with your doctor to fine tune your dosage of supplemental vitamin D to one that will, in 2–3 months, raise your blood levels to at least this amount.

Many medical experts involved in vitamin D research now feel that *optimal* blood levels of vitamin D should run between 50–80 ng/mL (or 125–200 nmol/L) year-round.[249] As mentioned earlier, the Vitamin D Council (www.vitamindcouncil.org), a nonprofit organization whose directors are among the foremost vitamin D experts in the world, recommends simply taking 5,000 IU of vitamin D daily for 2–3 months, then having your blood levels of vitamin D checked.*

What to Look for in a Supplement

Supplemental vitamin D is available in two forms, ergocalciferol (D_2, a plant-derived form) and cholecalciferol (D_3, the form found in fatty fish, which is also the form that is produced naturally when the cholesterol in human skin cells is exposed to ultraviolet light). Both D_2 and D_3 are technically referred to as "provitamin D" since humans can convert both forms into the most active form of vitamin D, which is called calcitriol $[1,25(OH)_2D_3]$. (Remember, we do this via a two-step process that starts in the liver and is completed in the kidneys, so both organs need to be functioning properly.) However, D_3 is a better supplement choice than D_2 since D_3 is much more biologically active.

In humans, vitamin D_3 has been found to be two-and-a-half times more effective than vitamin D_2 in raising and maintaining blood levels of vitamin D, and D_3 also has a 40% greater ability to bind to the vitamin D receptor (VDR) on our cells, which is the way in which vitamin D exerts all its effects. [250]

Safety Issues

You may see misleading information about how much vitamin D is safe to take. The reason for the confusion

---

* See "Getting Any . . . Sunshine?," page 119.

is that the Upper Tolerable Intake Levels (ULs), which tell us how much of a nutrient we can take daily without risk of toxicity, were set for vitamin D by the National Academy of Sciences back in 1997. At that time, the UL for vitamin D intake in adults, including pregnant and breastfeeding women (for whom recommended nutrient intakes are often higher) was set at just 2,000 IU per day.

We now know that this UL is way too low. Clinical research has clearly shown that vitamin D supplementation in the range of 1,000–2,000 IU per day is not high enough to restore vitamin D health in most individuals with chronic vitamin D deficiency—and this means most Americans, since the vast majority of us are deficient in vitamin D.

If the UL for vitamin D that was set in 1997 were correct, we would all become vitamin D toxic every summer! Just being outside in the summer sunshine for an afternoon can provide an adult with an amount of vitamin D equivalent to taking 10,000 IU/day. And a significant body of clinical research has now shown that prolonged intake of 10,000 IU/day of vitamin D_3 is unlikely to cause any adverse effects in almost all individuals in the general population, which is the criterion used to set the UL.[251]

Although you are highly unlikely to see any adverse effects from taking vitamin D, it's best to know what the symptoms of too much vitamin D (vitamin D toxicity) are. These include loss of appetite, nausea, vomiting, high blood pressure, and kidney malfunction. In addition, individuals with *primary hyperparathyroidism* (an overactive parathyroid gland whose over-activity is not caused by vitamin D deficiency) are at increased risk for vitamin D toxicity and should not take supplemental vitamin D without consulting with a physician.

You should monitor your vitamin D status within 2–3 months of beginning to take supplemental vitamin D to ensure you are taking enough, but not more vitamin D than you need. Ask your doctor to re-order the lab test that checks your blood levels of 25(OH)D_3. This is the major circulating form of vitamin D in the blood, and the form of the vitamin that is the true barometer of your vitamin D status. Adequate supplies of vitamin D are indicated by blood levels of 25(OH)D_3 of *at least* 30 ng/mL (nanograms per milliliter) or 75 nmol/L (nanomoles per liter), depending upon which form of measurement, ng/mL or nmol/L, the lab running your blood test uses to report these results.

VITAMIN K

What It Does

Vitamin K plays a number of life-saving roles in our bodies, among which helping our blood to clot is the most critical. Without vitamin K, specifically, the K_1 form of this nutrient, we would bleed to death from even a tiny cut. In its K_2 form, vitamin K is responsible for ensuring that calcium is deposited in our bones— and not in our arteries!

Vitamin K_1 (phylloquinone), the type of vitamin K found in plants (phyllo = plant), especially leafy greens, can be converted by health-promoting bacteria in our intestines into vitamin K_2 (menaquinone). Vitamin K_2 activates osteocalcin, the protein required for calcium to be deposited in bone. Once activated by K_2, osteo-calcin can attract calcium molecules and anchor them into the hydroxyapatite crystals that form our bone matrix. K_2 also activates another protein called matrix-Gla protein, which prevents calcium from depositing in and "calcifying" soft tissue, such as our heart, arteries, breasts, or kidneys.

Vitamin K, in both its K_1 and K_2 forms, also greatly lessens the body's production of a wide range of pro-inflammatory compounds (including interleukin-6, tumor necrosis factor, and C-reactive protein) and, by doing so, lowers overall inflammation. This is important for bone health because when inflammation increases, this signals the body to also increase production and activation of osteoclasts, the cells that break down bone. Before menopause, estrogen puts a damper on women's production of pro-inflammatory compounds, but as estrogen levels drop with menopause, the body's production of pro-inflammatory molecules increases. Vitamin K is especially important for postmenopausal women since it helps keep inflammation, and therefore the production of osteoclasts, under control.[252]

Not eating lots of leafy greens (not supplying your body with plenty of vitamin K) results in impaired calcium deposition in bone (and increased likelihood of calcified arteries) because, without enough vitamin K around, neither osteocalcin, which puts calcium in bone, nor matrix-Gla protein, which keeps calcium out of soft tissues, can be activated.[253]

Although you probably haven't heard about it, vitamin K's importance for bone health has been known for a long time. For more than 20 years, human studies have demonstrated that vitamin K insufficiency increases risk of osteoporotic fracture. Research published in 1984 found that patients who suffered osteoporotic fractures had vitamin K levels 70% lower than age-matched controls, an association that has been repeatedly confirmed.[254] One trial involving almost 900 men and women found a 65% greater risk of hip fracture in those with the lowest blood levels of vitamin K compared to those with the highest levels of the nutrient, who averaged an intake of K_1 of 254 micrograms per day.[255]

Other human research has shown that vitamin K_2, specifically, is an effective treatment against osteoporosis, even in individuals taking corticosteroids, patent medicines well known to have the adverse side effect of greatly accelerating bone loss. Over a two-year period, the rate of vertebral fractures in patients taking corticosteroids who were also taking vitamin K_2 was 13.3% compared to 41% in the patients taking corticosteroids but no K_2.[256]

K_2 has also been shown to rebuild bone in patients with osteoporosis. In a 24-week study, 80 patients with osteoporosis were given either 90 milligrams per day of vitamin K_2 (the menaquinone-4 form)—don't worry, what this means is explained below (starting on page 182)—or placebo. In those taking K_2, bone mineral density (BMD) increased in the second metacarpal (the middle bone in the index finger) an average of 2.2%. In those given the placebo, BMD decreased an average of 7.31%.[257]

A review study that looked at the results of all randomized controlled human trials lasting at least 6 months that evaluated the use of vitamin K_1 or K_2 to lower fracture risk found 13 trials that met this criterion. All but one showed that both vitamin K_1 and vitamin K_2 reduced bone loss, but vitamin K_2 was significantly more effective, reducing risk of vertebral fracture by 60%, hip fracture by 77%, and all nonver-tebral fractures by 81%.[258]

Numerous other recent studies have also shown that supplementation with vitamin K, particularly vitamin K_2, improves bone mineral density, helps protect against osteoporosis, and helps women with osteoporosis rebuild healthy bone.[259]

FOOD SOURCES OF VITAMIN K_1[260]

FOOD	SERVING	MICROGRAMS OF VITAMIN K_1	AMOUNT IN MICROGRAMS POTENTIALLY CONVERTED TO K_2 (MK-4 FORM)
Kale, raw	1 cup, chopped	547 mcg	32 mcg
Swiss chard, raw	1 cup	299 mcg	18 mcg
Parsley, raw	1/4 cup	246 mcg	15 mcg
Broccoli, cooked	1 cup, chopped	220 mcg	13 mcg
Spinach, raw	1 cup	145 mcg	9 mcg
Watercress	1 cup, chopped	85 mcg	5 mcg
Green leaf lettuce, raw	1 cup, shredded	63 mcg	4 mcg
Soybean oil	1 tablespoon	25 mcg	2 mcg
Canola oil	1 tablespoon	17 mcg	1 mcg
Olive oil	1 tablespoon	8 mcg	0.5 mcg
Mayonnaise	1 tablespoon	4 mcg	0.2 mcg

Latest Research States, "Treatment with Vitamin K, Especially MK-7, Effective Enough to Reduce Bone Resorption."

A landmark study published April 2012 in *Calcified Tissue International*, a leading journal for research on the structure and function of bone, compared the effects of vitamin K_1 to those of vitamin K_2 (as MK-7) on a number of indices of bone resorption (breakdown) and formation in 173 postmenopausal women.[261]

For this 12-month study, the women were randomly divided into four groups:

- A group of 38 women given 800 mg of calcium and 400 IU of vitamin D_3 per day (called the CaD group)

- A group of 38 women given 800 mg of calcium, 400 IU of vitamin D_3, and 100 mcg vitamin K_1 per day (the $CaDK_1$ group)

- A group of 39 women given 800 mg of calcium, 400 IU of vitamin D_3, and 100 mcg K_2 as MK-7 per day (the $CaDK_2$ group)

- A control group of 58 women (CG)

The first three groups received their supplements via milk and yogurt that had been fortified. No dietary intervention was delivered to the control group, who just continued with their usual diet.

What Happened?

- **Blood levels of 25(OH)D increased significantly in the $CaDK_1$ and $CaDK_2$ groups.**

  25(OH)D is the form of vitamin D circulating in the bloodstream and the most reliable indicator of body stores. By the end of the study, both groups given vitamin K averaged much greater levels of vitamin D than the group given only calcium and vitamin D (CaD) or the control group. However, in the group receiving vitamin K as K_2/MK-7, blood levels of vitamin D were more than 30% higher than in the group receiving vitamin K_1. The change in vitamin D levels was -0.7 in the control group, +1.6 in the CaD group, +2.5 in the $CaDK_1$ group, and +3.6 in the $CaDK_2$ group.

- **Blood levels of IGF-I increased significantly only in the $CaDK_2$ group.**

  IGF-1 is an anabolic (tissue building) hormone-like peptide. Recent studies show IGF-1 stimulates bone formation in postmenopausal women, primarily by signaling the precursor cells for osteoblasts to mature and become active. Blood levels of IGF-1 were -6.5 in the control group, +5.8 in the CaD group, +5.9 in the $CaDK_1$ group—and a whopping +11.9 in the $CaDK_2$ group.

- **Blood levels of UnOC (uncarboxylated osteocalcin) dropped in $CaDK_1$ and $CaDK_2$ groups, but $CaDK_2$ had almost double the drop in UnOC.**

  UnOC is the inactive form of osteocalcin, which is unable to deposit calcium in bone. Both the $CaDK_1$ and $CaDK_2$ groups had much lower levels at follow-up compared to the CaD and CG groups, but in the $CaDK_2$ group, which was given MK-7, the drop in UnOC was -23.6, almost double the -13.3 drop seen in the $CaDK_1$ group, which was given K_1!

- Urine levels of the bone breakdown byproduct deoxypyridinoline (D-Pyr) dropped in $CaDK_1$ and $CaDK_2$ groups, but the drop in $CaDK_2$ was triple that seen in $CaDK_1$.

  Osteoclasts' activity leads to the release of bone breakdown products, including pyridinium cross-links, such as deoxypyridinoline (D-Pyr). This is what the Pyrilinks-D urine test for bone loss measures. High levels of D-Pyr indicate excessive osteoclast activity and thus, excessive bone loss. Lower levels show the opposite—less osteoclast activity, less bone removal.

  Women in the CaDK1 group experienced an average -3.4 drop in D-Pyr. In women in the $CaDK_2$ group, the average drop in D-Pyr was -9.6!

- Both forms of vitamin K exerted beneficial effects on the RANKL/OPG ratio.

  What's the RANKL/OPG ratio? To explain this, we need to take a little trip "behind the scenes" for a look at these two molecules, one of which, RANKL, initiates a series of events that results in the production of osteoclasts ready to remove old bone, and another one, OPG, that shuts down this process.

  When RANKL, which stands for "receptor activator of nuclear factor-kappaB ligand," binds to a cellular receptor called RANK (receptor activator of nuclear factor-kappaB), this turns on nuclear factor-kappaB (NFkappaB), a seriously pro-inflammatory messenger. NFkappaB moves inside your cells and goes right to your DNA, where it sets off the production of a whole bunch of inflammatory processes—one of which is the activation of osteoclasts. You may remember we've said that anything that promotes chronic inflammation promotes bone loss. RANKL's activation of NKkappaB, which in turn activates osteoclasts, is behind this connection.

If we want to keep our bones, we must keep RANKL under control. However, RANKL is not an altogether bad guy we can afford to totally eliminate (which is what denosumab, aka Prolia® does—it totally shuts down RANKL). RANKL's binding to RANK is also necessary for the activation of immune cells (our T and B cells, specifically), and we must have functional immune systems to survive. What good are great bones if we're easy prey for destruction by infections or cancer?*

So, how do we safely put a leash on RANKL? We send in its decoy receptor osteoprotegerin (OPG), which also binds with RANKL, and thus blocks the interaction between RANKL and RANK, and the activation of NFkappaB. Pretty nifty how our body has worked out this balancing act for us, huh? I envision RANKL as a Conan the Barbarian kind of guy, and see OPG as standing for "Oh, Pretty Girl!" Enough OPG around and RANKL will be tamed, not eliminated (so our immune cells will still mature), but tuned down.

So, what encourages this happy meeting of our cellular characters, RANKL and OPG? You guessed it—vitamin K! (And so does soy, specifically, a bioactive isoflavone compound in

---

* More on this in the discussion of why you do not want to take denosumab (trade names Prolia® and Xgeva®) can be found on pages 52–66.

whole soyfoods called genistein, which is well known to lessen inflammation. Now we know genistein is doing so by increasing OPG and decreasing RANKL.* [262]

The study we're discussing here also showed that both vitamin K_1, and K_2 as MK-7, impact RANKL and OPG. Both forms of vitamin K affect both of these cellular receptors, but vitamin K_1 lowers RANKL more than K_2/MK-7, while K_2/MK-7 increases OPG more than K_1.

So, now you have yet another reason to eat plenty of leafy greens, which are loaded with vitamin K_1, and to also take a vitamin K_2 (MK-7) supplement.

Vitamin K_2 Partners with Vitamin D_3

Another reason to take vitamin K_2 is that K_2 partners with vitamin D. Vitamin D increases the production of osteocalcin and matrix-Gla protein, both of which require vitamin K_2 to become activated. Vitamin D thus increases both the demand for vitamin K_2 and the potential for benefit from K_2-dependent proteins.

Not surprisingly, the combination of vitamin K_2 and vitamin D_3 has been shown to be more effective

---

* A two year-long placebo-controlled study of 389 osteopenic postmenopausal women in Italy found giving them genistein (an isoflavone in soybeans) resulted in lower RANKL and higher OPG levels by the end of the first year, with further improvements in the ratio of RANKL/OPG by the end of the second year. Genistein was given to 198 women; the remaining 191 women received a placebo. Both the supplement containing genistein and the placebo supplement contained calcium and vitamin D3, and all the women received the same information about healthy diet. A significant (-0.021) reduction in the RANKL/OPG ratio occurred in the women given genistein, while in the women receiving placebo, the RANKL/OPG ratio worsened (+0.004).

in preventing bone loss than either nutrient alone. In a study of 173 osteoporotic/osteopenic women, those given both K_2 and D_3 experienced an average 4.92% increase in bone mineral density (BMD), while K_2 alone resulted in an average BMD increase of just 0.13%.[263]

The combined use of K_2 and D_3 has also been found to be more effective than either nutrient alone in improving bone mineral density (BMD) in postmenopausal women. In a 2-year study, 92 postmenopausal women were assigned to one of four groups: K_2 (45 milligrams per day of the menaquinone-4 form), D_3 (3,000 IU per day), a combination of these dosages of K_2 and D_3, or calcium lactate (2 grams per day). In the women receiving only calcium, lumbar BMD decreased. Those given either D_3 or K_2 experienced a slight increase in BMD, but those taking both K_2 and D_3 fared much better, increasing BMD in the lumbar spine (the part of the spine between the diaphragm and the pelvis) by 1.35%.[264]

How Much Do I Need?

You may be wondering, "Can I get enough vitamin K_2 to produce healthy bones from the K_1 and K_2 in my diet?" Probably not, even if you eat several cups of leafy greens every day.

Here's why: because ensuring that your blood will clot is more important for your immediate survival needs than putting calcium into your bones (or keeping it out of your arteries), all the vitamin K_1 in the foods you consume will first be used to activate the proteins necessary for blood clotting.[265] Only after this need has been met will any K_1 that is left over be available for conversion to K_2. In a best case scenario, only about 6% of the K_1 in the leafy greens you eat will ultimately get converted to K_2, and this means not enough K_2 for healthy bones (for an estimate of just how little K_2 this is, see the table on the next page).

In addition, whether you can convert K_1 to K_2 also depends upon whether you have healthy intestines, well supplied with the probiotic bacteria that do this job. If you have any gastrointestinal problems, your ability to produce K_2 may be greatly reduced, even if you are eating lots of foods rich in K_1.

So, do you eat lots of leafy greens every day? If you do, and your digestive system is well supplied with probiotic bacteria, you may be providing your bones with a tiny amount of K_2. But here's where it gets a bit more complicated because vitamin K_2 comes in two different flavors, menaquinone-4 (MK-4), and menaquinone-7 (MK-7). Humans typically convert K_1 into the MK-4 form of K_2, producing, at best, microgram amounts. But the research shows that, for healthy bones, we need at least 45 *milligrams* of MK-4, or much less (1,000 times less!), 45 *micrograms*, of MK-7.[266]

Both forms of K_2, MK-4 and MK-7, are found in certain foods, but in amounts too small for us to rely on them to protect our bones. MK-4 is found in tiny amounts in the fat of some animal products (e.g., meat, cheese, and egg yolk). MK-7 is present, again in very small amounts, in dairy products, like cheeses, but also in much larger amounts in fermented foods, such as sauerkraut and a fermented soybean product available in Japan called "natto." Unfortunately, natto is the only food that contains enough MK-7 to meet our bones' needs (approximately 870 micrograms per 3 ounces).[267] I say "unfortunately" because not only is natto hard to find in the US, it is an acquired taste,

FOOD SOURCES OF VITAMIN K₁, MK-4, MK-7 (IN MICROGRAMS PER 100 GRAMS— ABOUT 3 OUNCES)*

FOOD	K_1	MK-4	MK-7,8,9
Meats	0.5-5	1-30	0.1-2
Fish	0.1-1	0.1-2	—
Green vegs	100-750	—	—
Natto	20-40	—	900-1,200
Cheese	0.5-10	0.5-10	40-80
Other dairy	0.5 15	0.2-15	0-35
Eggs	0.5-2.5	10-25	—

even in Japan, due to its slimy texture and, for many people, pungent, unpalatable flavor.

In the US, our dietary intake of all forms of vitamin K combined (K_1 and all types of K_2) is only about 80 mcg/day, largely because we consume so few green vegetables. In the Netherlands, the Rotterdam study found dietary vitamin K intakes among those consuming the highest amounts of vitamin K averaged 370 mcg/day for K_1 and 45 mcg/day of menaquinones (MK-7, MK-8, MK-9), which corresponds to consumption of 100 grams (~3 ounces) green vegetables and 100g (~ 3 ounces) of cheese, respectively.[268]

Thus, to ensure the health of your bones, it is simplest and safest to take a supplement that supplies K_2, either in the form of MK-4, for which you will need to take 45 milligrams (15 mg, three times per day), or in the form of

---

* Adapted from Schurgers LJ, Geleijnse JM, Grobbee DE, et al. Nutrtional intake of vitamins K_1 (phylloquinone) and K_2 (menaquinone) in the Netherlands. *J. Nutr. Environ. Med.* June 1999;9(2):115–122. DOI: 10.1080/13590849961717.

MK-7, for which *at least* 45 micrograms is recommended. Higher doses, ranging from 180 micrograms to 865 micrograms, have been shown, in several recent studies, to be more effective. A randomized, double-blind study conducted on 35 lung and 59 heart transplant recipients during the first year after organ transplantation (transplant recipients are at greatly increased risk for osteoporosis) found a 180 microgram per day dose of MK-7 helpful in protecting lumbar spine bone mineral density (BMD).[269] And, a recent review of research on food factors shown to prevent osteoporosis found that people consuming 1.5 ounces of "reinforced natto" that provided 865 micrograms of MK-7 per day had much higher levels of activated osteocalcin than people consuming regular natto, which contains about 435 micrograms of MK-7 in 1.5 ounces.[270]

In January 2001, the US Food and Nutrition Board of the Institute of Medicine established an adequate intake (AI) level for vitamin K_1 of 90 micrograms per day for women and 120 micrograms per day for men.[271] The published research has shown this is way too little to promote optimal bone health.

What to Look for in a Supplement

The research shows that for healthy bones, we need 45 milligrams of MK-4 but less than 1 milligram of MK-7 daily. Why? What's the difference between these two forms of vitamin K_2?

Commercially available MK-4 is produced synthetically. This is the form that has been most widely used in the research. However, although it is well absorbed and gets into the bloodstream quickly, MK-4 has a half-life of only 6–8 hours. For this reason, high pharmacological doses (typically 45 milligrams per day, divided into 3 daily doses of 15 milligrams each) are necessary. This not only makes it inconvenient to take, but such high doses necessitate medical supervision in patients on blood-thinning medications (e.g., warfarin).

MK-7, a natural compound derived from natto, is also very well absorbed, and as little as 45 micrograms per day has been found to activate sufficient osteocalcin for bone health, although recent studies indicate doses ranging from 180 micrograms to 865 micrograms per day may be more effective. Less MK-7 is needed because this form of the vitamin hangs around a lot longer than MK-4; MK-7 has a serum half-life of 3 days, which enables the body to build up a buffer that can supply vitamin K_2 to all tissues 24 hours a day. MK-4 has a serum half-life of 6–8 hours. Even the highest dose of MK-7 shown effective in the research (865 micrograms/day) is much smaller than the dose required for MK-4 (45 mg, which, in the studies, is taken as three 15 mg doses throughout the day). The smaller dose not only makes MK-7 easier to take, but renders it highly unlikely to interact negatively with blood-thinning medications.[272]

Yet Another Reason Your K_2 Supplement Should Include the MK-7 Form: MK-7 Works with Vitamin D3 to Prevent Cardiovascular Disease

A number of recent studies have now indicated that reduced bone mineral density is a risk factor for cardiovascular disease.

One example is the MORE study, which included 2,576 postmenopausal women whose average age was 66.5 years. Those with osteoporosis (a total hip BMD T score < or = -2.5) had a 3.9-fold increased risk for cardiovascular events (like a heart attack) compared to those who only had osteopenia. However, even an osteopenic BMD (a T score between -2.5 and -1) was associated with a 2.1-fold or more than double increase in risk for a "cardiovascular event."

Furthermore, the presence of one or more vertebral fractures versus no vertebral fractures at baseline was associated with a 3.0-fold increase in risk. The greater her number of vertebral fractures, the greater a woman's risk for a heart attack.[273]

Most recently, Gerber, et al. (July 2011) reported a striking association between heart attack and osteoporotic fractures in a case-controlled study involving 6,642 residents of Olmsted County, Minnesota. Those who had suffered a heart attack were found to have a 32% increased risk of fracture.[274]

Why Does Losing Bone Increase Our Risk for a Heart Attack?

As mentioned earlier,* vitamin K_2 activates not only osteocalcin, which helps deposit calcium in bone, but also matrix-Gla protein, which keeps calcium out of our arteries. Several recently published studies show that vitamin K_2 (specifically in the form of its longer-chain menaquinones (e.g., MK-7), but *not* in the form of vitamin K_1 or the short-chain menaquinone, MK-4, provides effective protection against cardiovascular disease as well as osteoporosis. This suggests that MK-7 does a better job of activating matrix-Gla protein than K_1 or MK-4.

A large study conducted in the Netherlands, whose results were published in 2009,[275] examined the

* See page 172.

relationship between dietary intake of K_1 and K_2—and also differentiated between the MK-4 and MK-7 forms of K_2—and the incidence of coronary artery disease. This was studied in a group of subjects called the Prospect-EPIC cohort, which consisted of 16,057 women aged 49–70 years. The women were free of cardiovascular disease when the study began and were then followed an average of 8.1 years.

The women's average dietary intake of vitamin K_1 was 211.7 mcg/day, and their average dietary intake of vitamin K_2 was 29.1 mcg/day. Their K_1 intake was *not* found to be protective against cardiovascular disease, even though any K_1 not used up to activate clotting factors in the liver is converted to MK-4, *if* the healthy bacteria that do this are present in the intestines. (If your intestines are not happy, for example, if you have irritable bowel disease or if you have wiped out all of your intestinal flora by taking antibiotics and then not taken probiotics to restore your healthy bacterial population, all bets are off. This is one of the reasons why irritable bowel disease has been linked with osteoporosis.)[276]

A highly protective effect against coronary heart disease was seen, however, when the women's dietary intake of vitamin K_2 was high, specifically, when their consumption, not of MK-4, but of the longer-chain menaquinones, MK-7, MK-8 and MK-9 (which are primarily supplied by cheeses and other dairy products in the Netherlands), was high. The Rotterdam study, an earlier study whose results were published in 2004, also reported a strong inverse association between vitamin K_2 intake and coronary artery disease, but a much less significant association for K_1.[277]

Another recent study from the Netherlands, an area that has been a hotbed of vitamin K research for decades, also showed that higher dietary intake of the longer-chain menaquinones (e.g., MK-7) reduces calcification of the heart's arteries.[278] This research looked at coronary (heart) artery calcification and vitamin K intake in 564 postmenopausal women. While vitamin K_1 was not protective, women whose diets supplied the most K_2, which in the Netherlands is primarily the long chain menaquinones (e.g., MK-7 in cheeses), had a 20% lower risk of coronary calcification.

This growing research evidence helps explain why population studies conducted in the US that looked at whether vitamin K was protective against coronary artery disease showed little benefit. The US studies looked only at dietary consumption of K_1, but did not collect any data on K_2.[279]

Why Your Body May Prefer MK-7 to MK-4— or Vice Versa

As previously discussed,* two forms of supplemental vitamin K_2 are available: MK-4 and MK-7. MK-4 is used and cleared from the body within about 6–8 hours, while MK-7 remains active in our systems for much longer—around 3 days. For most people, MK-7's longer half-life is a very good thing—it results in our being able to take far less (just 100 micrograms per day is effective) and keeps K_2 available 24 hours a day to activate osteocalcin and matrix Gla proteins (plus the many other health-protective things vitamin K_2 does for us).

I (Lara) have heard from a few people, however, that in their bodies, MK-7 produces a stimulating

---

* See pages 182–185.

effect that interferes with sleep, while the MK-4 form, which is usually cleared out of our systems much more quickly and does not accumulate to provide a reserve, suits their physiology just fine. (If you take MK-4, the dose shown in the research studies to benefit bones is 15 *milligrams* [which equals 15,000 micrograms] taken 3 times daily [ideally, every 6–8 hours] for a total of 45 milligrams per day.)

In medical studies whose combined participants add up to hundreds of thousands of people, no side-effects from taking MK-7 have been reported, but the real people writing me had done their own unofficial "clinical trials." When they stopped taking MK-7, their symptoms went away. When they began taking it again, their symptoms returned. I discussed this at a recent medical conference (Institute for Functional Medicine's 2012 symposium) with a highly respected cardiologist who has used MK-7 in thousands of patients and never seen any side-effects. His comment, "They must have taken a bad batch or they are mistaken." I checked on the brands the women who wrote me were using (and they were reputable companies), so a bad batch of MK-7 was unlikely. And I was certain these individuals were not "mistaken" about the effects of MK-7 on their own bodies! Obviously, something was going on! I was very intrigued. Why might MK-7 be excessively stimulating for some people?

An explanation has recently been provided in a paper published in *Advances in Nutrition*, March 2012. This latest paper from three giants in the field of vitamin K research, Drs. Martin Shearer, Xueyan Fu, and Sarah Booth, is entitled, "Vitamin K Nutrition, Metabolism, and Requirements: Current Concepts and Future Research."[280]

Studies have now explored the associations between genetically inherited differences in the activity of key enzymes involved in vitamin K metabolism and an individual's vitamin K status. It turns out that common single nucleotide polymorphisms (SNPs) in several genes that direct the production of key enzymes involved in vitamin K metabolism (specifically, APOE, VKOR, and CYP4F2, explained below)[281] affect how quickly an individual metabolizes vitamin K and therefore how much vitamin K that person will require for optimal functioning. It's the genetic version of the Goldilocks tale: what would be the "just right" form and dosage of vitamin K for one may be "too little" or "too much" for another.

APOE Polymorphisms Affect How Much Vitamin K YOU Need

APOE stands for "apolioprotein E." Apolipoproteins are proteins that bind lipids (oil-soluble substances like fats, fat-soluble vitamins [one of which is vitamin K] and cholesterol) to form lipoproteins (lipo = fat, so these molecules are fat + protein combos). Apolioproteins act as transport vehicles for lipids through our lymphatic and circulatory systems.

Our body's different uses for vitamin K_1, and the MK-4 and MK-7 forms of vitamin K_2, are reflected in their being transported by different lipoproteins. Vitamin K_1 and the MK-4 form of vitamin K_2 share a similar structure, so both are primarily transported in lipoproteins carrying triglycerides. Triglycerides are one of the ways in which our bodies package unused fat calories, both from unsaturated fats (vegetable oils) and saturated fats (animal derived fats). Sent from our digestive tract to the liver, triglycerides are quickly broken down to release vitamin K, so it can be used to activate the vitamin K-dependent proteins required for blood coagulation. This prevents us from bleeding to death from even a paper cut, but can leave little vitamin K for use in the rest of our body.

The MK-7 form of vitamin K_2 is also initially taken up in triglyceride-carrying lipoproteins, from which it is rapidly removed by the liver, but unlike vitamin K_1 or the MK-4 version of vitamin K_2, MK-7 gets repackaged into LDL cholesterol. LDL cholesterol is the major carrier of vitamin K_2 from the liver to the rest of the body.

The result is that both vitamin K_1 and the MK-4 form of vitamin K_2 are typically used up in a matter of hours, while MK-7 has a much longer half-life: several days in comparison to 6–8 hours for K_1 and MK-4. MK-7's longer half-life results in its accumulating seven to eight fold higher levels in the body during prolonged intake and producing more stable blood levels than MK-4. However, for the five to ten percent of people whose apolioprotein E (APOE) genetic inheritance causes them to clear vitamin K_2 much more slowly than most people, MK-7's ability to remain active in the body longer may not make this form of vitamin K_2 their best fit.

APOE occurs in three "flavors"—its three isoforms, apoE2, apoE3, and apoE4. These differ from one another by just a single amino acid, but this tiny difference has a big impact on how those of us who have inherited one of these genetic "flavors" carry LDL cholesterol to our cells and how quickly our cells take up and use that LDL (and the vitamin K_2 within it). Individuals who are carriers of apoE4 remove LDL from the bloodstream the fastest, followed by carriers of

apoE3 and lastly, carriers of apoE2, in whom cholesterol is cleared more slowly.

What this means is that individuals who have apoE4
are going to use up their vitamin K_2 quickly; those who
have apoE3 will keep K_2 around the "average" amount
of time, and in those who have apoE2, K_2 will remain
active in their system for longer than "normal." Most
people (sixty to seventy percent of us) are carriers of
apoE3, fifteen to twenty percent carry apoE4 (so they
need *more* vitamin K than the "average" person), and
a few of us, five to ten percent, carry apoE2. Those of
us who have apoE2 are the individuals who may find
MK-7 builds up in their bodies to levels that cause difficulty sleeping.

Lab testing to check your apoE "flavor" is readily
available. A Google search will bring up many labs.
Here's one offering direct-to-consumer testing: http://
labtestsonline.org/understanding/analytes/apoe/tab/
test. (I have no financial or other connection to this or
any other lab.)

VKOR and CCGX—Key Enzymes in the Vitamin K-Epoxide Cycle

The vitamin K-epoxide cycle is the way in which our
bodies both put vitamin K into the form in which is
used to carboxylate (activate) the vitamin K-dependent
proteins (those involved in normal blood clotting, so
we don't bleed to death, as well as osteocalcin, which
puts calcium into bone, and matrix Gla-protein, which
keeps calcium out of our arteries) *and* recycle vitamin
K, so our cells can use it over again. Two enzymes play
key roles in this vitamin K cycle: g-glutamyl carboxyl-
ase (GGCX) and vitamin K epoxide reductase (VKOR).

If they both work quickly and well, we are better at activating vitamin K-dependent proteins and at recycling vitamin K, so we may need less, which would make the MK-4 version of vitamin K_2 a potentially better fit for us. If one or the other of these enzymes is slow to do its job, we will not be as good at activating our vitamin K-dependent proteins or at conserving vitamin K, so we are likely to need more for optimal health and to be better off with the MK-7 form, which naturally sticks around longer.

Several common SNPs have been found in the genes that direct whether our bodies produce fast or slow VKOR and GGCX enzymes. Although testing of VKOR and GGCX SNPs is not currently available outside the rarified world of high-tech research, a readily-available-at-virtually-any-lab test you could request to gain insight into how quickly your VKOR and GGCX recycle vitamin K would be a blood test called the prothrombin time (PT) and its derived measures, prothrombin ratio (PR) and international normalized ratio (INR). This test, also called "Pro-Time INR" and "INR PT," is used to determine the clotting tendency of blood, to check adequacy (or excess) of warfarin dosage, liver damage, and your vitamin K1 status.

A mid-to-high INR indicates your blood is less likely to clot excessively. An INR below the therapeutic range indicates increased risk of unwanted blood clot formation. The reference range for prothrombin time is usually around 10-14 seconds, and the INR in absence of warfarin use is 0.8-1.2. The target range for INR in individuals prescribed an anticoagulant (e.g., warfarin) is 2 to 3. If you are not taking warfarin, a normal INR suggests your VKOR and GGXX are doing a reasonable job for you; a low INR may suggest you need more vitamin K, both as K_1 and MK-7.

Vitamin K does not increase risk of bleeding; to the contrary, K_1 is used to activate clotting factors. Nor does it increase your risk of excessive blood clot formation; once your needs for clotting factors are taken care of, any extra vitamin K will be sent out into the bloodstream as K_1 and/or converted to MK-4 and delivered to meet vitamin K needs in the rest of your body—e.g., in your bones and arteries.

If you have consumed K_2 in the form of MK-7, your liver will put this form of vitamin K into LDL cholesterol and send it out to the rest of your body via your bloodstream.

CYP4F2 Affects How Quickly You Excrete Vitamin K

Humans excrete vitamin K (both K_1 and K_2, including MK-4 and MK-7) using a common prepare-for-elimination pathway in the liver. This pathway begins with the action of an enzyme called cytochrome P450 4F2 (CYP4F2). After CYP4F2 works it magic, the products that result are made water-soluble by being combined, mainly with glucuronic acid, a process called glucuronidation. Once made water-soluble, they can be excreted via bile (which goes into feces) or urine.

By now, you've probably figured out that the CYP4F2 enzyme does not work at the same speed in every one of us. How quickly—or slowly—your CYP4F2 enzyme works will affect the rate at which YOUR body eliminates vitamin K, and thus how much vitamin K YOU need.

If your genetic inheritance includes a slow version of the CYP4F2 enzyme, you will excrete vitamin K more slowly than the "average" person. Your needs for supplemental vitamin K will be lower than "average," and this may mean that MK-4 is a better "fit" for you than MK-7.

If you're taking warfarin, and you have the slower version of CYP4F2, you will require about 1 millligram/day *more* warfarin than individuals who have the speedier version of CYP4F2. The impact of CYP4F2 on vitamin K excretion was discovered by researchers trying to figure out why some patients needed a higher dosage of warfarin than others. Carriers of the slower CYP4F2 enzyme required higher doses of warfarin because their CYP4F2 enzyme did not process vitamin K for excretion as rapidly, so vitamin K remained present in higher concentrations in their livers.

The slower version of the CYP4F2 enzyme is present in about 30% of Caucasians and Asians, but in only around 7% of African-Americans. Carriers of this slower version of CYP4F2 should require less vitamin K than non-carriers to maintain an equivalent vitamin K status.

Genetic testing will likely soon be available to consumers who want to find out whether they have inherited a fast, slow, or average CYP4F2 enzyme, but in the meantime, once again, insight into your CYP4F2 status could be gained from your prothrombin time (PT) and its derived measures, prothrombin ratio (PR) and international normalized ratio (INR). If your INR is at the low end of the range, this would suggest your excretion of vitamin K is slower than "average," so you may need less vitamin K than the "average person" and may find MK-4 works well for you. If your INR is normal or at the high end of the reference range, MK-7 would most likely serve you best.

At this time, no research has shown that vitamin K_2 in its MK-7 form might have a stimulating effect that would result in sleep disturbance in sensitive individuals. However, recently, an article in *Science* reported a new discovery: in human cells, vitamin K_2 is involved in the production of energy (ATP) in our mitochondria (the energy production factories in our cells). Perhaps, in those whose genetic inheritance results in their keeping vitamin K_2 around longer, MK-7's effect of optimizing energy production neurons (the cells in our brain) might result in more brain activity, but impair our ability to tune down and sleep? Just speculation. We'll be following the vitamin K research closely for new developments.[282]

Bottom line: We are each unique! While the majority of us (somewhere around 85-95%) will find vitamin K_2 in its MK-7 form the most helpful for all the reasons discussed fully in *Your Bones*, if you are among the much smaller number of individuals whose genetic inheritance enables them to keep vitamin K around far longer than "average" and recycle it for re-use more quickly, you may find that MK-4 form of vitamin K_2 works best for you.

Safety Issues

Except for people on anticoagulant (blood thinning) medication, e.g., warfarin (Coumadin® is the most popular brand name for this patent medicine), vitamin K is extremely safe. No adverse events have been shown in humans given doses of MK-7 greater than 800 mcg/day. No adverse effects have been reported for higher levels of vitamin K intake from food and/or supplements, and there are no documented toxicity symptoms for vitamin K. In animal studies, vitamin K in amounts as high as 25 micrograms per kilogram of body weight per day (the equivalent of 1,750 micrograms of vitamin K for an adult human weighing 154 pounds) has produced no noticeable toxicity. Thus, when the Institute of Medicine at the National Academy of Sciences published its health recommendations for this nutrient in 2001, the experts chose not to set a Tolerable Upper Limit (UL) for vitamin K.[283]

Those taking warfarin can still take vitamin K, but will need to do so under the care of their doctors, who can work with them to calibrate a dose that will not disturb their international normalized ratio (INR).

An INR that is too high indicates high risk of bleeding and lessened ability to produce the blood clots needed to prevent you from bleeding to death from even a tiny cut, while an INR that is too low suggests the potential for excessive blood clot formation, so your doctor will want to increase your dose of warfarin to protect against this. The key factor here is maintaining a stable intake of vitamin K against which your doctor can calibrate the amount of warfarin YOU require.

Also, if you have been prescribed warfarin because you have heart failure, you may be able to discontinue it and use aspirin instead. Again, you must work with your doctor on this! Research presented at the American Stroke Association's International Stroke Conference in New Orleans, February 5, 2012, showed that aspirin is just as effective as warfarin for heart failure patients.[284] This study, which involved 2,305 heart failure patients, found no overall difference in risk of death or for either form of stroke (intracranial hemorrhage or ischemic stroke) between those who received aspirin and those who received warfarin. Researchers also noted warfarin had a higher risk of causing bleeding. The lead author of this study, Dr. Shunichi Homma, is quoted as stating, "Given that there is no overall difference between the two treatments and that possible benefit of warfarin does not start until after four years of treatment, there is no compelling reason to use warfarin, especially considering the bleeding risk."

Since warfarin is also well known to increase your risk of both developing osteoporosis and calcifying your arteries, ask your doctor to at least help you take vitamin K_2 if you must remain on warfarin.

If you are taking warfarin, the following information may help your doctor establish the right dose of vitamin K_2 for you:

It's well known that supplemental (and dietary) vitamin K can interfere with the anticoagulant action of coumarin derivatives, but lower doses appear to be safe. Experiments have shown that only at a dose of 315 mcg/day did K_1 affect INR, decreasing it from 2.0 to 1.5. MK-7 is more potent, causing a comparable decrease in INR at an intake of 130 mcg/day. For this reason, Schurgers, et al. recommend an upper safety limit of 50 mcg/day for supplemental long-chain menaquinones (i.e., MK-7) in patients on oral anticoagulant treatment.

This dose is comparable to the menaquinone content of 75 to 100 grams of cheese, and research evaluating the effect on INR of gradually increasing doses of MK-7 indicates 50 mcg/day would lead to a disturbance of the INR value of no more than 10%. Because of the 96 hour half-life of MK-7, regular intake of MK-7 in combination with properly adapted coumarin doses results in *more stable INR values*.[285] Thus carefully monitored patients on coumarin derivatives may be able to take a higher daily dose of MK-7, a preferable prescription given the greatly increased risk of vascular calcification with coumarin use.

B VITAMINS (B$_6$, B$_{12}$, FOLATE, AND RIBOFLAVIN)

What They Do

As mentioned earlier in the section "'Bs' for Better Bones,"* the B vitamins are needed to prevent levels of homocysteine, a nasty middleman compound in a very important cellular process called methylation, from accumulating.

Collagen is the main protein component in our bones. Collagen proteins link together, forming the organic part of the bone matrix. Homocysteine interferes with collagen cross-linking, causing a defective bone matrix and increased bone fragility.[286] In cell studies, homocysteine has been shown to trigger the self-destruct sequence (called *apoptosis*) in the cells that build bone (osteoblasts), and to increase the formation and activity of the cells that break down bone (osteoclasts).[287]

In addition to these directly harmful effects on bone, elevated homocysteine also promotes chronic inflammation, which triggers osteoclast production and activity, a significant contributing factor to bone loss in older individuals, particularly postmenopausal women. (Osteoclasts are the target of the bisphosphonate patent medicines, which were designed to help maintain bone mass by poisoning osteoclasts, and of denosumab, which prevents osteoclasts from ever maturing into potentially active cells.)

---

* See page 99.

Also as mentioned earlier,* estrogen helps lessen inflammation, which is one of the key reasons its decline during menopause results in increased bone loss.[288] When adequate supplies of the B vitamins are present, homocysteine is quickly metabolized into a harmless compound.

What to Look for in a Supplement

The following amounts should be present in a day's recommended dose of your multiple vitamin. Note that a daily dose of some multiple vitamins may be 2, 3, or even as many as 6 capsules. The *total* amount of the B vitamins provided by the daily dose should be at least:

- B_6: 50 milligrams
- B_{12}: 500 micrograms
- Folate: 1,000 micrograms
- Riboflavin: 50 milligrams

Safety Issues

- **B_6**: Nervous system imbalances have been shown to result from very high levels of vitamin B_6 intake—more than 2 grams (2,000 milligrams) per day. The tolerable Upper Intake Level (UL) set for vitamin B_6 for adults 19 years and older by the National Academy of Sciences is 100 milligrams per day.

- **B_{12}**: No toxicity symptoms have been reported for B_{12}, even in long-term studies in which subjects took 1,000 micrograms daily for 5 years,

---

* In the "What It Does" section for vitamin K, page 172.

so the National Academy of Sciences has set no UL for B_{12}.

- **Folate**: At doses greater than 1,000–2,000 micrograms, "inactive synthetic folate" (the fully oxidized, inactive "folic acid" form of folate obtained from supplements and/or fortified foods) can trigger nervous system-related symptoms, including insomnia, malaise, irritability, and intestinal dysfunction. The UL set for folic acid by the Institute of Medicine at the National Academy of Sciences is 1,000 micrograms for adults 19 years and older. As this is being written, most suppliers of multivitamins are switching from the inactive folic acid to the active methylfolate and folinic acid (or calcium folinate) forms. If at all possible, use one of these.

- **Riboflavin**: No toxic side effects have been documented for riboflavin, so the National Academy of Sciences has not set a UL for riboflavin.

VITAMIN C

What It Does

As noted earlier in the section " 'C' Your Way to Stronger Bones,"* vitamin C is essential for the development and maintenance of strong bones because 90% of the protein in the bone matrix is collagen, and vitamin C is an essential cofactor required for collagen formation. Vitamin C stimulates the production of osteoblasts (the cells that build bone), and is also one of the body's key antioxidants and thus helps lessen inflammation, which, if

---

* See page 105.

uncontrolled, results in increased production and activation of osteoclasts, the cells that break down bone.[289]

What to Look for in a Supplement

Vitamin C, ascorbic acid, is very inexpensive and readily available. Your main concern is dosage. In postmenopausal women, greater bone mineral density has been reported when vitamin C intake from supplements increased from 0 to 500 to 1,000 milligrams per day. Higher intake of vitamin C has also been associated with significantly higher BMD (less bone loss) in older men who had never smoked.[290]

Look for a supplement that will allow you to take at least 1,000 milligrams per day, preferably 2,000 milligrams per day, without having to swallow several large hard pills. Capsules containing vitamin C powder, a jar of vitamin C powder, or a product like Emergen-C® (which provides vitamin C in 1,000-milligram packets, comes in a variety of flavors, and makes a pleasant tasting fizzy drink), may be better absorbed and easier to swallow than large, hard tablets. You can even use your Emergen-C® drink as the liquid with which to swallow your other supplements. Vitamin C powder will add a lemony tang to a glass of water, fruit juice, or cup of tea.

A very few individuals experience loose stools, gas, or even diarrhea, when taking a single 1,000 milligram dose of vitamin C. If you are one of them, you have two options: you can try taking a "buffered" version of vitamin C or you can take your vitamin C in divided doses. Buffered vitamin C powder usually combines ascorbic acid with minerals like calcium, magnesium, or potassium. When buffered vitamin C powder is mixed with water, the result is a reduced-acid solution that effervesces for a short while—a plus if you enjoy fizzy drinks—and won't irritate a sensitive stomach or intestinal lining.

Another option, Ester-C®, is a complex of ascorbic acid combined with several of its naturally occurring metabolites, including dehydroascorbate, threonate, and aldonic acids. Ester-C® is significantly more expensive than plain old ascorbic acid, but it may be worth the additional cost. A test tube study found that cells treated with this vitamin C complex produced more collagen and mineralized tissue than cells treated with ascorbic acid alone, suggesting that Ester-C® may be more effective in helping to promote bone regeneration than ascorbic acid.[291]

Safety Issues

In 2000, the National Academy of Sciences set a Tolerable Upper Intake Level (UL) for vitamin C at 2,000 milligrams (2 grams) for adults 19 years or older. This UL is probably too low.

Very few research studies document vitamin C toxicity at any level of supplementation, and no toxicity effects have ever been documented in relation to vitamin C from food in the diet. As mentioned, some persons react to high supplemental doses, typically involving 5 or more grams of vitamin C, by developing loose stools or diarrhea. This type of diarrhea is called "osmotic diarrhea" because it results from an excess of fluid concentrating in the intestine as the body attempts to dilute the amount of vitamin C present. The magnesium in Milk of Magnesia® has the same effect.

Vitamin C can increase a person's absorption of iron from plant foods, such as spinach. Usually, this is beneficial, given that approximately 1 in 24 Americans or 11.2 million people in the USA, including 20% of premenopausal women and 2% of adult men, are iron-deficient.[292] However, those at risk of having excess free iron in their cells (e.g., men who eat a lot of red meat) may want to have their iron levels checked and donate blood or consider avoiding high supplemental doses of vitamin C.

Key Bone-Building Minerals

CALCIUM

What It Does

One of the most abundant minerals in the human body, calcium accounts for approximately 1.5% of total body weight, and approximately 99% of that calcium is stored in our bones and teeth.[293] The remaining 1%, however, is needed for numerous actions required for our physical bodies to continue to function. For example, calcium is necessary for blood clotting, neurotransmitter release, nerve conduction, and muscle contraction (including the contraction of the heart muscle—our heartbeat). Calcium regulates enzyme activity and cell membrane function, which determines what gets into and out of our cells.

Because these physiological activities are essential to life, our body has developed complex regulatory systems that tightly control the amount of calcium in the blood to ensure enough calcium is always available for them. When we don't consume enough calcium to maintain these essential blood levels, our body will draw on calcium stashed in our bones to maintain normal blood concentrations. Just like with any banking system, too many withdrawals without enough deposits leads to bankruptcy, which in the case of our bones, after many years, equals osteoporosis and bone fractures.

Calcium is best known for its role as the primary component that gives our bones strength and density. To mineralize bone, calcium joins with phosphorus, forming calcium phosphate, which then serves as the major component of the mineral complex—called *hydroxyapatite*—that provides structure and strength in bones.

Numerous studies have shown that calcium supplementation improves bone density in perimenopausal women and slows the rate of bone loss in postmenopausal women by 30 to 50%, significantly reducing the risk of hip fracture.[294] However, the most recent Cochrane Review (the gold standard in medical research) found that calcium supplementation *alone* has only a small positive effect on bone density.[295] This is the key point we are trying to make in this book! Healthy bones are the result not of just one, two, or even several compounds, but of more than a dozen nutrients derived from a healthy diet, supplements when optimal amounts of specific nutrients are difficult to get from the diet, and a healthy lifestyle that includes regular exercise.

What to Look for in a Supplement

Despite calcium's widespread availability in a variety of foods, most Americans are not getting enough to support healthy bones for life.* Thus, to ensure bone health, it's best to supplement. But how do you choose which of the many different available forms of supple-

---

* For a discussion of food sources of calcium, see "Are You Sure You're Getting Enough Calcium?," page 86.

mental calcium will best serve you? Here's what you need to know to decide.

Naturally Derived Calcium

May appear on labels as bone meal, oyster shell, limestone, or dolomite (clay). Since naturally derived calcium supplements have been found to contain concentrations of lead far exceeding the most recent criteria established to limit lead exposure (>1.5 µg/g), these forms are best avoided.[296]

Calcium Carbonate

The most commonly used form in calcium supplements, and that used in OTC antacids (e.g., Tums®, Rolaids®, Maalox®) is less expensive, but not nearly as well absorbed as the forms of calcium discussed below, chelated calcium, hydroxyapaptite, or calcium derived from sea-algae.

If you choose calcium carbonate, it is very important that it be taken with meals when you will be secreting hydrochloric acid. Why? Calcium is absorbed in the small intestine where normally, the pH balance is not acidic; therefore, stomach acid is needed not to absorb calcium, but to dissolve the delivery form—which in the case of calcium carbonate is essentially a piece of chalk.

Of concern is the fact that people with low stomach acid absorb only about 4% of an oral dose of calcium carbonate, and studies have found that about 40% of postmenopausal women are deficient in stomach acid. Obviously, if you do not have adequate stomach acid, antacids will not provide an effective means of delivering supplemental calcium to your bones![297]

FOODS RICH IN CALCIUM [298]

FOOD	SERVING SIZE	CALCIUM (IN MILLIGRAMS)
Yogurt, low-fat	1 cup	447 mg
Sardines	1 each	351 mg
Sesame seeds	1/4 cup	351 mg
Goat's milk	1 cup	325 mg
Cow's milk	1 cup	297 mg
Spinach	1 cup	245 mg
Cabbage, shredded, cooked	1/2 cup	239 mg
Mozarella cheese, part-skim	1 oz	183 mg
Cottage cheese, 2%	1 cup	155 mg
Blackstrap molasses	2 teaspoons	118 mg
Mustard greens, steamed	1 cup	104 mg
Tofu	4 oz	100 mg
Broccoli	1 cup	75 mg
Cinnamon, dried, ground	2 teaspoons	56 mg
Thyme, dried, ground	2 teaspoons	54 mg
Oranges	1	52 mg
Oregano, dried, ground	2 teaspoons	47 mg
Romaine lettuce	2 cups	40 mg

What might cause you to have too little stomach acid? Two very common possibilities are infection with *Helicobacter pylori*, the pathogenic bacterium that promotes ulcers, and self- or doctor-prescribed medication with H2-blockers [e.g., cimetidine (Tagamet®), ranitidine (Zantac®), famotidine (Pepcid®), and nizatidine (Axid®)] or proton-pump inhibitors for heartburn

or gastroesophaegal reflux (GERD) [e.g., esomepra-
zole (Nexium®), omeprazole (Prilosec®), lansoprazole
(Prevacid®), pantoprazole (Protonix®), rabeprazole
(AcipHex®)].

About 25% of the population in the western world,
including North America, is infected with *H.pylori*. In
developing nations, *H.pylori* infection is much more
common, affecting upwards of 80% of the populations.[299] If you are taking any of the acid-blocking patent medicines listed, your likelihood of not having
enough stomach acid to absorb the calcium from calcium carbonate is quite high.

Another common cause of low stomach acid is simply
getting older. By the time both men and women reach
age 60, half of us don't make enough acid in our stomachs
to optimally digest all our food—and that includes dis-
solving the carbonate form of calcium. Other less common causes of low stomach acid include food allergy
(especially wheat and dairy), overindulgence in alcohol,
and the aftereffects of some viral illnesses.*

Chelated Calcium

Chelated calcium will appear on the label as calcium
citrate, calcium malate, calcium gluconate, calcium
aspartate, etc. In these chelated forms, calcium is
bound to either an organic acid (e.g., citrate, malate,
gluconate) or amino acid (aspartate).

The resulting compounds are optimal calcium-deliv-
ery agents. They are 22% to 27% better absorbed than
calcium carbonate; degrade almost completely even

---

* For a complete discussion of low stomach acid, see *Your Stomach* by Dr.
  Wright, Praktikos Books: Mt. Jackson, VA, 2009.

when stomach acid is relatively low (so they can be taken without food and are the supplement of choice for individuals with low stomach acid and those using stomach acid-blocking patent medicines), and do not contain lead or other toxic metals. Chelated forms have been shown to increase absorption of not only calcium, but other bone-building minerals such as magnesium.[300]

Hydroxyapatite

Hydroxyapatite sometimes appears as MCHC (microcrystalline hydroxyapatite). The most expensive form of calcium, hydroxyapatite is a complex crystalline compound in which calcium is linked with phosphorus in a preformed building block of the bone mineral matrix.

MCHC contains hydroxyapatite plus bone-derived growth factors and all the trace minerals that comprise healthy bone. Although research on hydroxyapatite as a source of calcium is limited, two studies have shown it to be more effective in the prevention of osteoporosis caused by taking corticosteroid patent medicines.[301] And a recent meta-analysis of 12 well controlled trials comparing hydroxyapatite to calcium carbonate to prevent bone loss found hydroxyapatite increased bone mineral density 102% more than calcium carbonate![302]

Algae-Derived Calcium

AlgaeCal® is a recently developed *plant-based* calcium supplement derived from marine algae, which contains high levels of calcium, magnesium, and other minerals involved in the production of healthy bone. Several studies have now shown that AlgaeCal® is more effective at building bone than other supplemental forms of calcium. This is big news since, until quite recently, it has been "a given" that all elemental calcium—i.e., the cation Ca2+ disassociated from its salt (e.g., the carbonate or citrate portion of calcium carbonate or calcium citrate, respectively) has the same effects in the body. We now know this may not be true. Research conducted by AlgaeCal®, pitting its algae-derived calcium against calcium carbonate and calcium citrate in head-to-head studies—a human osteoblast study and two human studies—demonstrates it.

The osteoblast study revealed that AlgaeCal® produced 200–400% greater proliferation and mineralization of these bone-building cells than did calcium carbonate or citrate.[303] In this study, human osteoblast cells were treated with AlgaeCal®, calcium carbonate or calcium citrate—with and without also giving vitamin D_3. After four days, the osteoblasts treated with AlgaeCal® were found to have produced much greater amounts of an enzyme called alkaline phosphatase, compared to the cells that had been treated with either calcium carbonate or calcium citrate, regardless of whether vitamin D_3 was also given. This is significant because alkaline phosphatase plays a key role in osteoblasts' mineralization of bone.

In AlgaeCal-treated cells, levels of PCNA (proliferating cell nuclear antigen, a protein involved in DNA synthesis and repair) and DNA synthesis were also much greater (4.0-fold greater than control, 3.0-fold greater than calcium carbonate, and 4.0-fold greater than calcium citrate). The end result was that more calcium

---

* 72 mg naturally occurring plus magnesium carbonate

(Ca2+) was deposited in AlgaeCal-treated cells (2.0-fold more than controls, 1.0-fold more than calcium carbonate, and 4.0-fold more than calcium citrate-treated cells). When vitamin D_3 was also added to the treated osteoblasts, the results were even better.

AlgaeCal® was also found to significantly reduce oxidative stress in the osteoblasts after just 24 hours. (Remember oxidative stress promotes inflammation, which then triggers osteoclasts, the specialized cells that break down bone, to spring into action.) Algae-Cal® reduced oxidative stress in human osteoblasts by 4-fold compared to controls (untreated cells), 2-fold compared to calcium carbonate, and 2.5-fold compared to calcium citrate.

COMPONENTS OF BONE-HEALTH SUPPLEMENTS PROVIDED TO ALGAECAL 1 GROUP AND ALGAECAL 2 GROUP

INGREDIENT OR COMPONENT	ALGAECAL 1	ALGAECAL 2
Strontium Citrate (mg of elemental strontium)	680	680
AlgaeCal Bone-health Supplement	2,400	2,520
Trace Minerals in AlgaeCal (mg)	1,608	1,688
Calcium (mg)	720	756
Magnesium (mg)*	72	75
Magnesium from magnesium carbonate (mg)	0	275
Vitamin D-3 (IUs of Cholecalciferol)	800	1,600
Vitamin K-2 as MK-4 (mg)	1.5	0
Vitamin K-7 as MK-7 (mcg)	0	100
Boron (mg)	0	3
Vitamin C (mg)	0	50

Table adapted from Michalek, et al. *Nutrition Journal* 2011 10:32 oi:10.1186/1475-2891-10-32.

These promising results lead to two human studies using AlgaeCal®. In the first study, 158 adults agreed to follow an open-label bone-health plan for six months after taking a DXA test to evaluate their bone density, a 43-chemistry blood test panel, and a quality of life inventory (AlgaeCal 1). Two weeks after the last subject completed the six-month trial, a second group of 58 subjects was enrolled and followed the identical plan, but with a slightly different (and improved) bone-health supplement (AlgaeCal 2, the version now available to the public.)[304]

Bone mineral density improved in both groups (AlgaeCal 1 and AlgeCal 2) significantly compared to what normally happens—a loss in BMD is what is expected. The "conservative" (least) expected drop in BMD for women aged 41–55 is a loss of -0.5%/year, for women 56 and older, a loss of -1.0%/year, and for men, a loss of half these amounts. However, population-based longitudinal studies suggest that these loss estimates are not high enough. Minor bone loss starts at age 40, increasing to 0.5% to 0.9% a year in peri-menopausal women and to above 1% after menopause, after which the yearly loss in BMD remains about 1%. Other studies suggest that after midlife, in men as well as women, there is an age-related yearly loss of bone of 1%, which, for women, accelerates to 2% for up to 14 years around the age of menopause (which typically occurs around age 52). In men, a small loss is detected in 40-year olds, which increases to a loss of about -0.8% per year into old age.

Compared to the most conservative estimate for annual bone loss given above, AlgaeCal 1 had a positive mean annualized percent change (MAPC) in BMD of a gain of +1.15%. AlgaeCal 2 had a positive MAPC of +2.79%! With no negative side effects! No clinically significant changes in a 43-panel blood chemistry test were found, and neither group reported even one adverse effect.

So, what supplements did these study participants receive that produced such bone-building benefits? As the table on the next page reveals, the women in the AlgaeCal 2 group (who received the nutrients and dosages now used in AlgaeCal's AlgaeCal Plus® and Strontium Boost® supplements) were given twice as much vitamin D_3 (1,600 IU instead of the 800 IU in AlgaeCal 1) and vitamin K_2 in its MK-7 form rather than as MK-4. Also note that the dose of MK-7 (100 micrograms/day) is much lower than that of the MK-4 form (1.5 milligrams—the equivalent of 1,500 micrograms per day). As explained in our discussion of vitamin K (pages 172–199), the MK-7 form of K_2 is not only more effective, but does the job at a much lower dose than MK-4.

Upon completion of this initial study, a second study was done to look at the effects of three different versions of an AlgaeCal® bone-health supplement program.[305] In this study, 176 women over 40 years of age followed one of three different bone-health programs: Plan 1 used a bone-health supplement with vitamin D_3 (800 IU), AlgaeCal's plant-sourced form of calcium (720 mg), and vitamin K as MK-4 (1.5 mg) for one year. The other two Plans also used AlgaeCal's plant calcium, but in differing amounts (750 mg in Plan 2, 756 mg in Plan 3), and with differing amounts of vitamin D_3 (1,000 IU in Plan 2; 1,600 IU in Plan 3) and other bone health ingredients. Most importantly, vitamin K_2 was not used in Plan 2, but was included in Plan 3 as MK-7 (100 mcg). The table below lists the nutrients and dosage amounts provided in the three different plans.

COMPARISON OF THREE ALGAECAL
BONE-HEALTH SUPPLEMENT PLANS

INGREDIENT OR COMPONENT	PLAN 1	PLAN 2	PLAN 3
Strontium Citrate (mg)	680	No	680
Trace Minerals in AlgaeCal (mg)	1,608	1,682	1,688
Plant-sourced Calcium (mg)	720	750	756
Magnesium (mg)*	72	65	350
Vitamin D-3 (IUs of Cholecalciferol)	800	1,000	1,600
Vitamin K-2 as MK-4 (mg)	1.5	0	0
Vitamin K-7 as MK-7 (mcg)	0	0	100
Boron (mg)	0	0	3
Vitamin C (mg)	0	0	50

Table adapted from Kaats GR, et al. A comparative effectiveness study of bone density changes in women over 40 following three bone health plans containing variations of the same novel plant-sourced calcium.Int J Med Sci. 2011 Mar 2;8(3):180-91. PMID: 21448303.

Study participants in Plans 1 and 3 were also given a "health literacy booklet" containing information that could be used to choose better quality, low glycemic foods and a pedometer-based physical activity program.[306]

Using self-reports of adherence, subjects were categorized as "compliant" (if they regularly followed the bone-building program) or "partially compliant." Comparisons were also made between the three treatment groups and two theoretical groups: a non-intervention "control" group (no supplements), for which the

---

* 72mg + naturally occurring magnesium carbonate.

statistics were derived from the results of numerous previously conducted studies published in the peer-reviewed medical literature, and a group of calcium supplement users (e.g., calcium carbonate, calcium citrate) whose outcomes were derived from looking at the results of previously published studies using non-plant sources of calcium. Results for all subjects were shown as the percent their BMD changed after a year from baseline.

To really put what happened into perspective, you should know that a wealth of prior research has shown that just taking calcium and vitamin D does *not* increase BMD—this combination alone only slows down bone loss.

Calcium and Vitamin D₃ Slow Bone Loss, but Do Not Increase BMD

Much of the evidence supporting the value of calcium supplementation for preventing osteoporotic fractures has been summarized in an exhaustive meta-analysis of randomized trials involving 63,897 subjects 50 years of age and older, most of whom were healthy postmenopausal women with an average age of 67.8 years.[307] This meta-analysis includes 23 trials, involving 41,419 subjects, in which changes in BMD were measured. None of these studies show that calcium supplementation increased BMD over the study period. Although in the 17 trials, involving 52,625 women, that reported fracture as an outcome, supplementation was associated with a 12% risk reduction in all types of fractures, still the overall finding was that—with or without vitamin D₃—calcium supplementation was only associated with a "reduced rate of bone loss." *A yearly age-related decline of -0.1% in BMD is what is expected when taking only vitamin D$_3$ and non-plant sources of calcium.*

Algae-Derived Calcium Increases BMD

All three AlgaeCal® Plans tested produced *increases* in BMD—a marked improvement over just slowing the rate of age-related bone loss! In all three treatment groups, study participants with above average compliance had significantly greater increases in BMD compared to the losses seen in the two expected-change reference groups. Women in the Plan 3 group, the group receiving the most nutritionally comprehensive supplement program, gained significantly more BMD than the other two groups. Subjects in all three plans had an increase in BMD: Plan 1 = +1.20%, Plan 2 = + 0.33%, and Plan 3 = +2.5%! Again, no adverse effects were reported nor were any seen in the comprehensive blood chemistry tests run on study participants.

Why is AlgaeCal® a More Effective and Safer Form of Calcium for Building Bone?

In contrast to calcium supplements extracted from rock (calcium carbonate, which is derived from limestone or marble, or calcium citrate, in which citrate is combined with calcium that has been extracted from rock), AlgaeCal® is produced by milling a marine plant called *algus calcareus*. This sea-algae draws not only calcium, but 70 other minerals from the water in which it grows, metabolizing them into bioactive form for its own use, similar to the way in which vegetables and fruits absorb and utilize minerals from the soil.

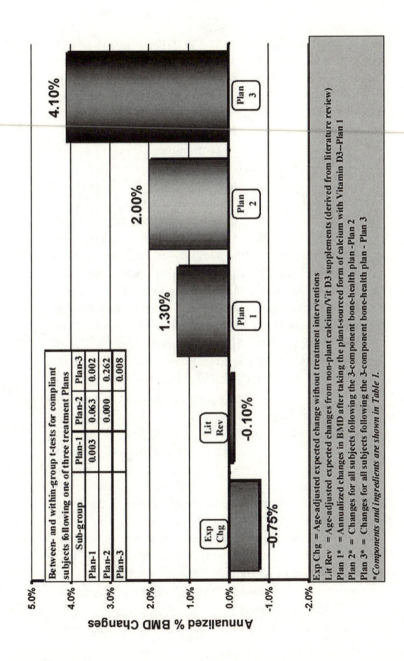

Exp Chg = Age-adjusted expected change without treatment interventions
Lit Rev = Age-adjusted expected changes from non-plant calcium/Vit D3 supplements (derived from literature review)
Plan 1* = Annualized changes in BMD after taking the plant-sourced form of calcium with Vitamin D3—Plan 1
Plan 2* = Changes for all subjects following the 3-component bone-health plan - Plan 2
Plan 3* = Changes for all subjects following the 3-component bone-health plan - Plan 3
*Components and ingredients are shown in Table 1.

Between- and within-group t-tests for compliant subjects following one of three treatment Plans

Sub-group	Plan-1	Plan-2	Plan-3
Plan-1	0.003	0.063	0.002
Plan-2		0.000	0.262
Plan-3			0.008

Annualized % BMD Changes

-0.75%
-0.10%
1.30%
2.00%
4.10%

Organic certification attests to both the purity and the sustainability of this algae.

It has long been recognized that a plant-rich diet helps maintain a bone-healthy calcium balance, not only because it results in a more alkaline body chemistry (remember, acidic body chemistry results in calcium being withdrawn from bone to restore a more alkaline pH), but also because numerous other essential bone nutrients are present in high-calcium plant foods. Calcium from plant sources was found to be highly protective against osteoporosis in postmenopausal women in the Korean National Health and Nutrition Examination survey. Koreans, who typically consume very little milk, cheese or other dairy foods, but large amounts of dark green vegetables (like collards, spinach, mustard leaves, broccoli, and cabbage), get their calcium from plant foods. Korean women eating the most calcium-rich plant foods had the highest BMD.[308] *Algus calcereus* is so-named because this sea plant is exceptionally rich in calcium.[309]

Furthermore, dietary components act in concert, which translates to the sum of their effect being greater than that of the parts.[310] This "law of Nature" explains numerous instances in the research where a single nutrient, given at high doses, has produced mixed results. A perfect example of this is vitamin E. In all the studies looking at dietary consumption of vitamin E, this nutrient has consistently been shown to exert significant cardioprotective effects, but in research using supplemental vitamin E (virtually always in the form of just one of the 8 constituents of the vitamin E family called α-tocopherol), outcomes range from positive to indifferent to negative.

The reason for this is that vitamin E-rich foods contain much more than just α-tocopherol! As found naturally in foods, vitamin E is a family of eight structurally unique compounds (four tocopherols: α-, β-, γ-, δ- tocopherol and four tocotrienols: α-, β-, γ-, δ-tocotrienol), each of which has unique as well as complimentary biological actions. And γ-, not α-tocopherol, is the form of vitamin E found in the highest levels in foods rich in this nutrient. For this reason, supplemental vitamin E should always be taken in its whole form, which will appear on the label as "mixed tocopherols and tocotrienols."[311] In addition, vitamin E-rich foods (e.g., almonds, spinach, Swiss chard, whole wheat) contain a bunch of other heart-healthy nutrients, including magnesium, zinc, copper, and B vitamins. Vitamin E-rich leafy greens also serve up vitamin K_1, vitamin C, and too many other beneficial nutrients to list here. The situation with calcium supplements is completely analogous!

Supplements that contain calcium derived from rock deliver calcium. *Algus calcareus* is a nutrient-dense, calcium-rich plant, so AlgaeCal® delivers not just calcium, but calcium in a balanced matrix of naturally present bone-supportive phytonutrients, magnesium and trace minerals, including boron, zinc, manganese, copper, silica, and strontium. AlgaeCal Plus® also contains vitamin D_3 *and* vitamin K_2 (in its most effective MK-7 form), and in amounts demonstrated in the published research to be effective. These inclusions, particularly of vitamin K_2, are quite important. Here's why:

Much press has been given recently to two studies suggesting that calcium supplements, taken with or without vitamin D, may increase risk for heart attack.[312] Supplementation with calcium and vitamin D has also been suggested to increase risk of kidney stones.[313] Both of these highly undesirable outcomes are signs that the body is not utilizing calcium appropriately. And both are explained by the fact that calcium absorption, which is increased by vitamin D, *must* be balanced by vitamin K, the nutrient required to activate the proteins that put calcium into bone and keep it out of arteries, kidneys, and breasts. Lara has summarized the research discussing this relationship among calcium, vitamin D_3, and vitamin K_2 in two medical journal articles published in *Longevity Medicine Review*, the first citing 193 PubMed studies and entitled, "Vitamin D and Vitamin K Team Up to Lower Cardiovascular Disease Risk," and the second, a review of the latest research on vitamin K_2 covering 84 more studies, entitled "Vitamin K_2: Optimal Levels Essential for the Prevention of Age-Associated Chronic Disease."[314] AlgaeCal® delivers calcium in a balanced matrix along with not just vitamin D_3, but the vitamin K_2 necessary for calcium's beneficial use in your body.

After coming across AlgaeCal's studies in the course of my normal scanning of the research related to bone health, I, Lara, decided to give AlgaeCal® a try and began using AlgaeCal Plus® in July 2011. In May 2012, I had my annual DXA run at the same medical office where my 2011 DXA had been done and using the same Hologic machine, since using the same brand of machine gives more reliable results.

On the next page is a graph showing the changes in my DXA and my progress back to healthy bones since my big drop in bone density during the years from 1998 to 2002. My BMD drops significantly from 1998 to 2002, then levels out (this was when we figured out that I need lots more vitamin D than the average person), then starts to slowly, but consistently climb back up beginning in 2003 as I learned about other essential bone nutrients, e.g., vitamin K_2 in its form as MK-7.

LARA'S DXA RESULTS 1998 THROUGH 2012

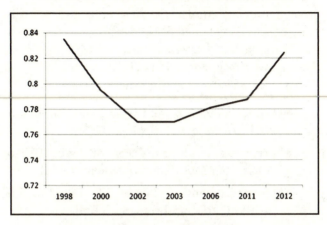

In June 2011, I began taking AlgaeCal®, and the effect, as illustrated by the graph line, has been dramatic. Since the only thing that changed in my personal bone-building program from 2011 through 2012 was switching to AlgaeCal Plus® as my calcium supplement (I had been taking another strontium citrate product for more than a year), I believe that sea-algae derived calcium has been a significant contributing factor to my dramatic improvement.

I, Lara, have been doing a lot of thinking about why the AlgaeCal Plus® product has been more effective for me than taking all these same nutrients via a number of other supplements. I think it may be because AlgaeCal® is supplying calcium in the matrix of all the other minerals the sea-algae used to build itself. Thus, AlgaeCal Plus® contains a number of trace minerals we may not be getting elsewhere that might be just the missing link our bones need to really get with it and build. We know from studying human physiology—and from countless studies—that nutrients work as a team in the human body, and the effects are often synergistic. Perhaps some trace mineral provided in AlgaeCal Plus® enhanced its calcium's effect on my bones' BMD? I expect more research will be conducted to determine precisely what's going on here; if I win the lottery, I'll fund it!*

Lara has improved significantly in all areas:

- Whole body BMD went from T score of -0.4 in 2011 to a T score of -0.2 in 2012

- Hip/femur went from T score of -1.7 in 2011 to -1.5 in 2012 (a 3.2% improvement in BMD)

- Spine went from T score of -1.9 in 2011 to -1.5 in 2012 (a 6% improvement in BMD)

- Bottom line: Lara is still slightly osteopenic, but is clearly, very rapidly rebuilding bone.

Safety Issues

Consuming more than 3,000 milligrams of calcium per day could result in elevated blood levels of calcium, a condition called *hypercalcemia*. If blood levels of phosphorus are low when calcium levels are high, or if insufficient vitamin K_2 is available,† hypercalcemia can lead to calcification of soft tissues, including the arteries, heart, breasts, and kidneys. The Tolerable Upper Intake Level (UL) set for calcium, by the National Academy of Sciences in 1997, is 2,500 milligrams per day.

---

* In addition to using AlgaeCal Plus® and Strontium Boost®, Lara has written blogs reporting the breaking research related to all aspects of bone health, which are posted on AlgaeCal's website. Dr. Wright has no connection with AlgaeCal®.

† See "Vitamin K," page 172; also page 219.

BORON

What It Does

Boron has been shown in numerous studies to have beneficial effects on bone architecture and strength.[315] Boron is a "trace mineral" meaning our bodies need just a trace to function properly; in boron's case, this is just 3–5 milligrams a day. But our bones really need that little bit because boron is required for the conversion of estrogen into its most active form, 17-beta-estradiol, and this is the form in which estrogen increases our bones' absorption of magnesium. Another key mineral in our bones, magnesium,* along with calcium and phosphorus, forms the crystal lattice structure of our bones.

Boron is also necessary for the reaction that occurs in the kidneys in which vitamin D is converted into its most active form [$1,25(OH)_2D_3$]. Estrogen increases the activity of our bone-building cells, the osteoblasts, and vitamin D is necessary for calcium absorption.[316]

When the US Department of Agriculture conducted an experiment in which postmenopausal women took 3 mg of boron a day, boron reduced the women's excretion of calcium by 44%, and also resulted in the activation of the bone-building forms of estrogen and vitamin D.[317]

What to Look for in a Supplement

Boron is one of the micronutrients your bones need for which a supplement is your best option. Although present in some foods, including raisins, hazelnuts, almonds, dried apricots, avocado, dates, peanuts, prunes, and walnuts, the amount of boron, even in

---

* See "Magnesium," page 224.

these foods in which this trace mineral is most concentrated, is really small. Raisins are the richest food
source of boron, and you'd have to eat 3 ounces of
raisins (185 calories worth) to gain 4.5 mg of boron.
Three ounces (6 tablespoons, which deliver 570 calories and 48 grams of fat) of peanut butter will give you
less than 2 milligrams of boron. Eat this amount of
peanut butter every day and you can forget zipping up
your jeans. Supplementation is obviously a more practical and less "weighty" means of receiving the daily
3–5 mg of boron you need for optimal bone health.

Safety Issues

None. Elemental boron and borates are nontoxic to
humans, animals, or fish. The *LD50* (which is the dose
of a compound high enough to kill 50% of animals
tested) is about 6 grams per kilogram of body weight.
Substances whose LD50 is greater than 2 grams are
considered nontoxic. In humans, intake of 4 grams
per day was reported to cause no incidents, and medical dosages of 20 grams of boric acid have caused no
problems. The Tolerable Upper Intake Level (UL), the
maximum dose at which no harmful effects would be
expected, is 20 mg per day for adults and pregnant or
breastfeeding women over 19 years of age.[318]

MAGNESIUM

What It Does

Magnesium is classified as a "macro-mineral" because
it plays so many roles in our bodies that we need several hundred milligrams every day. Magnesium activates
more than 350 enzymes, is involved in the production

of ATP (the energy currency of the body), and serves as a key compound in the crystal latticework matrix that gives structure to our bones. One of the enzymes activated by magnesium is involved in the conversion of vitamin D into its most active form—the form in which vitamin D greatly increases our ability to absorb calcium.

About two-thirds of the magnesium in our bodies goes into our bones, which serve as the body's bank account for magnesium, just as they do for calcium. When we are under stress—a not uncommon occurrence in our modern, excessively busy lives—our bodies use up magnesium at a very rapid clip.[319] Our hectic, stressful lives may translate into a need for more magnesium than the Adequate Intake (AI) recommended in 1997 by the Institute of Medicine at the National Academy of Sciences, which was a daily 360 milligrams for women or 400 milligrams for men. Among women in the US, the average dietary intake of magnesium is only 68% of this possibly insufficient AI, which means that a very large proportion of American women are deficient in magnesium.[320]

The Latest Research Indicates that 48% to 60% of Americans Do Not Consume Sufficient Magnesium![321]

Why? Magnesium is concentrated in foods many Americans don't eat very often, such as leafy greens, pumpkin seeds, beans, and fish. Happily, chocolate is also a decent source of magnesium (as if you needed another reason for a daily dose of chocolate; now you can say it's medicinal). Those chocolate cravings, particularly in premenopausal women, are a sign you need more magnesium. Estrogen levels build during a woman's monthly cycle, and estrogen pulls magnesium into our bones, lowering

FOODS RICH IN MAGNESIUM[322]

FOOD	SERVING SIZE	MAGNESIUM (IN MILLIGRAMS)
Pumpkin seeds	1/4 cup	185 mg
Spinach, steamed	1 cup	157 mg
Soybeans	1 cup	148 mg
Swiss chard, steamed	1 cup	150 mg
Halibut	4 oz	121 mg
Salmon, Chinook	4 oz.	138 mg
Navy beans	1 cup	107 mg
Almonds	1/4 cup	99 mg
Pinto beans	1 cup	94 mg
Cashews	1/4 cup	89 mg
Scallops	4 oz	77 mg
Tuna, yellowfin	4 oz	73 mg
Flaxseeds	2 tablespoons	70 mg
Summer squash	1 cup	43 mg
Beets, cooked	1 cup	39 mg
Broccoli, steamed	1 cup	39 mg
Brussels sprouts	1 cup	31 mg
Green beans	1 cup	31 mg
Banana	1 medium	29 mg
Whole wheat bread	1 slice	28 mg
Kiwi fruit	1	22 mg
Tomato, ripe	1 cup	20 mg

levels elsewhere throughout our bodies.[323] Those of us who are postmenopausal chocoholics can blame it on stress, which causes magnesium to be lost in urine.

Since, as noted above, magnesium is the mineral cofactor required to activate more than 350 enzymes, it's easy to see why the research is now discussing many ways in which suboptimal magnesium intake directly contributes not only to osteoporosis, but to a long list of other chronic degenerative diseases including type 2 diabetes, metabolic syndrome, elevated C-reactive protein (a marker of inflammation in our blood vessels), hypertension, atherosclerotic vascular disease, sudden cardiac death, migraine headache, asthma, colon cancer, and premature aging.[324] Restless leg syndrome and muscle spasms in the calves and feet may indicate magnesium insufficiency.[325] A key reason for muscle cramping during or after strenuous exercise is that magnesium is lost in sweat. (The perfect reason to have that piece of dark chocolate after your workout.)

Surveys conducted over the last 30 years show adults in the US are consuming increasingly more calcium in comparison to magnesium both in the foods we eat and from supplements, which typically provide at least twice as much calcium as magnesium. Just during the years from 1994 to 2001, the ratio of calcium-to-magnesium consumed in food rose from less than 3.0 to more than 3.0, with the result that at least half the US population has chronic latent magnesium deficiency, but our magnesium status is rarely checked or the test run is inappropriate, so we are assumed to be healthy.[326]

Are YOU Low in Magnesium?

If you are interested in checking to see if YOU are low in magnesium, the best test to assess your magnesium status is the Buccal Smear Intracellular Magnesium; the next best test available is the RBC (Red Blood Cell) Magnesium. In the Buccal Smear test, epithelial cells will be swabbed from the inside lining of the cheek and then evaluated via ionic magnesium measurement or elemental x-ray analysis. The RBC test involves a blood draw. Either of these tests provides a much better indication of the body's magnesium levels than the standard test, which checks magnesium levels in serum.

Here's why.

Blood is made up of a fluid portion (serum) and cells (including red and white blood cells). The test most doctors run checks serum levels of magnesium, but a serum test gives a very inaccurate appraisal of your actual magnesium status because only about 1% of your body's magnesium is stored in serum; the remaining 99% is found inside your cells where it does its work. Thus a normal blood serum magnesium does not necessarily mean you are not magnesium deficient.

Also because keeping magnesium levels up in the blood is so essential to survival, the amount of magnesium in serum is very tightly regulated by the body. (Actually, the way the body ensures that we have enough magnesium in serum by withdrawing it from our cells is similar to the way we withdraw calcium from our bones when our calcium intake is too low to maintain adequate blood levels.) You can have apparently adequate levels in serum, but be seriously deficient inside your cells. Only very severe cases of magnesium deficiency will show up in blood serum.

In contrast, the Buccal Smear test will show you how much magnesium was inside your cells working for you when the sample was taken. Cells that contain a nucleus and are metabolically active, such as the cells that make up soft tissue like the epithelial lining of the inside of your cheek from which the Buccal Smear is taken, give the most accurate reflection of your functional magnesium status. For this reason, a white blood cell (WBC) magnesium test is more accurate than the RBC magnesium because white blood cells, unlike red blood cells, have a nucleus and are metabolically active. Unfortunately, the WBC magnesium is quite complicated to run, so very few labs perform it. While red blood cells do not contain a nucleus, RBC testing will still provide a much better indication of the average amount of magnesium that has been present in nucleated cells over the prior four months than serum testing.

You will need to ask your doctor to order Buccal Smear testing[327] as this is not yet provided by direct-to-consumer labs. You can order a Red Blood Cell magnesium test directly from a number of on-line labs.[328]

Magnesium Insufficiency Promotes Bone Loss

When our magnesium levels drop too low, so do our blood levels of the most active form of vitamin D $[1,25(OH)_2D_3]$, which plays a key role in our ability to absorb calcium.[329] In addition, an increase occurs in a compound called "skeletal substance P," which promotes inflammation and bone breakdown.[330]

Magnesium is also necessary for regulating the secretion of parathyroid hormone and calcitonin—the two hormones responsible for maintaining the proper concentration of calcium within our bloodstream. When calcium levels are too low, parathyroid hormone stimulates osteoclasts to break down bone, thus increasing blood calcium levels. When calcium levels are too high, calcitonin suppresses the activity of osteoclasts, the cells that break down bone.

Thus, not having enough magnesium on board translates into impaired ability to absorb calcium and regulate its levels in the bloodstream, which leads to an increase in bone loss, plus a reduction in our body's ability to form new bone. Not surprisingly, women with osteoporosis have been shown to have a lower level of magnesium in their bones and to have other indications of magnesium deficiency compared to people without osteoporosis.[331]

And last, but certainly not least, magnesium deficiency triggers calcium-activated inflammatory cascades inside our cells that would normally only be activated in response to injury or pathogens. By now, you probably recognize why this is bad for our bones: chronic inflammation, regardless of its cause, activates osteoclasts.

In contrast, getting adequate magnesium from food and supplements has clearly been associated with higher bone mineral density in older men and women. A study involving 2,038 men and women (aged 70–79 years) revealed a direct correlation between higher whole body BMD and magnesium intake.[332]

Researchers are now saying it is imperative that we update the recommended daily requirements for magnesium, and that understanding how low magnesium status and rising calcium-to-magnesium ratios are contributing to the rising incidence of not only osteoporosis, but type 2 diabetes, metabolic syndrome, cardiovascular diseases, cancer, and other inflammation-related disorders is a research priority. Don't wait until they figure it out. Just be sure now that YOUR magnesium status is adequate.

Vitamin D Supplementation May Increase Your Needs for Magnesium

A final consideration—supplementing with vitamin D may increase your magnesium needs. Calcium and magnesium counterbalance one another in numerous cellular activities. If you are taking vitamin D, you will be absorbing more calcium, so you will also need more magnesium to maintain the balance between these minerals, both of which are vitally important for your overall health as well as that of your bones.

Symptoms of magnesium insufficiency include migraines and tension headaches, muscle weakness, leg cramps, restless legs, elevated blood pressure, transient ischemic attacks, and arrhythmia. If you are going to regularly be taking more than 2,000 IU/day of vitamin D, an amount that the latest research shows most of us need to maintain healthy blood levels of this vitamin, then you should consider supplementing with magnesium.

What to Look for in a Supplement

For the same reasons that choosing a supplement providing calcium in a chelated form is recommended above,* a chelated form of magnesium will serve you best. Look for products containing magnesium citrate, magnesium malate, or magnesium aspartate. Take 250 milligrams, twice daily.

In the unlikely event that you develop loose stools from supplementing with magnesium, try taking 25 milligrams of *pyridoxal-5-phosphate* (P5P) along with the magnesium. P5P is the activated form of vitamin B_6 and is responsible for ferrying magnesium inside your cells. In some people, the enzyme that converts B_6 into P5P is underactive, either because of their genetic inheritance or because they are lacking in riboflavin, which is also involved in this conversion. In either case, this can result in difficulty absorbing magnesium, which can be remedied by taking P5P.[333]

---

* See "Chelated Calcium," page 208.

Safety Issues

Intake of high levels of supplemental magnesium may cause diarrhea. This symptom has been noted in research studies in which doses of magnesium ranged from 1–5 grams (1,000–5,000 milligrams) but, as noted above, diarrhea can occur at lower supplemental doses.

If this happens, it may be due to impaired conversion of vitamin B_6 to its active form, P5P, which is responsible for bringing magnesium inside our cells. Supplying P5P by taking a P5P supplement providing 25 milligrams may greatly improve the body's ability to absorb magnesium. The upper tolerable limit set for supplemental magnesium by the National Academy of Sciences in 1997 is 350 milligrams per day for individuals 9 years or older.

ZINC

What It Does

Zinc is a trace mineral that is an essential micronutrient required for many cellular processes, especially in the cells that make up our immune system. Zinc signaling is necessary for immune cell activation, so a deficiency of zinc significantly impairs the function of both arms of our immune system—our innate and adaptive immune responses.*

---

* The innate immune system is the body's first line of defense against infection by other organisms. It is comprised of cells that recognize and respond to pathogens in a generic way, unlike the adaptive immune system, which creates an immunological memory of a specific pathogen after the first encounter and then can quickly mobilize cells targeted to formerly seen pathogens, thus giving us long-lasting protective immunity.

   The cells of our innate immune response include a variety of white cells (mast cells, phagocytes macrophages, neutrophils, dendritic cells, basophils, eosinophils, and natural killer cells) that identify potential threats,

Why is this a problem for our bones? Poor immune function results in systemic (all over the body) low grade inflammation. In addition, zinc is involved in our cells' ability to respond to insulin, a hormone that moves sugar from the bloodstream into our cells. Without enough zinc around, our cells respond less well to insulin, so sugar remains in the bloodstream where it causes bones' arch enemy: chronic inflammation. For these and many other reasons, zinc insufficiency is associated with the development of many chronic diseases, not just osteoporosis.[334]

In addition to causing inflammation, which turns on osteoclasts, zinc deficiency delivers a double whammy on our bones by also hindering our production of osteoblasts. How does zinc insufficiency result in suppression of osteoblasts' production and activity? The production of osteoblasts from their precursor cells is a process that is dependent on the activity of a major cellular DNA transcription factor called Cbfa-1/Runx-2 (for the technically inclined, "core-binding factor-1/runt-related transcription factor-2"). Who comes up with these names? Fortunately, we don't have to remember this one—the point here is that zinc is required to activate Cbfa-1/Runx-2, so not enough zinc means Cbfa-1/Runx-2 does not get

---

act as a chemical barrier to infectious agents, recruit other immune cells to sites of infection, and activate the adaptive immune system through a process called antigen presentation.

The adaptive immune system is composed of highly specialized cells, e.g., T and B lymphocytes, which recognize specific pathogens and mount stronger attacks each time the pathogen is encountered. [As discussed on pages 52–66, the RANKL inhibitor denosumab (trade names, Prolia®, Xgeva®) interferes with the development of T and B cells as well as osteoclasts.]

FOODS RICH IN ZINC:

FOOD	SERVING SIZE	MILLIGRAMS OF ZINC (PER SERVING)
Oysters, steamed Wild Eastern	3 ounces	154.0
Alaska King Crab	3 ounces	7.6
Flounder or sole	3 ounces	0.5
Veal liver, steamed or fried*	3 ounces	12
Roast beef (shoulder, shank, chuck)*	3 ounces	10
Lamb*	3 ounces	4.2–8.7 (depending on the cut)
Sesame butter (tahini)	3 ounces	10
Hummus (chickpea & tahini)	3 ounces	4.6
Whole sesame seeds	3 ounces	7.8
Roasted pumpkin seeds	3 ounces	10
Unsweetened baking chocolate	3 ounces	9.6
Cocoa powder	1 tablespoon	0.3
Milk chocolate	3 ounces	2.3
Toasted wheat germ	1 tablespoon	1.2
Peanuts, chopped	1 cup	8.8
Peanuts, dry roasted	1 ounce	1.0
Cashews, dry roasted	1 ounce	1.6
Almonds, dry roasted	1 ounce	1
Cheddar cheese	1 ounce	0.9
Mozzarella	1 ounce	0.8

* Be sure to buy only meat from grass fed animals. Meats from animals fed corn or grains are high in pro-inflammatory omega-6 fatty acids. Inflammation promotes bone loss.

FOOD	SERVING SIZE	MILLIGRAMS OF ZINC (PER SERVING)
Kidney beans	1 cup	1.9
Green peas	½ cup	1.5
Mushrooms, button & crimini	3 ounces	1.8

switched on, and does not stimulate osteoblast prolif-eration and differentiation.[335]

National surveys indicate that many older individu-als do not consume enough zinc, and a decline in zinc levels is very often observed with age.

If you have white spots on your fingernails, you need zinc; but even if you don't, you still may need zinc! One easy way to add zinc to your bone-building diet is to snack on pumpkin seeds or sprinkle a handful over your leafy green salad. You can eat them unroasted (more total nutrients) or roasted (some like the taste better). It is best to roast pumpkin seeds yourself as this is less expensive, and you can control the oven temperature (too high damages the healthy fats in pumpkin seeds) and not add lots of oil or salt. Toss a cup of raw (organic) pumpkin seeds with one table-spoon of organic olive oil, spread on a cookie sheet, and bake at 250 degrees for 20–30 minutes. You can add a teaspoon of wheat-free organic tamari sauce to the olive oil if you like a more salty flavor.

How Much Zinc Do YOU Need?

The current public health recommendations for zinc—the Recommended Dietary Allowances set in 1999 by the Institute of Medicine at the National Academy of Sciences—are:

- Females 19 years and older: 8 milligrams
- Pregnant females 18 years or younger: 12 milligrams
- Pregnant females 19 years and older: 11 milligrams
- Lactating females 18 years or younger: 13 milligrams
- Lactating females 19 years and older: 12 milligrams
- Males 14 years and older: 11 milligrams

These recommendations don't take into consideration that many of us don't absorb zinc as well when we're older. Hypochlorhydria (low stomach acid) and "hidden" gluten sensitivity (an inflammatory reaction to gluten, much less noticeably severe than full blown celiac disease, but an adverse reaction that causes chronic systemic low grade inflammation) are both strongly associated with osteoporosis.

By the time we're 60, approximately 50% of us have varying degrees of hypochlorhydria, which is often associated with subnormal digestion and absorption of zinc, calcium, magnesium, and many other minerals. A "hidden" sensitivity to gluten—a protein present not only in products that contain wheat, but spelt, emmer, faro, oats, and rye, as well—is often discovered in individuals with early-onset osteoporosis, because gluten sensitivity also interferes with the absorption of a wide range of minerals and other nutrients. Especially if you're in the "osteopenia" stage, please check with a physician skilled and knowledgeable in natural and nutritional medicine for a recommendation about how much zinc you personally need.

Safety Issues

With zinc, you can get too much of a good thing. Zinc toxicity has been reported in the medical literature, so in 2000, the National Academy of Sciences set a tolerable upper limit (UL) of 40 milligrams/day of zinc for individuals aged 19 years and older. While some experts agree with this upper limit, others point out that some of us—especially men, who get osteoporosis, too, but usually a decade or so later—may need more, especially men with prostate problems. Once again, it's best to check with a physician skilled and knowledgeable in natural and nutritional medicine for a personal recommendation.

Signs you are consuming too much zinc include: a metallic, bitter taste in your mouth, stomach pain, nausea, vomiting, cramps, and diarrhea. Although in Dr. Wright's more than 30 years of medical practice, during which he has treated thousands of patients and spoken at medical conferences around the world, he has never seen or heard of any of these symptoms from anyone taking zinc.

Zinc consumed in amounts greater than 40 mg per day can impact the body's use of other nutrients, including calcium and copper, but only if foods or supplements supplying adequate amounts of these nutrients are not included in your bone-building regimen. As you can see from the "Foods Rich in Zinc" table following, unless Wild Eastern oysters are a standard item in your diet, you are not at great risk of consuming too much zinc from food. Do take a look at your supplements, however, to be sure you are not getting more zinc than is desirable.

Zinc's "Special Relationship" with Copper

Zinc supplements taken in higher quantities or for months to years can actually lead to a copper deficiency! (And copper under the same circumstances can cause a zinc deficiency, but many fewer individuals take copper as a single supplement.) When there's too much zinc and not enough copper, the total cholesterol can go up, the HDL ("good") cholesterol, can go down, and the heart can even skip beats. (Fortunately, this potential effect from excessive amounts of zinc has never been reported as fatal!) Although there's not been controlled research about the best "balance" between supplemental zinc and supplemental copper, most physicians skilled and knowledgeable in nutritional and natural medicine recommend a 15:1 zinc/copper ratio.

What to Look for in a Supplement

Both zinc oxide, one of the most commonly sold zinc supplements in the United States, and zinc carbonate are insoluble and poorly absorbed.[336]

Research conducted in 1987 found that zinc picolinate was better absorbed than zinc gluconate or zinc citrate.[337] According to Dr. Joe Pizzorno,* one of the authors of the research paper cited here, the reason for zinc picolinate's greater absorption is that our bodies secrete picolinate (which is metabolized from the essential amino acid tryptophan) specifically for its use in enhancing the absorption of zinc from foods, not just into the bloodstream, but into cells. Thus, zinc picolinate is the form in which our bodies preferentially absorb and utilize zinc.

---

* Yes, Dr. Pizzorno is Lara's husband.

Zinc picolinate has since been shown to be significantly better absorbed than other forms when used in the treatment of individuals with alcoholism, to be effective in treating patients with taste deficiency disorders (loss of taste is one of the symptoms of zinc deficiency), to be an effective treatment for acne vulgaris when applied to the skin in a gel, and to significantly improve levels of superoxide dismutase, a potent anti-inflammatory antioxidant, in the lung tissue of patients with chronic obstructive pulmonary disease (COPD).[338]

Given this research and the fact that picolinate is produced by our bodies to assist in zinc absorption and its use by cells, zinc picolinate is recommended. However, one small study (involving 12 young women) that compared four zinc complexes (oxide, picolinate, gluconate, and glycinate) for acute uptake (within 4 hours) into the bloodstream, found zinc glycinate had the best acute uptake.[339]

STRONTIUM

What It Does

In just the last five years, more than 500 articles have been published in the peer-reviewed medical literature on the bone-building effects of strontium. One of the most abundant minerals on earth, strontium is present in the soil, air, water, fish, and most plant foods, especially cabbage, beets, and Brazil nuts. Worldwide, humans' estimated daily intake of strontium is 1–5 milligrams per day.

Chemically similar to calcium, strontium is absorbed in comparable amounts. Once in bone, strontium beneficially affects both aspects of the bone remodeling process: it not only slows down the development of osteoclasts, thus lessening bone removal activity, but also enhances the development of osteoblasts, thus increasing bone-forming activity.

Since pure strontium is chemically unstable, it is found in Nature in the form of salts, such as strontium citrate, strontium chloride, strontium carbonate, strontium gluconate, or strontium lactate. Strontium ranelate, a recently created, new-to-nature patentable form, has been the subject of a number of large, double-blind, placebo-controlled trials (further discussed below), which have confirmed strontium's effectiveness in halting and reversing osteoporosis. Strontium ranelate combines strontium with a synthetic compound called ranelic acid, which is supposed to be very poorly absorbed. This patentable form of strontium is currently being marketed in Europe (trade name Protelos®) for the prevention and treatment of osteoporosis.

Strontium's ability to prevent early postmenopausal bone loss was evaluated in a 24-month double-blind placebo-controlled study of 160 postmenopausal women. All the women were given calcium (500 milligrams per day). Those who also received strontium ranelate (1 gram per day) increased their lumbar BMD by an average of 5.53% compared to the women who were given a placebo. After two years, bone mineral density in the femoral neck (the neck-shaped area near the top of the femur) had increased 2.46% and BMD in the hip had increased 3.21% in women given strontium ranelate compared to those given the placebo. Plus, strontium was as well tolerated as the placebo.[340]

Strontium was also shown to greatly benefit postmenopausal women who had already had a vertebral osteoporotic fracture. In a two-year, double-blind, placebo-controlled trial involving 353 Caucasian women, study participants were given either strontium ranelate (0.5, 1, or 2 grams per day) or a placebo. All the women also received a daily 500-milligram supplement of calcium along with an 800 IU vitamin D_3 supplement. At the end of the study, the yearly increase in lumbar BMD in the women given 2 grams of strontium ranelate was 7.3%. During the second year of treatment, the 2-gram dose was associated with a 44% reduction in the number of patients who experienced a new vertebral fracture. Treating postmenopausal women who already had osteoporosis with strontium ranelate (2 grams daily for two years) resulted in an increase in these women's lumbar BMD of about 3% each year.[341]

The largest, most significant study of strontium to date was a five-year study that began in 1996 and included two clinical trials evaluating strontium ranelate's effects on women with osteoporosis: (1) the spinal osteoporosis therapeutic intervention (SOTI) study, which had a study population of 1,649 patients (average age was 70 years) and looked at strontium's effects on the women's risk of vertebral fractures, and (2) the treatment of peripheral osteoporosis (TRO-POS) trial, which included 5,091 patients (average age was 77 years) and looked at strontium's effects on nonspinal fractures. Both studies were multinational, randomized, double-blind, placebo-controlled trials that included two parallel groups: women with osteoporosis who were given strontium ranelate (2 grams per day) compared to a second comparable group of women with osteoporosis receiving a placebo.

After three years of follow-up, the SOTI study revealed that strontium caused a 41% reduction in the women's risk of experiencing a vertebral fracture compared to the placebo. Even in the first year, the women's risk of a new vertebral fracture was reduced 49% in the strontium group compared to the placebo. Lumbar BMD increased 11.4% in the strontium group, but decreased 1.3% in the placebo group. And strontium caused no adverse side effects.[342]

The TROPOS study, which looked at the effect of strontium on nonvertebral fractures, showed a reduction in risk of 16% in all vertebral fractures and a 19% reduction in risk of major nonvertebral osteoporotic fractures. In a subgroup of women at high risk of fracture—women 74 years of age or older who had a low femoral neck bone mineral density score—treatment with strontium was associated with a 36% reduction in risk of hip fracture.[343]

Strontium was also studied in 1,431 postmenopausal women with *osteopenia* (accelerated bone loss, an early warning signal for developing osteoporosis). In women with lumbar spine osteopenia, strontium ranelate decreased the risk of vertebral fracture by 41% (by 59% in women who had not yet experienced a fracture and by 38% in women who had already had a fracture). In women with osteopenia at both the lumbar spine and the neck of the femur, strontium reduced fracture risk by 52%.[344]

Most recently, a review found strontium was able to reduce vertebral fracture risk in patients with osteopenia, and to reduce vertebral, nonvertebral, and hip fractures in patients with osteoporosis aged 74 years and older.[345] A study involving 325 postmenopausal women with osteoporosis in mainland China, Hong Kong, and Malaysia, also confirmed strontium's benefits. After one year of taking either 2 grams of strontium or a placebo daily, bone mineral density in the lumbar spine, femoral neck, and hip in the women receiving strontium increased by 3–5% compared to those given the placebo.[346]

One more reason not to take a bisphosphonate: when a woman stops taking these patent medicines, bone remodeling remains suppressed for *at least* 6 months, which blunts bones' ability to benefit from strontium. A study published March 2010 in the *Journal of Bone Mineral Research* evaluated 120 women with osteoporosis in the United Kingdom, 60 of whom had taken bisphosphonates, and 60 of whom had not. All 120 women received strontium, calcium, and vitamin D. After one year, bone mineral density went up 5.6% at the spine, 3.4% at the hip, and 4.0% at the heel in the women who had *not* taken a bisphosphonate. In contrast, the women who had been on a bisphosphonate had only 2.1% increase at the spine and no increase in BMD at the hip or heel. Researchers do not know how long it will take for normal remodeling to begin again in the bones of the women who had used a bisphosphonate.[347]

What to Look for in a Supplement

How much strontium should you use? Based on the current research, it looks like somewhere between 340 and 680 milligrams of elemental strontium works best. The smaller quantities will help prevent bone loss from occurring while the larger doses can help treat osteoporosis.

In the US and Canada, natural strontium is available as an individual supplement, but you can also gain the benefits of strontium combined with other bone-building nutrients. Working with a company called Progressive Laboratories,* Dr. Wright has developed a formula called Osteo-Mins AM® that combines strontium with other bone-building nutrients including zinc, copper, boron, silicon, manganese, selenium, and molybdenum. Osteo-Mins®† is available through natural food stores, compounding pharmacies, and the Tahoma Clinic Dispensary.

Safety Issues

Strontium improves bone mineral density and strengthens bone in a normal, healthy way. This mineral is so safe that it is the key ingredient in toothpastes for sensitive teeth, such as Sensodyne®, which includes 10% total strontium chloride hexahydrate by weight. Strontium reduces tooth sensitivity by forming a barrier over microscopic tubules in tooth dentin in which nerve endings have become exposed by gum recession.[348]

However, since the quantities of strontium used in the studies are larger than those we might normally consume in our food each day, researchers wanted to check to be sure long-term use of strontium would not cause any alterations in the newly formed bone crystals or any other negative side effects. A number of studies have now addressed these concerns.

Strontium has been shown to improve vertebral bone density and strength in rats without altering bone stiffness, indicating that the improvement occurred without causing abnormal bone crystals. In

---

* 800-527-9512, www.progressivelabs.com.

† Osteo-Mins AM® is meant to be used along with Osteo-Mins PM®, which contains calcium, magnesium, and Vitamin D$_3$.

monkeys, strontium both decreased bone resorption (loss) and increased bone synthesis. And in cell cultures, strontium not only increased the reproduction of bone-forming osteoblast cells, but also enhanced and increased the synthesis of collagen (the major protein in the bone matrix).[349] In patients with postmenopausal osteoporosis, data from two large, double-blind, placebo-controlled, multicenter trials of 5 years' duration, strontium greatly reduced risk of fractures without causing any adverse side effects other than a very occasional case of nausea or diarrhea. Data on patients who continued to receive strontium during an additional three-year extension of these trials indicates that strontium continued to provide protection against new vertebral and nonvertebral fractures for the eight years of therapy, improving bone mineral density at numerous sites, and increasing markers of bone formation while decreasing markers of bone resorption.[350]

The only precaution—a very important one—is to make sure you're taking more calcium than strontium: much older research in animals shows that if strontium intake exceeds calcium intake over a long period of time, the animals develop bone deformities. Also, you will surely be at less risk for potential side effects if you take a natural form of strontium rather than the patent medicine form, strontium ranelate.

Don't Let Misleading Scare Tactics Prevent You from Reaping the Bone-Building Benefits of Natural Forms of Strontium!

After the first edition of *Your Bones* came out, we received many questions about strontium. Is it really safe? Does it really improve bone and reduce our risk of fractures? Having reviewed the published research conducted on both natural strontium and the patent medicine, strontium ranelate, we can confidently assure you that natural forms of strontium can provide a safe and highly effective contribution to the health—both the density and the tensile quality—of your bones. Strontium ranelate also improves bone density and quality, but at the cost of increasing your risk for a variety of adverse side effects, including deep vein blood clots and DRESS syndrome.

What's being said to dissuade us from utilizing strontium? It has been asserted that:[351]

- Strontium has a long list of undesirable side effects, commonly ranging from nausea to skin irritation, and less often (fortunately), blood clots and fainting.

- Since strontium is denser than calcium, it is difficult to assess actual bone improvement in a DXA scan.

- Several studies conclude that strontium causes the outer cortical bone to become thicker, actually reducing tensile strength. This increases the risk of fractures.

- Strontium competes with calcium absorption.

When confronted with the facts in the research, however, these apparent threats to one's health when taking supplemental natural forms of strontium either simply do not hold up or are revealed to be no problem at all. Let's take a closer, research-based look at each of them.

Natural Forms of Strontium, When Consumed in Lesser Amounts than Calcium, Are Very Safe

The side effects attributed blanket-fashion to all available supplemental forms of strontium have been seen with strontium *ranelate*, but *not* with any natural form of strontium, such as strontium citrate.

The *only* negative effects seen with natural strontium occurred in 1 animal study conducted in 1994 and 1 human study conducted in 1996.

In the animal study, immature lab rats (whose bones were still developing) were deliberately given a low calcium diet and supplemented with high doses of strontium. Not surprisingly, since calcium is the major mineral found in normal bone, and these animals were calcium-deprived, the rats developed ricket-like bone deformities.[352]

The human study was conducted in Turkey in 1996.[353] Before complete data analysis, it looked like there was a higher incidence of bone malformations (i.e., rickets) in young children in areas of Turkey with very high strontium concentrations in the soil. However, when the question of whether the children had been breastfed was taken into account, the risk for rickets no longer differed between people living in high strontium areas compared to those with low strontium. Why? Because breast milk provides the calcium and protein that prevents excessive incorporation of strontium into bone. In other words, only when much more strontium is consumed than calcium do bone formation abnormalities, e.g., rickets, occur.

According to the Centers for Disease Control's Agency for Toxic Substances and Disease Registry, which published a 161-page report [354] on the health effects of natural forms of strontium, e.g., strontium citrate:

There is no direct evidence that strontium is toxic to humans, but there is suggestive epidemiological evidence that the oral toxicity observed at high doses in juvenile laboratory animals may pertain to humans under special circumstances *[here, they are referring to the 2 studies discussed immediately above, which is why their following sentence emphasizes the importance of adequate calcium, phosphorus, and vitamin D]*. At low exposure levels, ingestion of stable strontium poses no harm to organisms with access to adequate calcium, phosphorus, and vitamin D. At higher exposure levels, especially under conditions of inadequate calcium, phosphorus, and vitamin D, stable strontium will interfere with normal bone development, causing "strontium rickets" of variable severity.

Adverse Side Effects Are Seen ONLY with Strontium Ranelate—Natural Forms of Strontium, Such as Strontium Citrate, Are Safe

In contrast, following on the heels of data collected in a number of other studies,[355] the most recent research—a three year study conducted in France whose results were published in October 2011[356]—confirms that the *patented unnatural form of strontium, strontium ranelate* has a number of potential side effects, at least two of which are very serious: an increased risk for venous thromboembolism (VTE, deep vein blood clots) and DRESS syndrome.

Overall, the likelihood that you will be among the ones affected is argued to be small—although a review of the research on strontium ranelate published in 2005 states "Strontium [ranelate] caused a 50% increase in the risk of venous thromboembolism (including pulmonary embolism)." [357]

In the health information provided for medical professionals,[358] Servier, the pharmaceutical company with the patent on strontium ranelate (trade name Protelos®) states:

> In phase III studies, the annual incidence of venous thromboembolism (VTE) observed over 5 years was approximately 0.7%, with a relative risk of 1.4 (95% CI = [1.0 ; 2.0]) in strontium ranelate treated patients as compared to placebo.

What does this mean in plain English? Over a 5-year period in the Phase III studies, each year, 0.7% of those taking strontium ranelate developed VTE. Saying that those taking strontium ranelate had a relative risk for VTE of 1.4 compared to placebo means that strontium ranelate increased risk for VTE by 40%. In research dating back to the early 1909, strontium citrate has never been found to increase risk of VTE.[359]

The other serious side effect for which people taking strontium ranelate are at increased risk is DRESS syndrome. (Strontium citrate has never been found to increase risk of DRESS syndrome either.) Symptoms of DRESS syndrome typically begin 1–8 weeks after exposure to the offending patent medication. Classic symptoms include widespread rash, fever, and involvement of one or more internal organs. Approximately 50% of patients will have hepatitis (liver inflammation), 30% will have eosinophilia (high levels of white cells in the blood indicating immune system activation), 10% will have nephritis (inflamed kidneys), and 10% will have pneumonitis (inflamed lungs). DRESS syndrome is often severe and can result in death if not diagnosed early—thus the warnings to see your doctor immediately if you develop a rash after taking strontium ranelate.

In his excellent YouTube presentation on strontium,[360] Dr. Brunnel, discussing strontium ranelate, notes that "99–93% of the ranelic acid is excreted unchanged within a week." We have a question and a comment to make in regards to this. The question is, "What has happened to the up to 7% of ranelic acid that is *not* excreted from the body? What is it doing?" And the comment is that it is important to realize that just because something is excreted does not mean it did not do anything on its way through the body. Ranelic acid is a new-to-nature, never before seen by the human body, compound. Simply assuming it is inert and is not going to do anything inside the human body is questionable— and the side effects associated with the use of strontium ranelate suggest this assumption is incorrect.

The latest review of the evidence confirming strontium ranelate may produce potentially lethal adverse effects was recently published in *Prescrire International*, March 21, 2012. The title of this review: "Strontium ranelate: too many adverse effects: Do not use."[361]

Since VTE and DRESS syndrome are likely to result in death, why expose yourself to *any* increased risk for them when you can take strontium citrate, a natural, proven to be safe and effective form of strontium?

Strontium Citrate Is Not Only Safe, but Delivers an Important Added Benefit to Your Bones

While working my way through the last 30 years of research on strontium, I (Lara) mentioned to my husband, Dr. Joe Pizzorno, that I was looking into the safety and effectiveness of natural forms of strontium versus the patent medicine, strontium ranelate. His response was that the "citrate" form of natural strontium, specifically, should be the best.

The reason for this is that—unlike ranelic acid, a weird hydra-headed new-to-nature molecule—citrate actually helps make the body's pH more alkaline. This is very important because it helps prevent the low-grade metabolic acidosis—an overly acidic pH—that is caused by a diet too high in protein, is quite common in the US and Canada, and causes bone loss. In fact, this is such an important health issue that Joe recently wrote an article about it, which was published in the *British Journal of Nutrition* in April 2010.[362]

Data from US Third National Health and Nutrition Examination Survey (NHANES III) shows that the average American diet (i.e., the typical Western diet) is acid-producing and results in a state of chronic low-grade metabolic acidosis. This increases bone loss because an acid pH is a strong activator of osteoclasts, the cells that break down bone. In this case, the osteoclasts' activity is ramped up because when bone is broken down, calcium is released to restore a more alkaline pH. Taking strontium in its natural form of strontium citrate will help you maintain a more alkaline pH.

Strontium Produces Unreliable DXA Results

It is true that strontium affects DXA results. Strontium has a larger atomic number (Z=38) than calcium (Z=20). This causes the DXA BMD reading to be over-estimated. Here are the facts on this from the most recently published paper discussing this issue:

> If 1% of calcium atoms in hydroxyapatite are replaced by strontium, BMD measurements are increased by 10% although the net mass of bone mineral increases by only 0.5%. [363]

The key issue here, however, is "What is the *practical* importance of this for YOU?" What does this say about strontium's ability to help you maintain healthy bones and prevent fractures?

Bottom line: Strontium increases BMD. Well, what's wrong with that? Is the DXA still useful? Absolutely, an improvement in your DXA shows that you are responding positively to treatment with strontium, that your BMD is increasing, and your risk for fracture is decreasing.[364]

So, yes, BMD as measured by DXA will be over-estimated in people taking strontium, but what really matters here is that strontium treatment increases bone mass and reduces fracture risk. DXA is useful in that it shows whether you are responding (absorbing strontium well), and a better DXA score still correlates with lower risk for fractures.

Strontium Does NOT Increase Risk for Fractures— Quite the Opposite

Concerned women contacted me (Lara) after seeing the claim on the internet that "Several studies conclude that strontium causes the outer cortical bone to become thicker, actually reducing tensile strength. This increases the risk of fractures." Such assertions should be backed up with footnotes citing the studies noted, and they should be bona fide, peer-reviewed research papers accessible on PubMed.

When I looked at the website article in which this statement was made, I found no references had been provided to substantiate the claim, so I ran an exhaustive search on PubMed for these "several studies"—and could find nary a one. What I did find were papers showing the exact opposite.

In animal studies (discussed in the 161-page report on strontium by the Agency for Toxic Substances and Disease Registry cited above), strontium has been proven to improve BMD *without* altering bone stiffness. In fact, research analyzing the bones of animals fed strontium has shown that the bone crystal remains normal, and the flexibility is not lessened.[365]

Numerous papers reporting the results of the SOTI and TROPOS trials—large, multi-center human trials that together involved ~7,000 postmenopausal women (many of whom had already had an osteoporotic fracture when they began treatment with strontium)—show strontium greatly reduces risk of vertebral, femur and hip fractures in as little as 1 year. (There are way too many references to provide them all; but listed in this endnote are a few of the most significant papers.[366]) Other studies have produced similar results, but SOTI and TROPOS are the largest, and have been running the longest.

A key aspect of the SOTI (Spinal Osteoporosis Therapeutic Intervention) and TROPOS (Treatment of Peripheral Osteoporosis Study) trials was the advanced age of most of the subjects compared with many previous

osteoporosis trials: 23% of the combined study populations were aged 80 years or older at enrollment. In
women older than 80 years, strontium produced a 55%
reduction for vertebral fractures over the first year of
treatment and a 32% reduction over 3 years.

In the SOTI trial, which included 1,649 patients
whose average age was 70 years, at the end of the
first year, women taking strontium had a 49% lower
risk of a new radiographic (seen on x-ray) vertebral
fracture compared to women given a placebo. The
risk of a clinically symptomatic vertebral fracture
was 52% lower. After 3 years, the strontium group
had a 41% lower risk of a new radiographic fracture,
and the incidence of clinically symptomatic vertebral fractures was 38% lower. When the 4-year data
were reported, they showed a 33% reduction in radiographic vertebral fractures.

In the TROPOS study, an even larger trial with 5,091
patients whose average age was 77 years, strontium
produced a risk reduction of 16% in vertebral fractures
and a 19% reduction in risk of non-vertebral fractures
(e.g., hip, femur, wrist, ribs, etc.) In TROPOS, in the
subgroup of women at highest risk of fracture (women
74 years of age or older who had a low femoral neck
BMD score), strontium reduced the risk of hip fracture
36%. Over 3 years, the reduction in vertebral fracture
risk was 39% and was similar even for patients who
had already had a vertebral fracture when the study
began. The 5-year data showed a 24% reduction in vertebral fracture risk.

The most recent paper, published November 2011,
reports the results of *10 years of strontium use* in the postmenopausal osteoporotic women who, after participating

in the SOTI and TROPOS studies for 5 years, were invited to enter a 5-year extension, during which they received strontium ranelate at a dose of 2 grams/day. The results: vertebral fracture risk was reduced by 31%, nonvertebral fracture risk by 27%, major nonvertebral fracture risk by 33%, and hip fracture risk by 24%.[367]

Obviously, these results run counter to the claim that strontium increases fracture risk!

Strontium Competes with Calcium for Absorption

Yes, and calcium wins. "The simultaneous intake of strontium and calcium remarkably reduces the bio-availability of strontium."[368]

For this reason, it is best to take strontium and calcium at different times of day to get the most benefit from the strontium.

Strontium Citrate Has Much to Offer Your Bones!

We hope this discussion of the research findings helps put your mind at ease regarding strontium. Strontium has much to offer your bones! We now know that strontium not only lessens osteoclast production and bone resorption (however unlike the bisphosphonates, e.g. Fosamax®, Boniva®, or the latest osteoporosis patent medicine on the block, denosumab, e.g. Prolia®, strontium does not prevent healthy bone remodeling), but also boosts osteoblast production and bone synthesis.[369] What's not to like about that?

No adverse effects have been associated with the natural forms of strontium *when calcium and vitamin D are also supplied.*

The only precautions are: take more calcium than strontium, for best results take strontium at a different time of day from when you take your calcium, and take a natural form of strontium.

Bio-Identical Hormone Replacement Builds Bone

Both estrogen and progesterone play key roles in maintaining healthy bones. Estrogen suppresses the production of osteoclasts, the cells that break down bone; slows down the activity of already formed osteoclasts; curbs the production of inflammatory cytokines (small proteins secreted by immune system cells that promote inflammation-associated bone loss); and enhances the absorption of calcium and its retention in bone.[370]

As important as estrogen is to bone health, however, if you've read the earlier sections of this book, you know that simply lessening the rate at which bone is broken down or resorbed is only half of the equation. Maintaining healthy bones requires constantly rebuilding the bone that needs to be replaced—which is where progesterone comes in. Progesterone is responsible for boosting the production and activity of the cells that build new bone, the osteoblasts.

Progesterone levels begin to decline in women long before menopause—in some women, the drop in progesterone begins as early as their late 30s. By the time a woman reaches age 50, she may have lost as much as 75% of her youthful progesterone production.[371]

Even in young women, progesterone levels are normally low during the first half of the menstrual cycle. Progesterone production increases during the second half of the menstrual cycle (the luteal phase) after an egg is released from a follicle in the ovaries—an event called *ovulation*. After ovulation, the remains of the follicle join to form the *corpus luteum*, whose primary function is to secrete lots of progesterone, which prepares the uterine lining for the implantation of the egg, if fertilized. If no ovulation takes place—which happens more and more frequently as women enter perimenopause—no corpus luteum is produced, and only the small baseline amount of progesterone, which is made by the adrenal glands, is available.

Young women may also lack optimal levels of progesterone if they are using oral contraceptives (*aka* birth control pills).[372] Birth control pills come in two flavors—those containing only a patented version of estrogen, and those that combine the patented estrogen with another patent medicine, a new-to-Nature analog of progesterone called a progestin.* Both types of birth control pill work by inhibiting follicular development and preventing ovulation. Thus, both types of birth control pills inhibit young women's natural production of progesterone.[373]

One of the most recently developed contraceptives, now being used in women as young as 14 years of age, is an IUD containing a progestin called levonorgestrel that is marketed under the trade name, Mirena®. This IUD is so potent that it not only prevents ovulation, but causes amenorrhea (cessation of menstruation) in many of the young, premenopausal and perimenopausal women in whom it has been inserted. As discussed earlier,† progesterone is primarily produced as a

---

* (The dangers of progestins are outlined in the section following: "Why Bio-identical Hormones Rather than Conventional, Patent Medicine Version of HRT?")

† See page 6.

result of ovulation and is required for the development of osteoblasts. A recent meta-analysis has estimated a BMD increase of 0.5% per year in women with normal ovulation, but a decrease in BMD of 0.7% per year in young women with ovulatory disturbances (anovulation or short luteal phase). The progestins inhibit ovulation. Since the span of years from adolescence when menstruation begins through our early 30s are the years when women are supposed to be building up our peak bone mass, use of the progestins may be setting up young women for early and severe osteoporosis.[374]

In addition, cadmium, a toxic compound in cigarette smoke,* disrupts the ovaries' production of progesterone.[375] For these reasons, even young or perimenopausal women may be at risk of producing too little progesterone to promote healthy bone remodeling. In the Canadian Multicentre Osteoporosis Study, oral contraceptive users had bone mineral density scores 2.3% to 3.7% lower than women who had never used oral contraceptives.[376]

Symptoms of premenopausal progesterone insufficiency may include: heavy periods, premenstrual syndrome (PMS), migraine and other headaches, fibrocystic breasts, breast tenderness, decreased libido, water retention/bloating, anxiety, and depression.

Since progesterone balances estrogen, opposing estrogen's stimulation of cell growth, insufficient progesterone translates into an increased risk of breast, uterine, and endometrial cancer. Because progesterone is necessary for the production and activation of osteoblasts, having too little promotes bone loss.

---

* See earlier discussion on page 139.

Ready to look into finding out whether your levels of estrogen and progesterone are adequate to protect your bones' health? It's easy to do so. Just ask your doctor to order a 24-hour urine collection hormone test for you.

WHY BOTHER WITH A 24-HOUR URINE TEST WHEN SALIVA TESTS ARE COMMONLY AVAILABLE BY MAIL ORDER AND A BLOOD DRAW TAKES ONLY A COUPLE OF MINUTES?

Saliva test results are not reliable.[377] Blood tests are sometimes useful, but they only provide a snapshot of what's going on in your body at the moment the blood is drawn. 24-hour urine testing (yes, you collect your urine in a large bottle for a full 24 hours then transfer some samples to small vials for processing) is the preferred method of evaluating sex steroid hormone levels. It is the gold standard both because it is highly accurate and also because it provides way more information, including whether your hormones are being metabolized into helpful, safe compounds or into potentially cancer-causing ones. Neither saliva nor standard blood tests are able to measure many of these metabolites.[378]

One final caveat: be sure to work with a physician who will prescribe bio-identical hormone replacement for you if indicated.

WHY BIO-IDENTICAL HORMONES RATHER THAN CONVENTIONAL, PATENT MEDICINE VERSION OF HRT?

Why use bio-identical hormones rather than the patent medicines, Premarin® (horse estrogens derived from the urine of pregnant mares) and Provera® (medroxyprogesterone, a patented, lab-created progestin—not progesterone!)?

Chances are you are already thinking the answer to this question is obvious! The bodies of postmenopausal women, including their bones, do better when given hormones identical to those their premenopausal bodies produced than when given those produced by female horses (conjugated equine estrogens, trade name Premarin®) or some unnatural aberration concocted in a chemistry lab (medroxyprogesterone, trade name Provera®).

Not only are bio-identical hormones more effective, but numerous studies have demonstrated that patented HRT is extremely dangerous. Perhaps the most widely publicized of these trials has been the Women's Health Initiative (WHI). It was impossible to keep it quiet in 2002, when the WHI was halted early (after 5.2 years instead of its planned 8.5 years), because risks for both breast cancer and cardiovascular disease (heart attack, stroke, blood clots) went way up in the women who were receiving conventional HRT (Premarin® and Provera®).[379]

It's true that horse estrogens (conventional HRT) were found to offer a very small degree of protection against osteoporosis—5 to 7 fewer hip fractures per 10,000 women compared to a placebo.[380] But because patented HRT (Premarin®, Provera®, Prempro®—the last one being a pill that combines conjugated equine estrogens with medroxyprogesterone) have been definitively shown to increase your risk of cancer, heart disease, and stroke, conventional HRT is now primarily used to treat hot flashes and is prescribed at the lowest possible dose for the shortest amount of time possible.

One very positive result of the WHI's exposure of the risks of taking conventional HRT: its use—even short term for hot flashes—quickly plummeted by more than 50%. And as a result of this drop in the numbers of women taking HRT, the incidence of breast cancer fell 8.8% in women ranging in age from 40 to 79![381]

Safety Issues

Too much estrogen—even bio-identical estrogen—can overstimulate cell growth in the lining of the uterus or breast. If you decide to investigate BHRT, read Dr. Wright's latest book on the subject, coauthored by Lane Lenard, PhD, *Stay Young & Sexy with Bio-Identical Hormone Replacement, the Science Explained*, and work with a physician well versed in this area.*

Prescriptions for bio-identical hormone replacement are not cookie cutter items. You will need to be tested to determine the estrogen dosage your body requires; a compounding pharmacy will then formulate a prescription specifically for you, and your doctor will monitor you using blood and urine tests at regular intervals to ensure you are getting all the benefits without increasing cancer risk.

Your doctor will also help you determine how much bio-identical progesterone is optimal for you. Unlike estrogen, bio-identical progesterone is not a growth stimulator. During the short period in which your dose may need adjusting, too much might make you sleepy, but will not cause any unpleasant or dangerous side effects.

---

* For help finding a physician in your area, see in Resources section: "Where Can I Find an 'Integrative' Doctor Who Will Help Me Build and Keep My Bones Strong, Naturally?"

In contrast, the patent medicines containing progestins (Provera®, Prempro®), which are given with conjugated equine estrogens to supposedly help lessen the risk of unopposed estrogen, may not only cause breast tenderness, skin irritations, depression, breakthrough bleeding, swelling, and hirsutism (excessive hairiness in atypical areas, e.g., a mustache on a woman), but also contribute to conventional HRT's increased risk of asthma, stroke, heart disease, and breast, ovarian, and endometrial cancer.[382]

The claim to fame of the latest, fourth-generation progestins (e.g., drospirenone, dienogest), which are used in birth control pills, is that they have been designed to be closer in activity to the bio-identical progesterone (which raises the obvious question: why not just use bio-identical progesterone?), but their potential for causing coronary heart disease and breast cancer still remains an open question.[383]

No perimenopausal woman desiring to take progesterone to help prevent accelerated bone loss during the years immediately prior to menopause should have to subject herself to these risks when she can take bio-identical progesterone. For the reasons previously discussed, young women, particularly those at increased risk for osteoporosis,* may also wish to consider using alternative means of birth control, e.g., a cervical cap, diaphragm, or condom.

---

* See Chapter 1, page 5.

The Bone-Building Diet (I Can Eat My Way to Strong, Healthy Bones?)

You've probably heard the saying, "You are what you eat." It's true, particularly in relation to your bones. If you want strong, healthy bones for life, you've got to *eat real food, mostly plants, preferably organic.*

Conveniently, this healthy way of eating that creates and maintains strong bones for life is essentially the same diet that will lower your risk not only for osteoporosis, but for all chronic degenerative diseases, including cancer, diabetes, heart disease, and Alzheimer's.

Among all modern, technologically advanced Western societies, the lowest incidence of osteoporosis is found in the countries along the Mediterranean Sea, a fact attributed to the eating pattern in this area. If you want to put a label on it, you can call it the Bone-Building Mediterranean-Style Diet.[384]

It includes *lots of fresh vegetables* accompanied by:

- Beans
- Wild-caught fish
- Free-range eggs
- Low-fat dairy products, like yogurt, and a little cheese, often from goat's milk
- Small amounts of other animal protein, e.g., organically-raised free-range chicken, turkey, beef, pork
- Nuts and seeds
- Whole grains like brown rice, whole wheat pasta or bread, oats, quinoa
- Extra virgin olive oil as the primary source of added fat

- A wide variety of herbs and spices as seasonings
- Fruit, preferably fresh, for snacks and dessert
- If desired, one to two daily 4-ounce servings of red wine

In his book, *In Defense of Food*, Michael Pollan sums up how to follow the healthiest way of eating by saying: "Eat food. Not too much. Mostly plants."[385] To spotlight bone health, we just need to shift the emphasis to *what* rather than *how much*.

Happily, "*how much*" becomes a nonissue anyway since it's virtually impossible to consume too many calories when eating "real food, mostly plants, preferably organic"—unless you make like a squirrel preparing for hibernation and really pack away those nuts. A small handful of nuts, about an ounce a day, is the amount you should enjoy and not risk gaining too much weight.

You also need to limit your alcohol consumption. One or even two 4-ounce glasses of red wine is a good idea. Red wine contains a bone-building, longevity-promoting phytonutrient called resveratrol, which has been shown to significantly promote osteoblast production and to prevent bone loss caused by estrogen deficiency.[386] However, if you drink more than 2 daily glasses of wine, as explained earlier, your bones will not be fine.*

---

* See "More Than Two Drinks of Liquor Makes Bone Loss Much Quicker," page 143.

SO, WHAT DO THE THREE CATCH-PHRASES—EAT REAL FOOD, MOSTLY PLANTS, PREFERABLY ORGANIC—ACTUALLY MEAN?

Eat Real Food

Eat food as close to its natural state as possible. This means buy mostly food that is unprocessed, unpackaged, and unadulterated. This kind of food is found along the perimeter of the grocery store in the refrigerated sections.

Real food has to be refrigerated because, unlike the stuff in boxes in the aisles, it is not loaded with preservatives, fake flavoring, color additives, salt, sugars, etc., etc. Instead, real food is loaded with literally thousands of health-building nutrient compounds and enzymes that will quickly spoil on the shelf, but are needed to prevent our bodies, including our bones, from spoiling. These compounds are removed from the highly processed food-like items in the non-refrigerated aisles in our grocery stores to extend their "shelf life." If you prefer to extend your life, don't eat these.

Real food takes a little more time to prepare, but costs a lot less, even when organic. If you don't believe this, just compare the price of organic, thick-cut, rolled oats (1/4 cup will cook up into a large bowl of delicious hot oatmeal in about five minutes) to that of a packet of highly processed, sugar-and-chemical-laden instant oatmeal. Or compare the price of a large organic Russet potato to a bag of potato chips; if thinly sliced, tossed with a tablespoon of olive oil, spread on a cookie sheet, and baked, one potato will deliver the equivalent of a whole bag of potato chips, but for far fewer calories.

Eating home-baked potato chips instead of that bag of overly processed, excessively greasy potato chips will shrink your waistline as well as your food bill. Plus, the olive oil you'll use to flavor them at home is good for your heart. The cheap, omega-6-rich (and therefore pro-inflammatory) oils used to process store-bought potato (and other) chips is not. Avoid pro-inflammatory, processed foods if you want to protect not only your heart and brain, but your bones.

If you have the space, consider planting a vegetable garden. Once you experience the taste of a just-picked snap pea, carrot, or vine-ripened tomato, or a tossed salad made from greens out of your own garden, you will be hooked. If you plant a vegetable garden, even if you pay more to buy vegetable starts rather than a packet of seeds, an investment of about $25 will provide an abundance of fresh produce from late spring through fall. You'll eat better, get a little exercise walking outside to the garden, and spend less.

A great resource for learning all you need to know to make choosing, storing, and cooking real food easy, practical, and delicious is the nonprofit, totally free, no-advertisements website, The World's Healthiest Foods: www.whfoods.org.

Mostly Plants

Eat *at least* three cups of vegetables every day. Four to six cups would be good. Eight to ten cups would be better.

Eat lots of leafy greens. At the very least, one cup daily.* Going green every day helps keep osteoporosis away. An

---

* See "Greens Give the Go-Ahead for Great Bones; Their Absence Slams the Brakes on Bone-Building," page 98.

absence of greens in your daily diet slams the brakes on bone-building. For virtually no calories, green leafy vegetables deliver vast amounts of the minerals and vitamins your bones need, including calcium, magnesium, folate, vitamin C, and vitamin K_1. Fill up on leafy greens, and you will build up your bones, not your belly, hips, or thighs. And let's face it—you want not just great bones, but a great body, right? Greens will help you get both. Although green vegetables actually contain less calcium than many animal proteins, green vegetables contain very little if any phosphorus, which "offsets" the calcium. By contrast, animal proteins contain large quantities of phosphorus, which lead to excretion from our bodies of much of the calcium consumed in those animal proteins.

Not only do plant foods contain the nutrients necessary to build bone, but a diet rich in plant foods makes your body chemistry slightly alkaline, which is required for good bone health. As discussed earlier,* a diet high in animal protein promotes an acidic body chemistry. So does a diet high in refined sugars, including the high fructose corn syrup found in soft drinks and the vast majority of processed foods—yet another reason to avoid this junk. If protein or sugar dominates in your diet, your body will buffer the acidic chemistry produced by withdrawing alkaline minerals, i.e., calcium, from your bones.

Skimp on the refined sugars, but don't skimp on protein. Don't overdo it either.† Bottom line, your best protein choices are low-fat dairy products; fish rich in

---

* See "Is Your Diet Leaching Calcium from Your Bones?," page 91.

† See "How Much Protein Do YOU Need?" on page 92 to find out. This section also lists bone-friendly sources of protein.

omega-3 fatty acids but low in mercury, such as sardines and wild-caught salmon; calcium-enriched tofu; omega-3-rich free-range eggs; and beans.

Preferably Organic

Calorie-for-calorie, organically grown foods contain more bone-building minerals and phytonutrients than conventionally grown foods.

Nutrient levels in most conventionally grown fruits and vegetables have steadily declined, primarily as a result of what is called "the dilution effect." Conventionally grown crops grow bigger and faster as a result of the use of nitrogen fertilizer. Faster growing crops have less time to extract nutrients from the soil and move them up from the roots up the stalks and into the portions of the plant that are eaten.[387]

In addition, because they are protected by pesticides and constant irrigation from the stress caused by insects, fungal invasions, and drought, conventionally grown crops spend little energy on generating phytochemicals, including the vitamins and hundreds of health-promoting phenolic compounds plants can produce. Why? Because plants create these in response to their needs for self-defense. Less need = less self-defense nutrients in your food.[388]

Research confirms this. A review, released March 2008 by The Organic Center, identified 97 peer-reviewed studies published since 1980 that compared nutrient levels in organic and conventionally grown foods.[389] These studies were then rigorously analyzed for scientifically valid "matched pairs" of organic/conventionally grown produce. Two hundred and thirty-six matched pairs were found and evaluated for nutrient content.

(To qualify as a matched pair, plants had to be grown nearby one another, in similar soils and climate, to have similar plant genetics, irrigation systems, nitrogen levels, and harvest practices.)

Organically grown fruits, vegetables, and grains were found to contain higher levels of eight of the eleven nutrients assayed, including higher levels of polyphenols and antioxidants. Overall, organically grown foods were 25% more nutrient-rich than conventionally grown varieties.

Not only was this difference found to be sizable enough to conclude organically grown foods can be counted upon to provide more nutrients, but Neal Davies, a Washington State University professor and a coauthor of the report, noted that "the nutrients in organically grown foods are often in a more biologically active form," which translates to more beneficial activity from the nutrient. In other words, the same amount of nutrient delivers more bang for the buck if consumed in an organically grown food.

In September 2009, a rebuttal to this study appeared in the *American Journal of Clinical Nutrition*. This paper, another review, discounted the claim that organically grown foods are nutritionally superior to conventionally grown. However, it wasn't a very good review. The reviewers did not use matched pairs and did not include antioxidant capacity in the compounds evaluated, in part because they relied upon much older studies starting back in 1958. These older studies analyzed plant varieties that are no longer even being cultivated and did not contain data on phenolic antioxidant compounds because they were just starting to be discovered!

Furthermore, the authors of this review made no allowance for the fact that since the 1950s, breeders and growers of nonorganic plants have used practices that have consistently increased yield but have lead to the dilution (lessening) of nutrients in the crop, as noted above.[390]

Since February 2008, fifteen new studies have been published, most of which utilize the updated design and superior analytical methods used in the Organic Center March 2008 review. These newer studies generally confirm the findings of the 2008 Organic Center report, particularly in the case of nitrogen (which is higher in conventional crops, a disadvantage since it may be converted into cancer-causing nitrates in the intestines), and for vitamin C, total phenolics, and total antioxidant capacity, which are typically higher in organically grown foods.[391]

An earlier review of 41 studies comparing organic to conventionally grown foods, published in 2002, found organically grown foods contained 27% more vitamin C, 21.1% more iron, 29.3% more magnesium, and 13.6% more phosphorus.[392]

A number of other current papers published in the peer-reviewed medical literature confirm that organic foods contain significantly higher levels of nutrients (especially bone-building vitamin C, polyphenols, flavonoids, and minerals) and lower levels of pesticides.[393]

And you really want to minimize your exposure to pesticides because they promote inflammation in humans, which, among their numerous other nasty effects, can contribute to bone loss by triggering osteoclast production and activity, and by causing mutations in hematopoietic stem cells—cells in bone marrow that give rise to all the different types of blood cells.[394]

A study comparing organic to conventionally grown tomatoes found organic tomatoes contained 4.52%

more vitamin K, 129.81% more calcium, and 65.43% more zinc than conventionally grown tomatoes.[395]

Another, looking at celery, showed organic celery contained 70.22% more vitamin K, 47.93% more zinc, and 118.18% more vitamin C than conventionally grown celery.[396]

Yet another, analyzing the content of minerals and phenolic compounds in eggplant, found organic cultivation had such a positive effect on the accumulation of beneficial mineral and phenolic compounds that organically and conventionally produced eggplants could easily be told apart by looking at their nutrient composition profiles![397]

The nutritional profiles of a woman's diet—if she eats the high fat, high sugar, highly processed Standard American Diet (for which the shorthand is, aptly, SAD) or if she chooses a whole foods, mostly plants, mostly organic Mediterranean-style diet—will have a huge impact on what she will look and feel like at age 85. Don't be SAD! You can have strong, healthy bones for life. Eat a bone-building diet, and you will greatly increase your likelihood of standing tall and looking good when you turn 85.

Bone-Building Exercises

USE IT OR LOSE IT

Lack of weight-bearing and resistance exercise is a well-documented risk factor for osteoporosis.[398] Numerous studies show that not moving against gravity—whether as a result of being an astronaut on a space mission, in bed recovering from a surgery or illness, or life as a couch potato—leads to massive loss of bone minerals, as much as 1% of bone mineral mass per week![399]

On the other hand, consistent bone-building exercise is one of the most effective ways to decrease your fracture risk. In response to resistance exercise training (any type of exercise that puts real demands on muscle and thus its attachments to bone), a number of studies of postmenopausal women have shown that bone responds with increases in bone mineral density sufficient to move these women back toward the norm seen in healthy younger women.[400]

After a year of regular exercise, the typical gain in BMD is 1–3%. Doesn't sound like all that much—until you realize that, without exercise, after age 40, women start losing BMD at a rate of 0.3–0.5% per year. The rate of BMD loss increases after age 50 to about 1–1.5% per year, and frequently ramps up to more than 2% per year during the first 6–10 years after menopause, after which it slows back down to somewhere between 1–2% per year.[401]

If regular exercise can give you a gain in BMD of 1–3% per year instead of a loss of 1–2% a year, it's actually preventing a 1–2% loss plus adding another 1–3% in BMD—this translates into an actual gain in BMD from exercise of 2–5% per year.

However, exercise is definitely a "keep using it or keep losing it" situation. In studies in which postmenopausal women stopped exercising, the gains they made in spinal bone mineral density were lost after a period of inactivity.[402]

Why is Exercise Essential for Healthy Bones as We Age?

Our bones reach their full length (and we our full height) between the ages of 15 and 19, but bones retain the capacity to grow in width throughout the human lifespan. After mid-life, our bones begin to thin and become more porous. Despite the bone benefits from our needing to work against the force of gravity during normal activities, we still typically lose 30% of our muscle strength between the ages of 30 and 80.

Unless we actively combat it, we will lose somewhere between 0.5% and 2% of our BMD each year. The "conservative" (least) expected drop in BMD for women aged 41–55 is -0.5% per year; for women 56 and older, this loss doubles to 1.0% per year. Men also lose bone, although at a rate of about half these amounts. A number of studies indicate that, for women, bone loss accelerates to at least 2% for up to 14 years around the age of menopause (which typically occurs around age 52).[403]

Now for the good news: physical activity can counteract this! Get physical and you will continue to stimulate increases in the width of your bones and in their ability to absorb minerals throughout the rest of your entire life. And exercise-stimulated increases in bone width and strength can offset the negative effects that aging, if unopposed, is going to have on your bone tissue.[404] In addition, regular physical exercise strengthens your muscles and improves your balance, greatly reducing your risk of falls that can cause a fracture.[405]

The message is clear: being buff is essential for beautiful bones. Be physically active! If you don't use it, you will lose it!

Does It Matter What Kind of Exercise I Do?

Good question! Yes, it really matters what types of exercise you do. Not all exercises are equally good at building bone. Some, like swimming, are ineffective. (When you swim, the water is bearing your weight, not your bones.) Others, particularly in cases of osteoporosis, can actually increase your fracture risk (more about this and how to exercise safely, shortly).

What Kinds of Exercise Should I Consider and How Much Is Needed to Turn on My Bones' Mineral-Absorbing, Width-Building Action?

Unless you just love to exercise—yes, these people do exist—you want to know what kinds of movement signal your bones to buff up and how many moves you have to make, so you can choose an exercise program that will deliver the goods in the least amount of time.

Exercise physiologists now know that to build bone exercises must:[406]

- **Be Dynamic, Not Static**

  Bones are designed to provide resistance against the forces of muscle contraction and gravity when your body parts are moving. Rhythmic movement, such as dancing, strutting your stuff in a Zumba class, walking briskly, jogging, climbing stairs (or using a StairMaster or elliptical machine), riding a bicycle, lifting weights, performing squats and/or lunges, Pilates exercises (either in the form of mat exercises, such as the Pilates mat exercises described below, or exercises using the Pilates Reformer or Cadillac), cause intermittent muscle contractions that deliver brief stresses on your bones and increase blood supply to your muscles, increasing delivery of nutrients, hormones and oxygen. Such exercises send your bones a message: "You've been challenged. Buff up!"

A dynamic and precise exercise regime like Pilates is particularly good for preventing or combatting osteopenia or osteoporosis because it safely provides the necessary intermittent contractions and isolates muscles right at the spots where bone-building is needed. Because Pilates can be practiced anywhere you can place a mat (and your body) on the floor, we've included a full section about it in this chapter to give you an introduction to this bone-building exercise option. Contributed by Nancy Brose and Kristi Milner Quinn,[407] (two Stott Pilates expert instructors, who not only specialize in working with clients with or at risk for osteoporosis, but teach other Pilates instructors how to do so), this section introduces you to Pilates and explains how and why it is such a great bone-building form of exercise. (See "Pilates, the Perfect Exercise Plan for Building Bone—Beautifully.")

Static exercises—like holding a yoga posture, or floating on your back in the pool—while delivering other benefits, do not build bone. Even swimming, although dynamic, is virtually gravity-free, so won't help build bone either.

■ **Exceed a "Threshold Intensity"**

After menopause, to be effective in increasing bone mineralization, exercise has to be not only regular, but of sufficient intensity. Your bones have to get the "get buff" message! A leisurely stroll or window shopping at the mall won't send it. We're talking "brisk walk" here. Speaking of which, if you can talk non-stop—stop! Then rev it up and use your breath to ramp up oxygen and nutrient delivery to your muscles, so you can build bone.

In relation to weight lifting, if you can perform more than 4 sets of 8 reps of a bicep curl without feeling like your bicep muscle is on fire, you need to increase the weight. Same goes for your other muscles. Your leg and buttocks muscles (your quadriceps, hamstrings, gluteus maximus and medius, for the technically inclined) should be letting you know you've asked them to work hard by the time you're done with squats or lunges.

On the plus side here, working these muscles, especially your gluts, will restore your posterior to the position on your body it used to occupy when you were in your twenties and get you looking good in "skinny jeans." Nancy and Kristi will go into this further in relation to Pilates; fortunately, it's not as hard as you think. You do want to work your muscles, but you don't need to overdo it. You want to gently and consistently build, gain stability at a higher threshold, then increase the challenge to those muscles again.

While this may sound excruciating, trust us, this process is actually fun. You will feel so strong, so empowered—just think of yourself as Osteoporosis Avenger Woman, which you will, in fact, become. Don those superhero sweat pants and save your bones!

- **Exceed a "Threshold Strain Frequency"**

  The rate at which you contract your muscles counts. Increasing the frequency of your muscle contractions will increase your bone-building response. Using dancing as an example, you want an upbeat, high tempo cha cha—not a waltz. This is why a Zumba class may be your bone-building cup of tequila. You want to play tennis, not golf—well, golfing is okay if you forget the cart and walk really fast to the next spot where your ball ended up. (And carry your own clubs, too.) Get dewy—or just sweat. You can take a shower later.

- **Be Relatively "Brief and Intermittent"**

  A couple of shorter, but gung ho, exercise sessions each day are much better than spending hours at the gym a couple of days a week. In fact, dividing your exercise time in half and exercising twice a day, say a half-hour before leaving for work or at lunch, and then another half hour 6–8 hours later in the evening—remember, energetic dancing counts—produces a more "osteogenic" (bone-building) response than spending your entire lunch hour or half of Saturday slugging away. In other words, you can have a life, and still get enough exercise to make a real difference.

- **Impose an Unusual "Loading Pattern" on Your Bones**

  You have to do something that uses different movement patterns and thus stresses your bones in uncustomary ways from your normal activities. The take home message here is: Don't do the same exercise routine over and over until you can breeze through it on autopilot, thinking about something else.

Vary the order of the exercises or the way in which you work a muscle group. For example, if you lift weights, work a different muscle group first, use the machines in a different order, use free weights instead of machines, or find a different exercise than the one you usually do to work that muscle group. If you do Pilates, vary the order or the exercises that you choose. Be sure to read our section below to make sure you choose the best and safest exercises too! If you are taking classes at a gym, you'll notice the good instructors do this just to keep it interesting as well as more effective.

PILATES, THE PERFECT EXERCISE PLAN FOR BUILDING BONE—BEAUTIFULLY

Pilates can serve you as the perfect exercise regimen for building bone safely, effectively, beautifully. Here's why:

Pilates Is Precise and Efficient. Every Movement Counts, so You Get Maximum Bone-Building Benefits from Your Allotted Exercise Time

In our bodies, we have two main types of muscles: muscles that move us (our "mobilizing muscles") and muscles that support us (our "stabilizing muscles"). Our stabilizing muscles are also known as the "core" muscles.

In most athletic or everyday activities, our mobilizing muscles, which are typically bigger and stronger, tend to take over. When these stronger muscles take over, many smaller, weaker muscles get neglected. Not so good since these weaker muscles are often the "core muscles" that stabilize our spine and hip joints. And it is these stabilizing core muscles that most directly stimulate bone growth in the areas needed! Obviously, we need to target and strengthen these muscles. To do so, we must first isolate them, ensuring they do the work instead of letting our larger "go to" muscles take over.

With Pilates, You Work from Your Core Muscles Outward

To prevent fractures while boosting your bones' strength and flexibility, you want to increase your balance; strengthen the muscles that stabilize and extend (arch) your back; stabilize your hips (pelvic girdle); strengthen and increase flexibility throughout your hip area, your lower legs and your feet; and keep all your joints moving and open. (By "open," we don't mean excessively pulled apart, just freely filling all the space they were designed to occupy.)

And the good news is: all of these goals are accomplished by simply working from your center or core outward. This is why, in Pilates, you begin by learning how to strengthen your core muscles.

Your "core muscles" are the ones that support the trunk of your body and surround the space in which your organs reside. It's these core muscles that enable you to do things that require strength over time. For example, maintain an erect, graceful, and pain-free posture as you move throughout your day—or even while running a marathon (or, a more reasonable goal for most of us, run from store to store for an entire day of shopping at the outlet mall). Core strengthening focuses on muscles like your multifidi, transversus abdominus, internal and external obliques, and the psoas—these are the key muscle players that support your spine and pelvis. In the hip joint, your core muscles include your deep lateral hip rotators (such as the piriformis). In your rib cage and shoulder girdle, these core muscles include your serratus anterior and rotator cuff muscles.

Don't worry—you don't have to know all this technical stuff to get the benefits of Pilates exercises, but having the inside scoop, literally, on how and why Pilates will help you build bone can deepen your practice.

Pilates Helps You Activate the RIGHT Muscles

It doesn't matter how much weight you are bearing; what matters most when you want to build bone is that you are activating the right muscles.[408] When you walk, squat or do push-ups, for example, you are bearing up your own weight. But you may not be really zeroing in on the muscles that will most benefit your bones. When you begin a Pilates for Osteoporosis program, you will first have a postural analysis that identifies your unique needs, and this will serve as the foundation for the exercise plan created for you that ensures the exercises you do provide your optimal bone-building match.

WHAT ABOUT WEIGHT TRAINING?

You can certainly lift weights to help build bone strength, but Pilates can focus the bone-building load on your muscles more effectively. For one thing, Pilates helps you strengthen your stabilizing core muscles, so you can hold your body properly to get the most out of your weight training. You don't want to just lift weight. You

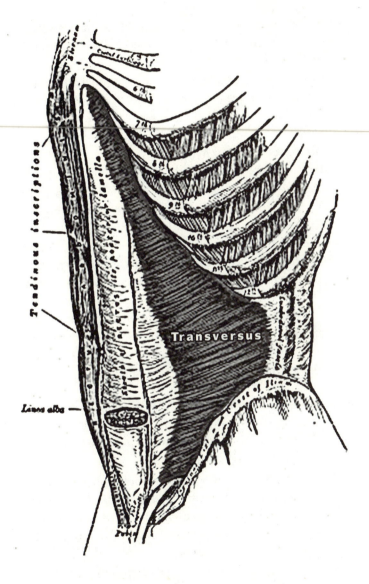

Transversus Abdominus, core muscle wrapping
front to back under the superficial muscles

do this carrying in the groceries. (And you can also compress your vertebrae or pull a muscle and injure yourself trying to carry in all the groceries in one trip—be less efficient or ask for some help!) Proper postural alignment and weight bearing on the right places is the key.[409]

It is important to understand the relationship between core muscle strengthening and most weight training exercises to make sure you get action on the part of your bones where you need to build.

Most weight training exercises are designed to build our mobilizing muscles. These movers are the muscles that help you jump, run, push, and climb. They are bigger, but more superficial (the outermost layers of muscle), than your core muscles, and they don't always attach at the parts of the bones you want to stimulate to grow to meet your goal of improving bone density and lowering fracture risk. These mobilizing muscles are very important, *but the stability and improved balance of your spine and hip depends on your stabilizing core muscles.*

For example, if you are doing a squat, the mobilizing muscles you will become immediately aware of are your quadriceps, the muscles on the front of your thighs. If you've tried doing squats, have you ever noticed that you feel a bit off balance unless you move quickly to keep up momentum (and get this exercise over with)? This is because the faster you move, the more easily your quadriceps can overcome a lack of strength in your deep hip stabilizers: your lateral hip rotators. And these lateral hip rotators are the muscles you really want to strengthen to stabilize your hip and prevent a hip fracture.

To make your hips a "fracture-free zone," you want to target bone-building at the top of your thigh bone (the upper portion of your femur, which is called the

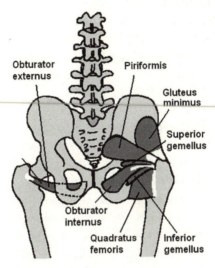

Deep lateral rotators of the hip

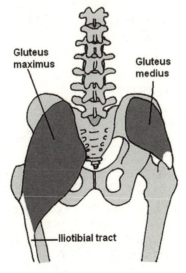

More superficial gluteal muscles

"femur neck"), because this is where osteoporotic hip fractures almost always occur.*

To build bone in the neck of your femur, you want to access and strengthen your lateral hip rotator muscles. In order to access these muscles and create the desired pull at the top of your thigh bone (when muscles pull on bone, this tells the parts of the bone being pulled on to get stronger), you want to stabilize your pelvis and spine. And what does this? Your core muscles. So, what you need for strong bones is exercise that really develops your core strength—in other words, Pilates.

If your core is unstable, your body will most likely compensate for you by arching your lower back too much (your fanny will stick out and your stomach will drop forward, not attractive!), or you will hike up one of your hips or put too much stress on your knees, all which make you vulnerable to injury. Most importantly for preventing fractures, however, any exercise that does not improve your core stability is not going to help you to improve your balance, avoid falls, and build spinal and hip strength.

WHAT ABOUT WALKING?

Walking is great; we absolutely recommend it. But by now, you probably realize that for building strong bones, there's more to it. Studies have shown that walking alone doesn't load our hips sufficiently to decrease our risk of fracture. You need to be able to do focused exercises, such as squats. When you squat down, your

---

* Unless you are taking a bisphosphonate or densumab, in which case, you are at risk for an "atypical femur fracture" which will occur a bit lower on your thigh bone. See discussion of "atypical femur fractures" compliments of bisphosphonates and denosumab on pages 41-47.

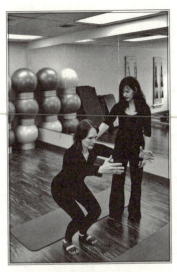

PHOTO 1
Hips loaded by body weight in a squat
moving from flexed hip joints . . .

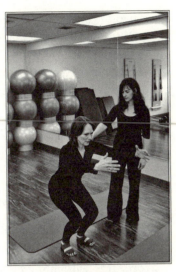

PHOTO 2
which while loaded are
extending and . . .

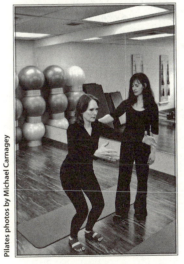

PHOTO 3
continuing up . . .

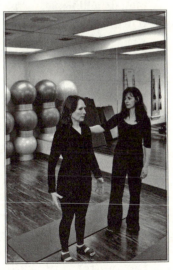

PHOTO 4
into fully extended hip joints
loaded by body weight

Pilates photos by Michael Carnagey

hip joints and your knee joints are flexed. To return to standing upright, you have to move through the full range of motion in your hip joints, and you do so by lifting the load of your own body weight. Both moves combined—squatting down and returning to standing—allow for full range of motion through your hip joint and utilize all your hip rotators, flexors, and extensors—precisely the muscles you want to activate to build bone in your femurs and hips.[410]

Okay, you may be feeling overwhelmed by now, but all you need to do is get the main point here. For maximal benefit, exercise must target the right muscles and their attachments to your bones; precision is the key. First, you need to balance and stabilize your core. This will help you ensure that you are properly putting the demand your legs—from your feet all the way up to your hip joint—so the right bone-building signals will be sent. Then you can squat, walk, move dynamically in the gym—and in your everyday activities—and be continually strengthening your bones just exactly where they need it. Integrate Pilates into your life, and your every move can help you build and maintain healthy bones—and do so beautifully!

FOCUS ON EXTENSION AND BALANCE— AVOID FLEXION EXERCISES

An exercise study conducted for 11 years (between 1989 and 2000) monitored four groups of women. Each group was assigned a specific exercise regimen. One group was given only extension (back arching) exercises to do; another was given only flexion (forward bending) exercises; a third group was given flexion and extension exercises, and the

EXTENSION EXERCISES LOWER BUT FLEXION EXERCISES INCREASE FRACTURE RISK

Exercise Group	Risk of Fracture Afterward
Extension Exercises Only	16%
Flexion Exercises Only	89%
Flexion & Extension Exercises	53%
No Exercise	67%

Adapted from Sinaki M, Mikkelsen BA. Postmenopausal spinal osteoporosis: flexion versus extension exercises. *Arch Phys Med Rehabil.* 1984 Oct;65(10):593-6. PMID: 6487063

fourth group, which served as a control, did neither form of exercise.

Extension exercises dramatically lowered risk of fracture to just 16%, while flexion exercises resulted in an 89% risk for fracture—an even greater risk than the 67% risk of fracture seen in the group doing no exercise. When flexion and extension exercises were combined, risk of fracture was 53%, significantly greater than the 16% risk seen with extension exercise only. The results of this study are shown in the following table:

You can see that the beneficial results of proper exercise can be significant—and so can the harmful results of improper exercise! This study shows it may be better to do no exercise at all than to do the wrong kind—i.e., flexion (forward-bending, spine-compressing) exercises.

Other studies have also shown that extension exercises, which result in stronger lower and upper back muscles, provide long-term risk reduction for vertebral (spine) fractures. A medical journal article describing one such study, entitled "Stronger back muscles reduce the incidence of vertebral fractures: a prospective 10 year follow-up of postmenopausal women," involved

50 healthy postmenopausal women aged 58–75 years, 27 of whom performed back-strengthening exercises for two years, while 23 served as controls and did no back-strengthening exercises. After the initial two-year period, the exercise program ceased. Eight years later, the women were re-evaluated. Among those who had served as controls, risk for compression fracture was 2.7 times greater than in the women who had performed back-strengthening exercises for two years.[411]

Why Avoid Flexion Exercises?

One of the most harmful postures for people with osteoporosis or osteopenia is "kyphosis," which means excessive flexion or rounding forward of the upper spine. Think of the little old lady with a dowager's hump. Excessive flexion puts the bones of the spine in a vulnerable position and promotes weakness and degeneration in the affected area.

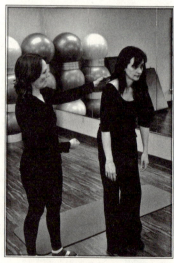

Why Are Extension Exercises So Great?

When you do exercises that extend your upper spine (require a backward arch in your thoracic area, the part of your spine surrounded by your rib cage), the demand on your back extensors causes them to strengthen.

PHOTO 5
Kristi is standing with her upper spine in flexion—this is called Kyphosis

What you don't want to do, in addition to flexing forward, is to overarch your lower back (the lumbar portion of your spine) because this may cause your back to ache. If you have a dull, aching pain in your low back, your body's telling you that you are using the wrong muscles.

As your upper back extensors strengthen, you decrease your risk of spinal compression fractures. These occur when the front of the vertebra collapse under pressure, resulting in what is called "vertebral wedging."

IMPROVE YOUR POSTURE

Statistics from the International Osteoporosis Foundation show that two out of five people over the age of 65 fall each year. The good news, also reported by the International Osteoporosis Foundation, is that "individually tailored exercise programs are proven to reduce falls and fall related injuries."[412] A qualified Pilates instructor, who has been trained to understand the use of Pilates exercises to lessen fracture risk and restore bone health in individuals with osteoporosis, can provide

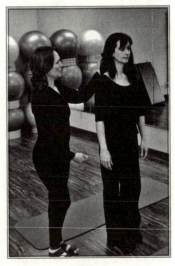

PHOTO 6
Kristi is standing with her upper spine in neutral, using strengthened back extensors

highly personalized programming that will ensure you are effectively using your muscles to stimulate bone strengthening where you need it most.

THE PILATES FOR OSTEOPOROSIS CURRICULUM

To most effectively utilize Pilates to build bone at specific sites, Nancy and Kristi developed a specific program now used by qualified STOTT PILATES® instructors that incorporates dynamic movement; allows you to access and strengthen your weaker core muscles; and emphasizes balance, strength, extension and weight bearing exercises.

Pilates for Osteoporosis Is a Safe and Effective Choice for bone-building and Fracture Prevention

The primary concept in Pilates is core strengthening. The Pilates Equipment (i.e., the Reformer and the Cadillac) were created to help injured soldiers recover from severe injury. Pilates equipment is designed to isolate and strengthen those weaker core/stabilizing muscles, while helping to safely support you and ensuring you work from your center outward.

Pilates places a good deal of emphasis on healthy spinal movement throughout its repertoire of exercises. Its careful, precise movements foster good posture and balance. Pilates's combination of core strengthening, improved balance and flexibility, plus the ability to target the specific muscular attachments to the bones most in need of strengthening, all reduce your likelihood of accidents and fracture in everyday life.

The added benefits of a beautifully erect posture, along with grace and joy in movement, makes Pilates a form of exercise you are sure to enjoy, right from your very first exercise session, and thus to continue throughout your life.

Safe Individual Attention and Tailored Exercises

You want to be sure you are working with an instructor who is knowledgeable about the best use of Pilates for osteoporosis. Individual attention and tailored exercises make Pilates for Osteoporosis a safer and more effective approach for building bone than the standard Pilates class.

Most "standard" Pilates classes include a number of forward bending/flexion exercises. Pilates for Osteoporosis takes the special factors related to osteoporosis into account and modifies your exercise regimen to ensure it safely and effectively helps you build bone. For example, the signature Pilates exercise called the "Hundred" flexes the upper body up off the floor, which would put you in a crunch position with your legs extended in

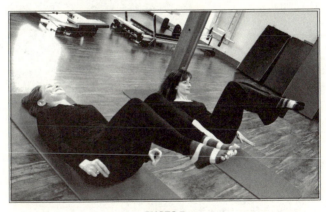

PHOTO 7
"The Hundred": Kristi has her head lifted with her upper back in flexion; Nancy has her head down modified for Osteoporosis

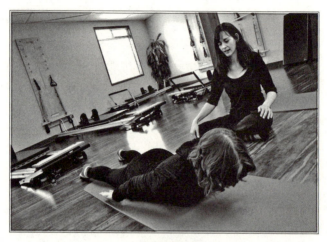

PHOTO 8
Nancy being taught Breast Stroke on the mat.

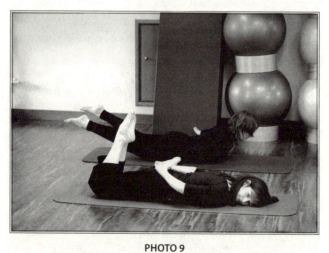

PHOTO 9
Nancy and Kristi showing extension that incorporates rotation
with the Double Leg Kick Series on the mat.

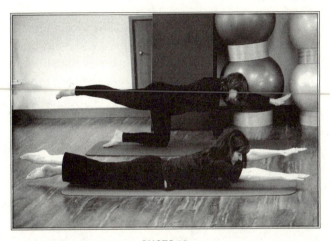

PHOTO 10
Progressions of the "Swimming Exercise": Kristi performs the full
exercise; Nancy is on her knees, modified to develop the stability
and strength needed to properly execute Kristi's exercise.

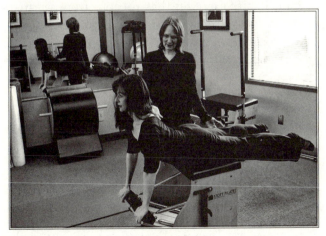

PHOTO 11
Kristi being taught the Swan Dive on the Pilates Chair.

the air. This is too much flexion for someone at risk of osteoporotic or compression fracture.

An instructor trained in Pilates for Osteoporosis will teach you how to do the Hundred with your head and shoulders resting on the mat, cueing you to lift not your rib cage, but only your legs into a right angle bent knee position by using your core, while maintaining a stable, balanced pelvis. By pumping your arms, you will dynamically challenge your abdominal muscles— without inappropriately also challenging your spine. As your core muscles strengthen, Pilates will continue to challenge you. You can hold weighted balls in your hands or extend your legs straight out at an angle of about 80 to 90 degrees. When this becomes easy— and it will—you can place a "Magic Circle" around the outside of your mid-to-lower calves. Pressing your legs out against the "Magic Circle" will add even more challenge and load.

Some Pilates exercises that are done from a seated position also normally flex the spine in a "C" curve forward. Again, Pilates for Osteoporosis modifies these exercises, so you maintain a more neutral, erect spine and hinge at the hip joint instead of curving (flexing) your spine forward. As a result of this adjustment, the spinal extensors in your back will be challenged as well as the muscles of your hip, safely promoting strong bones in both areas. Plus, mastering these exercises will give you a beautifully erect posture and lend grace and control to your every forward leaning movement.

Other Pilates exercises, such as the Breast Stroke, Swimming, Swan Dive, and Double Leg Kick, also include a progression to their performance that will strengthen your back extensors, further supporting your spine.

Some Pilates exercises, however, are best avoided by people with osteoporosis. Forward bending exercises, such as the Rollover, Jack Knife and Short Spine should be avoided—but not forever, just until your bone density has been restored!

A special cautionary note here: if on bisphosphonates or denosumab, even if bone density appears to have improved, do not add flexion exercises back in! Your bones may have the right density, but are likely to not have good strength and resiliency. Remember, these patent medicines work by preventing osteoclasts from doing their job of removing worn out, brittle bone. BMD goes up, but bone quality goes down. For this reason, flexion exercises are not advised!

Does It Matter How the Exercises Are Performed?

Absolutely! Proper execution is one of the most important, foundational tenets of Pilates. And more importantly, done incorrectly, any type of exercise could set you up for injury. Remember our discussion of squats?

Footwork, which is done on the Reformer, is a wonderful exercise for both your spine and your hips, two primary areas of your body compromised by bone loss. The Footwork exercises are basically load-bearing squats, but a special type of squat that you do safely, while fully supported and lying down, yet isolating your stabilizing muscles. Using the Reformer and learning how to ensure an optimal postural position, you will be able to focus upon and recruit the core muscles of your spine to stabilize your spine and pelvis. You will quickly become able to successfully engage your deep lateral hip rotators. Footwork done correctly pays big dividends for your efforts and will yield the most benefit to both your spine and hips.

It's impossible to see every aspect of your alignment, so it is extremely helpful to have a knowledgeable instructor observe your form, both initially and periodically thereafter. Your instructor's expert guidance will ensure that you are safely gaining the very best results from your exercises instead of losing potential benefits because of less than perfect moves.

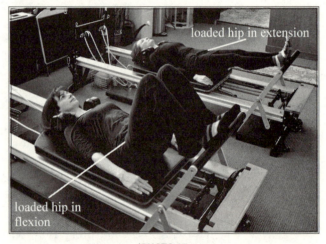

PHOTO 12
Nancy and Kristi doing footwork on the Reformer, loading the hip in a way that allows building deep lateral rotator strength.

Where Do I Find Someone Trained in Pilates for Osteoporosis?

Fortunately, many instructors have now taken courses on how to use Pilates to specifically focus on building bone in clients with osteopenia and osteoporosis. In the Seattle, Washington area, we teach a Pilates for Osteoporosis Instructor Certification program, and most of the nationally recognized Pilates Instructor Certification programs have or are developing programs.*

Getting Started Is Easy

Find a local Pilates studio with instructors trained in Pilates for Osteoporosis. (See "Resources," page 353)

Schedule a private session. You will learn about your body's specific postural alignment issues, and your instructor will design an individualized plan that's safe and most effective for you.

After you feel comfortable with what you are taught during your initial session, you will be able to take classes at the studio, at a local gym or community center, or even work with a mat program you can do at home since you will know how to modify the exercises for your best result.

Your instructor can also put together a home workout you can do in just a few minutes each day, so you can consistently stimulate your bones and move most quickly towards stronger, healthier bones. By doing as little as five different exercises (10 repetitions of each), you can strengthen your core, your back extensor muscles, and your gluteal muscles along with the deep lateral rotators that stabilize your hips and thighs. And you can do this even when you're away from home since all you need is your body and a mat or any kind of cushion for the floor. In a pinch, a doubled over towel, blanket or bedspread can transform your hotel room into your personal Pilates "studio."

Your instructor will teach you which exercises are best for you and how to modify any "standard" exercises, so

---

* See "Organizations Offering Pilates for Osteoporosis Training," page 357.

they safely support and maximally promote the health of your bones.

You'll notice a wonderful difference in just a few weeks. Then you'll want to check in with your personal instructor periodically for regular feedback on your posture (which will improve dramatically!), as well as to adjust your plan, so it continues to challenge you as you progress.

Consistency Is Essential for Success

You'll begin to notice benefits in weeks, but as you know, rebuilding bone takes time. This is why DXAs are run no more than annually. You must invest in yourself consistently and often.[413] Fortunately, Pilates exercises are so pleasant, and you will feel so wonderful after each session, that you find them a treat, not a chore.

LES MILLS BODYPUMP®—SERIOUS BONE-AND-BODY BUFFING EXERCISE

Once your bone density is back in the osteopenic range, LES MILLS BODYPUMP®, a lift-weights-to-music program, could be just what you need to compliment your Pilates exercises, restore your bones to better than normal—and keep them seriously buff.

Since its inception 20 years ago, BODYPUMP® has become the world's most popular lift-weights-to-music program. Women (and men) are now "BODYPUMP-ing" in 80 countries around the world, with certified BODYPUMP® instructors teaching this class in 12,700 clubs to millions of folks every week.

Why has BODYPUMP® become so popular? It is weight-lifting made easy, accessible and—no kidding, fun—even for us "lightweights" who have not yet (and thought they never would) try weight lifting.

What Can You Expect in a BODYPUMP® Class?

You'll be in a group class lifting weights to music, doing a workout choreographed by exercise-science experts and taught by certified, licensed instructors—so everything is designed to protect your bones and joints from injury. Instructors will help you start out with very light weights and learn correct technique and form, so you can safely get the best results from your workout, and they—and your weight-lifting sisters—will motivate you to keep coming back.

Lots of studies have confirmed that resistance training not only prevents bone loss, but actually helps rebuild strong, flexible bone. Problem is that women are put off by weight training. We think that even if it will help build our bones, it will transform us into little Arnold Schwarzenegger-ettes with large, bulging muscles. Not true for BODYPUMP®. This workout is scientifically proven and specifically designed to build long, lean muscle—not bulk. And although it is equally beneficial for men, globally well over half of "BODYPUMP-ers" are women.

Interested? More Details

LES MILLS BODYPUMP® is a 55-minute total-body workout that challenges all your major muscle groups and constantly changes the loading pattern while you squat, press, lift and curl (which will be fine for you to do once your BMD has moved back up to the osteopenic and well out of the osteoporotic range).

The key to BODYPUMP® is THE REP EFFECT™, which turns traditional thinking about lifting weights on its head. BODYPUMP® exercises muscles with light to moderate weights and lots of repetitions in a single workout. In a typical BODYPUMP® class, you perform 800 repetitions in 55 minutes (70 to 100 repetitions per body part). That's around four times the reps an average person can achieve on their own in a weight-training workout. If this sounds too dreadful to con-template, I (Lara) promise you won't notice; you'll be moving right along with the great music, and before you know it, each section of exercises will be done, and you'll be taking your break before starting in on the next body part.

BODYPUMP® is super time-efficient; you get a total body workout in just 55 minutes. It's much easier and more fun than going to the gym to work out alone. Not only do you get help and motivation from the instruc-tor—a professionally-led workout without having to pay fees to see a personal trainer—but you'll soon find you are on a very supportive team, lots of women like you getting stronger with every class.

Research conducted by Drs. Jinger Gottschall, Jackie Mills and Bryce Hastings of Pennsylvania State University—a study called "Get Fit Together: A Les Mills Group Fitness Intervention Study"—that was presented May 2012 to the annual conference of the American College of Sports Medicine—showed that a an exercise program of LES MILLS® classes increased pelvic bone density by 9% in (formerly) sedentary adults.

In this study, 15 women and 10 men between the ages of 24 and 40, completed a 30-week program. They started out with 6 weeks of learning the exercises, then 12 weeks during which they took 6 fitness classes per week (3 emphasizing cardiovascular fitness, 2 strength, and 1 flexibility), and a final 12-week block during which they added one more cardio class for a total of 7 weekly classes.

Granted, this is much more intense than would suit many of us; however, the results they earned are downright spectacular—very inspiring! Compared to their baseline measurements, participants' average:

- Oxygen consumption increased by 57%. Our bodies use oxygen to produce the energy that fuels everything—including the process of building our bones.

- Triglycerides dropped 16%. Triglycerides are fats in our bloodstream that are the first way we stash unused calories after we eat starchy and other high carbohydrate foods; high levels of triglycerides in our blood correlate with increased risk for insulin resistance, heart disease and stroke. All of these indicate chronic inflammation. Insulin resistance, in particular, is a sign that pro-inflammatory sugars are floating around in our bloodstream. And chronic inflammation, regardless of its cause, increases the production and activity of osteoclasts, the cells that break down bone.

- LDL cholesterol dropped 10%. LDL cholesterol is the type of cholesterol that, when it is at high levels and HDL cholesterol levels are low, and the body is in a state of chronic low level inflammation, increases risk for cardiovascular disease.

- Pelvic (hip) bone mineral density increased 9%!

- Total body fat mass decreased by 6%. (I read this and think, "Skinny jeans will fit and be comfy right out of the dryer!")

If visions of looking seriously buff in your jeans inspire you (and remember, you must be well out of osteoporotic ranges and just osteopenic to try this), you can learn more about BODYPUMP®, including where these classes are offered in your area, at http://w3.lesmills.com/global/en/classes/bodypump/about-bodypump/.

I (Lara) have been "BODYPUMP-ing" two to three times a week for almost two years now, but neither I nor Dr. Wright has any financial or other connection with the Les Mills company.

LAST, BUT CERTAINLY NOT LEAST, FOR BEST RESULTS, ANY EXERCISE REGIMEN YOU ADOPT MUST BE SUPPORTED BY ADEQUATE SUPPLIES OF BONE-BUILDING NUTRIENTS

While it is true that a postmenopausal woman's skeleton does not build bone as easily in response to exercise as that of a young woman, this is due primarily to the decline in female hormones (estrogen and progesterone) that occurs with menopause, and to inadequate intake of calcium, vitamin D, and the other nutrients involved in healthy bone formation (including vitamin C, vitamin K, the B vitamins, boron, magnesium, and strontium). Fortunately, with bio-identical hormone replacement, a healthy diet and supplemental bone-building nutrients, these lacks can easily be corrected.

A key reason for exercise's bone-building effects is that exercise improves the body's ability to utilize vitamin D and calcium to build bone. If these nutrients aren't available, then it's as if your bones got a call to go to a party, went to the closet and really had nothing to wear. To build and maintain healthy bones, postmenopausal women need both bone-building nutrients and exercise. Studies have shown that neither calcium supplementation without exercise nor exercise without sufficient calcium intake can increase bone mineral density. Combine the two, however, and women's spinal BMD goes up.[414] It will go up a lot more if your bones are also receiving a good supply of all the other bone-building nutrients discussed earlier.

CHAPTER 8

If I Follow These Recommendations, What Can I Expect? How Soon Will I See Results?

BIOCHEMICAL TESTS OF BONE resorption (bone loss) should be run every three months until a normal reading is obtained. (Remember, after age 40, it's normal for both men and women to lose a tiny amount of bone each year, but the loss should be so small that it does not compromise bone strength.)

Initially, you should expect your rate of bone resorption to, at the very least, greatly slow down. Once your rate of bone turnover has stabilized at the normal level, you will begin increasing your bone mineral density as you will be building new bone.

Improvements in laboratory tests of bone resorption (bone loss) are typically seen within three to six months. Improvements in the DXA usually take longer to manifest—one to two years.

APPENDIX A

Lab Tests For Your Bones

IF YOU'VE BEEN FAITHFULLY following the bone-building program outlined in *Your Bones* for several months, you can confirm that it's working by running one of the following lab tests.

LABS THAT CAN HELP CONFIRM YOU ARE NO LONGER LOSING EXCESSIVE AMOUNTS OF BONE

24-Hour Urine Calcium Excretion

This test checks the amount of calcium that your kidneys are removing from your body via urine. Excreting excessive amounts of calcium is a sign that you are losing bone. You collect all your urine over a 24-hour period; you're given a large, special container in which to do so. You typically follow your normal diet and drink fluids as you normally would. You may be told not to drink alcohol during the collection. If you are taking certain medicines, such as diuretics or antacids, these may affect your test results, so be sure to mention this to your doctor before running this test. Many labs, including direct-to-consumer labs, offer the 24-hour urine calcium test.[415]

TESTS FOR MARKERS OF BONE RESORPTION

Bone resorption ("medspeak" for bone breakdown) tests measure the amount of certain bone proteins in the urine or blood (serum) that have been released from bone as a result of osteoclast activity. There are currently three such tests available: NTx, Dpd, and CTX. The serum CTX appears to be the most reliable of the three.

NTx

The NTx (N-terminal telopeptide, the full name is "amino-terminal collagen crosslinks") is measured in either urine or serum. This test reflects bone resorption by cathepsin K, an enzyme expressed by osteoclasts, or by matrix metalloproteinase (MMP), a family of enzymes involved in tissue remodeling. The problem with NTx is that while levels do fluctuate in response to bone resorption, they can vary spontaneously, particularly in urine, dropping as much as 50% from day to day with no treatment. To help correct for this, ask to have several days' worth of samples run and request the serum rather than the urine NTx test.[416]

DPyr

D-Pyr (the full name is "deoxypyridinoline," and you may also see this test referred to as D-Pyrilinks, Pyrilinks-D, deoxyPYD) is one of two pyridinium cross-links that provide structural stiffness to type I collagen found in bones. The other is pyridinoline (Pyr). While both pyridinoline and deoxypridinoline are released during the breakdown of collagen and are excreted in urine, pyridinoline is present in not only bone, but cartilage matrix and other connective tissues (except skin), while deoxypyridinoline is found in only in bone and dentin (the inner portion of teeth, immediately below teeth's enamel and above their pulp), so provides a more specific indicator of bone loss. Urinary Pyr and D-Pyr are elevated in patients not only in osteoporosis, but in bone diseases such as rheumatoid arthritis, osteoarthritis, hyperparathyroidism, hyperthyroidism, Paget's disease, and osteomalacia.[417]

CTX

The CTX or C-terminal telopeptide (the full name is "carboxy-terminal collagen crosslinks") test measures a specific crosslink peptide sequence of type I collagen that is found in bone: the portion cleaved by osteoclasts during bone resorption. Serum levels of this peptide sequence are proportional to osteoclastic activity at the time the blood sample is drawn. The test used to detect the CTX marker is called the Serum CrossLaps, and current research indicates that it is more specific to bone resorption than the other currently available tests.[418]

Initially, urinary levels of CTX were measured, but this was found to be no more reliable than urinary NTx values—both tests suffered from large spontaneous fluctuations unrelated to therapy or intervention. In contrast, the newer serum test for CTX levels shows minimal spontaneous disruption and high accuracy. Research comparing CTX to NTx and to Dpd, has found CTX to be the most accurate. [419]

LAB TESTS THAT MAY HELP IDENTIFY YOUR CAUSES OF EXCESSIVE BONE LOSS

If—despite faithfully following the bone-building program provided in *Your Bones* for two to three months—you are still excessively resorbing bone, the following lab tests may help you identify (and thus be able to naturally ameliorate or eliminate) the cause(s) of your continuing bone loss.

Vitamin D: 25-hydroxyvitamin D

As explained earlier,* vitamin D is required for calcium's absorption from the intestines and its resorption from the kidneys. Calcium is absorbed in the small intestine with the help of calbindin, a vitamin D-dependent calcium-binding protein inside the cells that form your intestinal epithelium (the lining of your intestines). 25-hydroxyvitamin D [abbreviated 25(OH)D], which you may also see referred to as calcifediol and calcidiol on your lab report, is a precursor to the hormonal form of vitamin D, and is produced in the liver when an hydroxyl group gets added to vitamin D_3 (cholecalciferol, the form of vitamin D produced in your skin when 7-dehydrocholesterol is exposed to sunlight, and the form it is recommended you take as a supplement). 25(OH)D is then sent into your bloodstream

---

* See "Vitamin D," pages 168–172.

and delivered to your kidneys, where it is converted into calcitriol (1,25-(OH)2D3), the hormonal form of vitamin D in which it's biologically active.

25(OH)D is what is measured in blood and is considered the most sensitive indicator of a person's vitamin D status. Optimal levels of 25(OH)D are now thought to be in the range of 60–80 ng/mL (which is equivalent to 150–200 nmol/L). Levels less than 32 ng/mL (80 nmol/L) indicate vitamin D deficiency. Ideally, you should have your 25(OH)D levels checked every 4–6 months since our needs for supplemental vitamin D typically lessen during the spring and summer months (when the UV index is greater than 3 in temperate regions, even in more northern latitudes, so we can produce vitamin D from the exposure of 7-dehydrocholesterol in our skin to sunlight), but increase during the fall and winter (when exposure to UVB ultraviolet light with an index greater than 3 decreases). You may find you need a higher dose of supplemental vitamin D_3 during the latter part of the fall, winter, and early spring.

Most any lab, including numerous direct-to-consumer labs, now runs the serum 25(OH)D.[420]

Undercarboxylated (Also Referred to As Uncarboxylated) Osteocalcin (unOC)

This blood test will let you know if you are getting sufficient vitamin K_2 to activate the vitamin K-dependent Gla-proteins: osteocalcin, which is essential for bone health, and matrix-Gla protein, which prevents calcification of soft tissue, i.e., blood vessels and organs.

As discussed on pages 172–199, vitamin K_2 is an essential nutrient for bones, promoting healthy bone rebuilding in a number of ways. Only after osteocalcin's been carboxylated (activated) by vitamin K_2 can it latch on to calcium and bind it to the hydroxyapatite crystals forming the bone matrix. (Think of carboxylation as adding a trailer hitch to K_2, so it can link up with calcium, allowing it to be towed into and attached to bone.)[421] Vitamin K_2 also teams up with vitamin D_3, which increases the production of Gla-proteins, including osteocalcin in osteoblasts (the cells that build bone), while also inhibiting the production of osteoclasts (the cells that break down bone).[422]

A normal prothrombin time (the test for clotting activity that has been the standard used to check vitamin K_1 adequacy) is not sufficient indication that enough vitamin K_2 is present to maintain bone osteocalcin activity. Request an osteocalcin test, actually a test for undercarboxylated (or uncarboxylated) osteocalcin or unOC. This will measure how much inactive osteocalcin is present in your blood. High levels of undercarboxylated (or uncarboxylated) osteocalin indicate you don't have enough vitamin K_2 around to activate sufficient osteocalcin to promote optimal bone health. Similarly, high levels of undercarboxylated matrix-Gla protein (MGP) indicate that not enough vitamin K_2 is available to protect against vascular calcification.

And now you can see why you really need enough K_2 on board when you are taking calcium and vitamin D! This is one of the reasons why recent studies have accused supplemental vitamin D and calcium of increasing risk for cardiovascular disease.[423] This is precisely what one would expect; it's simply the rules of human physiology at work, nothing mysterious. Vitamin D increases your body's ability to absorb calcium and also increases your production of the vitamin

K-dependent Gla-proteins whose job it is to put calcium into bone and keep it out of arteries, etc. Vitamin D does nothing more to help your body use calcium appropriately. Putting calcium into your bones and keeping it out of your arteries—whether that calcium comes from the food you eat or from supplements—is the job of proteins whose expression is increased by vitamin D, but whose activation requires vitamin K_2. If you take calcium and vitamin D, you must also provide your body with K_2 or the extra calcium you will absorb is just as likely to end up in your arteries as in your bones.[424]

A lab test assessing your levels of either unOC or uncarboxylated Matrix-Gla protein will let you know about your vitamin K_2 status, but only unOC has recently begun to be offered by a few cutting edge labs.[425]

White Blood Cell Micronutrient Analysis

This test provides an assessment of how well 35 different nutrients are actually functioning inside an individual's cells. A number of vitamins essential for bone formation and integrity are evaluated by this test, including vitamin D_3 (cholecalciferol), vitamin K_2 (only the MK-4 form*), the B vitamins (B_6, B_{12}, folate), and vitamin E. Minerals tested include calcium, magnesium, zinc, copper, manganese, and selenium. Also tested are key antioxidants, including alpha lipoic acid, coenzyme Q_{10}, and glutathione.

Nutrients work synergistically—for example, as already noted, vitamin D_3 increases calcium absorption,

---

* If you are supplementing with MK-7, you will need to also run the unOC test explained above, for accurate information about your K2 status.

while vitamin K regulates calcium's use in the body—so a deficiency even in a single, but especially in multiple nutrients, can affect the impact of other nutrients on your bones. Unlike traditional serum or urine tests, the process used by this micronutrient test evaluates the functioning of these vitamins, minerals, and antioxidants inside your own white blood cells, so personal differences in age, genetics, health, prescription drug usage, absorption rate, and other factors are automatically taken into consideration.

The white blood cell micronutrient test, offered by SpectraCell Laboratories, can be ordered directly by consumers as well as by physicians; however, for it to be covered by insurance, it must be ordered by a physician, and whether it will be covered depends upon the insurance carrier and the diagnosis code.[426]

Intact Parathyroid Hormone—Plus—Ionized Calcium

Taken together, the results of these two blood tests—one to evaluate your circulating levels of intact parathyroid hormone (iPTH, the most frequently ordered parathyroid hormone test)[427] and another to check your levels of ionized calcium—can reveal whether you have hyperparathyroidism, a condition in which your parathyroid glands are working overtime and pulling excessive amounts of calcium out of your bones.[428]

You have four tiny parathyroid glands in your neck (each is about the size of a grain of rice). Their job is to keep the calcium in your blood up to the right level because calcium is crucial for a wide range of essential body functions. When the level of ionized calcium (the metabolically active portion of calcium not bound to proteins in your bloodstream) is adequate, your parathyroid glands should be "asleep"; they should only "wake up" when needed. So, if your ionized calcium level is at the high end of normal or above, your iPTH level should be *very* low since parathyroid hormone secretion into your blood should not be occurring unless your calcium levels are too low. If both ionized calcium and iPTH levels are higher than normal, it is certain that you have hyperparathyroidism.

However, even if your iPTH levels are within normal range, you might still have overactive parathyroid glands. If, despite iPTH levels within normal range, your parathyroid glands have gone crazy and are pulling calcium out of your bones when they don't need to do so, your kidneys will be working overtime to pee it out, and this will be shown by a high level of calcium in a 24-Hour Urine test (discussed above).

So, to be sure your parathyroid glands are not causing your bone loss, you need to run the tests to check ionized calcium and iPTH levels in your blood, plus a 24-hour urine calcium excretion test (explained above) to see how much calcium your kidneys are clearing out. Since your family doctor may not be familiar with the necessity to interpret all three of these tests together, it might be best to consult with an endocrinologist.

If these test results are abnormal, then the question becomes, is it primary or secondary hyperparathyroidism?

As explained on pages 114–117, primary hyperparathyroidism is relatively rare (prevalence of primary hyperparathyroidism has been estimated to be 3 in 1,000 in the general population, but as high as 21 in 1,000 in postmenopausal women. It is almost exactly three times as common in women as men.)[429] Most often, it is due to a benign tumor. Once the offending parathyroid tumor is removed, your bone density should quickly begin to improve since an overactive parathyroid will not be constantly draining calcium from your bones. For lots more information about hyperparathyroidism, an excellent resource is www. parathyroid.com.

Secondary hyperparathyroidism* may result from insufficient consumption of calcium, vitamin D deficiency, chronic kidney or liver disease, or hypochlorhydria (low levels of stomach acid, which is quite common after age 50, and may be caused at any age by other factors, such as a *helicobacter pylori* infection or the chronic use of acid-blocking drugs.[†]

If parathyroid hormone levels are within the normal range, despite vitamin D deficiency, this may indicate magnesium insufficiency. If you are deficient in magnesium, you may not produce parathyroid hormone in response to low blood calcium, even if your vitamin D level, and therefore your ability to absorb the calcium you consume from food or supplements, is very low.[430] To check, you can request one of the magnesium tests described next.

Buccal Smear or Red Blood Cell Magnesium

The best tests to assess your magnesium status are the buccal smear intracellular magnesium and the SpectraCell micronutrient test (discussed above); next best available test is the RBC (Red Blood Cell) Magnesium. The Buccal Smear test involves swabbing epithelial

---

* As explained beginning on page 114.

† See page 136.

cells from the inside lining of your cheek; the RBC test requires a blood draw.

The test most doctors run checks serum levels of magnesium, but a serum test gives a very inaccurate appraisal of your actual magnesium status because only about 1% of your body's magnesium is stored in serum; the remaining 99% is found inside your cells where it does its work. Thus, a "normal" blood serum magnesium does not necessarily mean you are not magnesium deficient. You can have apparently adequate levels in serum, but be seriously deficient inside your cells where it counts. Only very severe cases of magnesium deficiency will show up in blood serum.

The Buccal Smear test will show you how much magnesium was inside your cells working for you when the sample was taken. An RBC test for magnesium will provide an indication of the average amount of magnesium that has been present inside your cells over the prior four months.

You will need to ask your doctor to order Buccal Smear testing as this is not yet provided by direct-to-consumer labs.[431]

You can order a Red Blood Cell magnesium test directly from a number of online labs.[432]

Iodine

Iodine is required for the production of thyroid hormones. Under production of thyroid hormones (hypothyroidism) causes bone loss. So does overproduction of thyroid hormones (hyperthyroidism).

You have two good options to check your iodine levels: a 24-hour urine collection[433] or a finger prick blood test.[434]

Urinary iodine concentration (UI) is a sensitive indicator of recent iodine intake (days) since more than 90% of dietary iodine is excreted in the urine. Random urine sampling is often used, but a 24-hour urine collection is recommended since this will obviously provide a better evaluation. According to WHO standards, 50–99 mcg/L indicates mild deficiency, 20–49 mcg/L indicates moderate deficiency, and <20 mcg/L indicates severe deficiency.

A thyroglobulin (Tg) test may be an even better choice since it is a much more convenient, simple blood test (Tg can also be assayed on dried blood spots taken by a finger prick) and provides a good assessment of iodine status over weeks or even months. When you have enough iodine, small amounts of Tg are secreted into your bloodstream; blood levels of Tg are normally <10 mcg/L.[435]

BONE-BUILDING, AND POTENTIALLY BONE-BUSTING, HORMONES

The 24-Hour Comprehensive Urine Hormone Test[436]

In addition to parathyroid hormone (discussed above), a wide variety of other hormones and their metabolites, if out of normal range, can contribute to bone loss. This comprehensive lab test is the most accurate, simplest and cost-effective way to check, with just one test, your levels of all of them. Some of the key reasons why the 24-Hour Comprehensive Urine Hormone test is more accurate than blood or saliva testing are discussed below.[437]

Hormones that affect bone remodeling include the following:

Cortisol and Cortisone

Cortisol is a hormone (more specifically a glucocorticoid) produced by the adrenal glands in response to stress. Cortisol is part of our "fight or flight" response; it gets you ready to do combat with (or run away from) all the saber-toothed tigers in your life (whether they be emotional/mental [scary or worrying thoughts], or physical [including, you are attacked by the Standard American Diet—no kidding, subsisting on the processed "food-like" items sold in our grocery stores and fast food joints raises cortisol levels]).[438]

Cortisone is the inactive form of cortisol and serves as a "cortisol savings account" in your body. When you need more cortisol, you withdraw some of your cortisone "savings" and convert it into cortisol "cash."

Cortisol's primary functions are to increase your blood sugar (you might need to power up your muscles to run away); suppress your immune system (not essential when dealing with tigers); and aid in fat, protein, and carbohydrate metabolism (more energy sources for those muscles). It also decreases bone formation (an even longer term health issue than your immune function). High levels of cortisol suppress osteoblasts, preventing their synthesis of new bone, and interfere with absorption of calcium from the gastrointestinal tract. This is why, as discussed on pages 134–136, the various patent medicine synthetic forms of cortisol ("pseudo-cortisol"), used to treat a variety of diseases, so rapidly cause bone loss.

Chronic stress—unless you have healthful ways of neutralizing it (like exercise, meditation, prayer, snuggling with your sweetie, etc.)—can result in chronically elevated levels of cortisol, which will significantly increase your risk for osteoporosis. Eventually, you will have emptied all the reserves from your "cortisone savings account," so you won't be able to maintain normal levels of cortisol. This is called "adrenal exhaustion," and is unfortunately very common nowadays and also contributes to "low turnover" osteoporosis.[439]

In addition, cortisol affects thyroid metabolism. It's a "Goldilocks" kind of hormone; you want the right amount, not too much or too little. Either too much or too little cortisol inhibits, while normal levels promote, the conversion of the thyroid hormone thyroxine (T4) to triiodothyronine (T3). T4 is only about one-third as active as T3, so not having a cortisol level that would satisfy Goldilocks can significantly contribute to hypothyroidism. And lots of us middle-aged or older adults have subclinical hypothyroidism. Its reported prevalence in US adults is between 3.9 and 6.5% of the population.[440]

This leads us to thyroid hormone.

Thyroid Hormone

Thyroid issues are complicated, so bear with us here. Bottom line: the 24-hour comprehensive urine hormone test will provide your doctor with the information needed to help you.

The medical experts define subclinical hypothyroidism as a condition of "mild thyroid failure characterized by normal levels of T3 and T4 with moderately elevated serum TSH of between 5 and 10 mU/L." TSH, which stands for thyroid stimulating hormone, is the hormone that tells the thyroid gland to produce T4, and then T3, which stimulates the metabolism of almost every tissue in the body (including your bones). Many individuals with subclinical hypothyroidism are treated with thyroid hormone replacement (using the patent medicine, levothyroxine), but they are now finding that unless the dosage of levothyroxine is just right (Goldilocks again), this treatment can contribute to osteoporosis. If the dose is too low, you still have hypothyroidism. If the dose is too high, it's as if you had hyperthyroidism. Either situation contributes to bone loss.[441]

A blood (serum) test is the best option for checking your TSH levels because TSH is a protein and therefore does not show up in urine in significant quantities if your kidneys are functioning normally. Nonetheless, the 24-Hour Urine will give you a much better idea of whether your thyroid hormones are doing their work inside your cells than a blood test for TSH.[442]

Here's why.

T4 is the major form of thyroid hormone in the blood, but T3 is the active hormone (three to four times more potent than T4), primarily responsible for regulating the metabolic machinery inside your cells. The ratio of T4 to T3 released into the blood is roughly 20 to 1. In your 24-Hour Urine test results, you want to see higher levels of T3 than T4.

If your results are not optimal, here are some potential reasons why, which you can discuss with your doctor:

- *You may need more iodine.* Both T4 and T3 are formed from a combination of tyrosine plus iodine (to make T4, your body needs 4 iodine molecules, and 3 iodine molecules are needed for T3). If you are not getting enough iodine, your body will not be able to make thyroid hormones. To determine if this is an issue for you, you can ask your doctor to run one of the tests (discussed above under "Iodine") that check your iodine status.

- **You may need more selenium.** Even if your TSH is effectively signaling your thyroid gland to make hormones, and you have enough iodine to create them, the conversion of T4 to T3 may not be happening inside your cells for several reasons. T4 gets converted to the T3 inside our cells by enzymes in which the trace mineral, selenium, is an essential part. If you are not getting enough selenium, these enzymes won't work, so you will not be able to convert T4 to T3, and you will have functional hypothyroidism.

- **You may have been so stressed out for so long that your cortisol reserves are depleted.** As noted above, you gotta have cortisol to convert T4 to T3; long-term stress, which depletes your adrenal reserves of cortisone, will therefore cause inhibition of the T4 to T3 conversion. The 24-Hour Urine will let you know what your cortisol/cortisone status is.

- **If you've got a whole lotta chronic inflammation going on**, your body will be producing inflammatory messenger molecules (such as the cytokine, interleukin-2) that promote the formation of autoantibodies to the thyroid, and these will inhibit conversion of T4 to T3.

So, as you can see, despite having normal blood levels of thyroid hormones, a person can be functionally hypothyroid—and this can contribute to bone loss. If you have the 24-Hour Comprehensive Urine Hormone test run, you and your doctor will get a much better indication of what is happening inside your cells, so you can fix what's off (and causing your bone loss).

DHEA

Produced in the adrenals, DHEA is the most abundant steroid in the human body. Levels peak between 25 to 30 years of age and then decline. DHEA is first converted into androstenedione, and then may be used to produce testosterone and its metabolites (for which reason DHEA replacement may boost libido in women) or estrone, and thus other estrogens.[443]

DHEA helps build new bone tissue, primarily through its indirect elevation of serum levels of estradiol, and has been shown to significantly improve bone mineral density in older adults. Low levels are associated with increased risk of fracture and osteoporosis.[444]

Estrogens in Women

Women's bodies produce dozens of types of estrogens. The three types of estrogen often considered as "principal" or "classical" estrogens are estrone (E1), estradiol (E2), and estriol (E3). The 24-Hour Comprehensive Urine Hormone test evaluates levels of these three forms of estrogen plus many of their metabolites.

- **Estrone (E1)**: is one of the most potent estrogens and the most abundant estrogen in postmenopausal women. Estrone is a major source of local bioactive estrogen formation in bone and plays an important role in maintaining bone, especially in postmenopausal women.

  In our bodies, estrone is converted into metabolites that play both cancer-preventive and potentially cancer-promoting roles. Estrone's potentially cancer-causing metabolites are 4-hydroxyestrone (4-OH estrone, the most carcinogenic estrogen metabolite) and 16α-OH estrone (which we need in small amounts because it is involved in building bone). Estrone's protective metabolites are 2-hydroxyestrone (2-OH estrone), 2-methoxyestrone (2-CH₃O-estrone) and estriol (E3). Levels of all of these are checked in the 24-Hour Comprehensive Urine Hormone test. If your estrogens or estrogen metabolites are found to not be in healthful (bone-building but not cancer-promoting) balance, a knowledgeable physician can help you safely restore healthy balance naturally using diet, supplements and (if desired) bio-identical hormone replacement.

- **Estradiol (E2)**: is the most active estrogen and the primary "estrogen" used in conventional hormone replacement (HRT). [Actually, conventional HRT uses estrogens way more potent than human estrogens that are taken from the urine of pregnant horses, which is why this patent medicine is called Premarin® (pregnant mares' urine)]. In humans, estradiol is produced from both estrone and testosterone. Estradiol also readily converts to estrone. Small amounts of estradiol are also produced in the adrenal cortex, adipose (fat) tissue, brain, arterial wall and, in men, in the testes. Unless converted to estrone, estradiol is metabolized into protective 2-OH estradiol and 2-methoxyestradiol (2-CH₃0 estradiol).

- **Estriol (E3)**: Derived from estrone through the intermediate (bone-building but potentially cancer-promoting) 16α-OH estrone, estriol is one of the weaker estrogens, but has anti-proliferative (anti-cancer) effects in estrogen sensitive tissues (e.g., breast and uterus).

2/16α Ratio

The ratio of 2-hydroxyestrone (2-OH E1) to 16α-hydroxyestrone (16α-OH E1) is an indicator of an individual's risk of developing breast cancer (women) or prostate cancer (men). (To be very precise, the "2/16α" is associated with cancer risk in premenopausal women. It's likely also associated with cancer risk in postmenopausal women using BHRT but not yet proven to be so. In men, the "2/16α" approaches, but does not quite achieve statistical significance for prostate cancer risk; however, an elevated 16α-OH E1 does have statistical significance, for prostate cancer risk. 2-OH E1, a metabolite of estrone, has weak estrogenic activity and is associated with protection against breast and prostate cancer. 16α-OH E1, also an estrone metabolite, stimulates cell division and proliferation, and is associated with increased risk of breast, endometrial, and prostate cancer. However, as mentioned above, 16α-OH estrone is also involved in bone-building, so you need some. Very low levels indicate increased risk for osteopenia/osteoporosis in both women and men.

The ideal 2/16α Ratio range is 2 to 4. A 2/16α Ratio of >2 indicates increased risk for positive and negative estrogen receptor breast cancer, prostate cancer (as noted in the preceding paragraph), cervical cancer, ovarian cancer, and laryngeal cancer. A 2/16α Ratio of <4 indicates increased risk for osteopenia, osteoporosis.

Fortunately, the 2/16α ratio is highly modifiable with natural interventions. Estrone's conversion to (pro-carcinogenic) 16α-OH E1 is promoted by obesity, hypothyroidism, pesticides, alcohol, and cimetidine (another reason not to take this stomach acid blocker patent medicine, trade name, Tagamet®*). Conversion to (protective) 2-OH E1 is promoted by two phytochemicals in cruciferous vegetables, such as broccoli, cauliflower, etc.; Indole-3-carbinol (I3C) and 3,3'-Diindolylmethane (DIM) DIM, a compound derived from our digestion of crucifers containing I3C. In addition to the consumption of cruciferous vegetables, estrone's conversion to protective 2-OH-E1 is also promoted by exercise, flax, soy, and omega-3 fatty acids.[†]

Progesterone

Progesterone opposes, modulates and balances estrogen's effects, not only in the uterus but in our breasts, brain, bones, urinary tract, and skin. If unopposed by progesterone, estrogen can excessively stimulate cell growth in the breast and lining of the uterus, which can increase risk for cancer.

Among its many and widespread beneficial functions, bio-identical progesterone (but not the patent medicines called "progestins") activates osteoblasts to build bone, acts as a natural anti-depressant and diuretic agent, normalizes blood clotting and helps regulate thyroid function. Also, since progesterone is the precursor of the glucocorticoids (e.g., cortisol), low levels of progesterone can significantly contribute to adrenal fatigue. [445]

---

* The stomach acid-blocking patent medicines are discussed on pages 136–137.

† More reasons to eat the whole foods bone-building diet described in Chapter 3, "What You Don't Know Can Give You Osteoporosis."

In the 24-Hour Comprehensive Urine Hormone test, progesterone levels are evaluated by checking those of pregnanediol, an inactive progesterone metabolite whose levels in urine give an indirect (but accurate) measure of progesterone levels in the body. Pregnanediol is used since progesterone's structure prevents it from being eliminated in urine in significant quantities.

Evaluating levels of all of these hormones can also be very helpful in pre-menopausal women with a bone health concern. From our teens throughout the rest of our lives, not just our estrogens and progesterone, but our DHEA, cortisol, and thyroid hormones are very important to bone health. In menstruating women, low levels of estrogen or progesterone can hinder development of optimal peak bone mass. Premenopausal women with amenorrhea (no period) have lower estradiol levels and lower bone mineral density (BMD) and/or lose bone rapidly. Even premenopausal women with apparently "normal" menstrual cycles may not be developing optimal peak bone mass because they are not ovulating each month. Progesterone is produced by the corpus luteum, which forms *after* ovulation, so if a woman does not ovulate, her progesterone levels will be low. A number of studies have now suggested that progesterone supplementation may be indicated for pre- or perimenopausal women with regular, estrogen-sufficient menstrual cycles who, however, are also experiencing ovulatory disturbances [either not ovulating or having short luteal phase (the part of the menstrual cycle when progesterone is secreted) cycles]. A significant number of menstruating women (as many as 25% of premenopausal women in the US and Canada) may be experiencing subclinical ovulatory disturbances that result in their not producing progesterone despite having regular, asymptomatic menstrual cycles. [446]

Furthermore, some of the newer contraceptive options for premenopausal women, such as the Mirena® IUD, result in amenorrhea (lack of periods, which means lack of ovulation, which means lack of progesterone production, which means lack of osteoblast activation). This is of serious concern since young women are supposed to be building up their lifetime reserve of bone mass by their early 30s. This long-term side effect has not shown up in the published research *yet*. The young premenopausal women using this IUD are not going to quickly become osteopenic. It takes years for bone loss to result in osteopenia/osteoporosis, but since they are not going to be building up their maximal levels of bone mass, when they reach their late 40s to early 50s (the perimenopausal/menopausal years), these young women are going to be at significantly increased risk for osteoporosis. [447]

Men's Bone-Building Sex Hormones:
Testosterone, Estrogen

Low testosterone is a common cause of osteoporosis in men, and men's testosterone levels are usually checked if excessive bone loss is occurring. As previously discussed,* men's bones also require estrogen.

However, checking a man's testosterone levels in serum (blood) does not provide sufficient information. For example, if you are a man over age 50 and your serum (blood) test results indicate your total testosterone is at normal levels, you may still be experiencing an

---

* See page 88.

increased risk of not only osteoporosis, but cardiovascular disease and depression, along with loss of muscle and libido, prostate enlargement, and/or erectile dysfunction—if most of your testosterone is bound to sex hormone binding globulin (SHBG). This becomes increasingly likely after age 50, the age at which testosterone levels typically begin to decline, while levels of SHBG increase. The 24-Hour Comprehensive Urine Hormone test will let you know how much of your testosterone is free, and how much is conjugated (bound to SHBG).[448]

If your free testosterone is low, supplementing with bio-identical testosterone should be done cautiously in men with type 2 diabetes, a family history of type 2 diabetes, or with signs of symptoms of "metabolic syndrome," which include central obesity ("belly fat"), high cholesterol and/or triglycerides, high blood pressure, and osteoarthritis. If any of these apply, then testing for insulin resistance (also a part of "metabolic syndrome") is important before starting supplemental testosterone. An overactive "insulin signal"—the body's natural accompaniment to insulin resistance—is the principal cause of overactive conversion of testosterone to estrogen, called "hyper-aromatization." "Hyper-aromatization" can most often be reversed by diet and supplement changes to reverse insulin resistance and the high insulin signal. Excessive aromatization, in addition to its "feminizing" effects, can increase prostate cancer risk because estradiol can be metabolized to estrone, which can then be converted to either protective 2-hydroxyestrone (2-OH) Estriol (E3) or into potentially pro-carcinogenic 16α-OH estrone.

On the other hand, insufficient aromatization not only promotes bone loss in men since some 16α-OH is required for bone remodeling, but has recently been shown to promote prostate cancer by inhibiting the production of another testosterone metabolite called 3β-adiol. A 24-Hour Comprehensive Urine Hormone test will let your doctor know, not only your levels of free testosterone, but if you are producing enough, but not too much, 16α-OH for healthy bones.

For men's bone health, a little bit of testosterone should be being converted into estradiol, an even smaller amount of which should be metabolized into 16α-OH estrone. Production of either too much or too little estrogen (and therefore too much or too little 16α-OH estrone) is easy to correct with natural diet, supplement and exercise interventions. A full explanation of all of these will be provided to your physician along with the results of this test.

TESTS TO CHECK FOR EXCESSIVE INFLAMMATION

High Sensitivity C-Reactive Protein (hsCRP)

C-reactive protein (CRP) is a protein found in the blood, levels of which rise in response to inflammation (for the technically inclined, it's an acute phase protein our livers churn out in response to immune cells' production of pro-inflammatory cytokines like the interleukins IL-1, IL-6 and IL-8, and TNF-α.)

CRP is a known predictor of risk for cardiovascular disease, e.g., heart attack and stroke. Recently, studies have also shown a clear link between above normal levels of C-reactive protein and risk for fracture. In Japan, where women typically have substantially lower levels of CRP than their Caucasian counterparts, women whose CRP levels were above what is normal for the Japanese had more than double the risk for fracture (2.22, if in the medium quartile, and 2.40, if in the quartile with this highest CRP levels).[449]

There are two different tests for C-reactive protein, one called "CRP" and one called "hs-CRP". CRP is the standard test, which measures a much wider, higher range of CRP levels but does not do well in capturing the lower ranges, which are those you want to check to see if low-level, chronic inflammation is contributing to your bone loss. hs-CRP (high-sensitivity CRP) is the test that accurately detects these lower concentrations of C-reactive protein.

People with chronic inflammation, for example individuals with inflammatory conditions, like arthritis or periodontal disease, should have the CRP, not hs-CRP test run. Their CRP levels will be very high—often too high to be measured or meaningful using the hs-CRP test. Both tests measure the same molecule in the blood. The hs-CRP test is for apparently healthy people to determine if they have low-grade chronic inflammation. It measures CRP in the range from 0.5 to 10 mg/L. The standard CRP test measures CRP in the range from 10 to 1000 mg/L.

Hs-CRP usually is ordered as one of several tests in a cardiovascular risk profile, often along with tests for cholesterol and triglycerides since the best way to predict cardiovascular risk is to combine a good marker for inflammation, like hs-CRP, along with the lipid profile.[450] Research has now shown that "healthy" people whose hs-CRP results are in the high end of the normal range (above 3.0 mg/L) have 1.5 to 4 times the risk of having a heart attack compared to those whose hs-CRP values are at the low end of the normal range 1.0 mg/L or less.

Because the hs-CRP test serves as a marker for inflammation, it is important that you are not just getting over a cold, flu, other infection or injury when you run this test. As noted above, CRP is an acute phase protein, so levels dramatically rise in response to any recent illness, infection, or trauma (including dental work). For this reason, any acute inflammation will raise the amount of CRP and give a falsely elevated estimate of risk. Also, don't take a nonsteroidal anti-inflammatory drug (NSAID) as these patent medicines, like aspirin, ibuprofen, and naproxen, or taking statins may temporarily reduce CRP levels in your blood, giving a falsely lowered estimate of risk.

Women on conventional hormone replacement therapy with patent medicines such as Premarin®, Provera®, etc., (but *not* bio-identical hormone replacement therapy) have been shown to have elevated hs-CRP levels, yet another reason to use BHRT and not conventional HRT.

Homocysteine

A potentially bone-destroying amino acid, produced as an intermediate compound part way through an essential cellular process called methylation,* homocysteine is either immediately converted into other, harmless compounds with the help of the B vitamins, vitamin B_{12}, vitamin B_6 and folate—or accumulates inside cells, eventually spilling out into the bloodstream from which it goes everywhere in our bodies, causing damage to all it touches, including our bones.

For the technically inclined, the thiol groups in homocysteine undergo autooxidation, a process in which reactive oxygen species (a type of free radicals)

---

* Discussed on pages 99–101.

form and produce other free radicals that produce even more free radicals. The end result is an unhappy state for our bones (and everything else) called oxidative stress. The increase in oxidative stress leads to damage to the lining (endothelium) of our blood vessels, causing endothelial dysfunction, decreased blood flow to bone, reduced oeteoblast activity, increased osteoclast activity, and damaging interactions with extracellular matrix proteins (collagen). In sum, it's a metabolic pachinko game in which many threads of dysfunction come together to promote osteoporosis.[451]

Even mildly elevated levels of homocysteine have been shown to lower BMD in the femur.[452] If, despite consuming the amounts of B_{12}, B_6 and folate recommended for the mythical "average" person from your diet and supplements,* your homocysteine levels are still elevated, you most likely need more of these nutrients than "average." Or your genetic inheritance may include one or more slow enzymes for the conversion of these B vitamins into their activated forms, in which case, you may need to supplement with their activated forms.†

Many labs test homocysteine levels.[453]

Gluten Intolerance: Celiac Disease, Wheat Allergy, Gluten Sensitivity Tests

Not just full-blown, but "sub-clinical" celiac disease, wheat allergy, or even what is now being recognized as an unhappy response to wheat protein called "gluten sensitivity," causes inflammation in the intestine.

---

* Discussed on pages 99–105.

† Discussed on pages 346–347.

(For the technically inclined, celiac disease is an auto-immune condition; wheat allergy is an IgE-mediated adaptive immune system response; while gluten sensitivity invokes a response from our innate immune system.) In all three forms of gluten intolerance, however, an inflammatory cascade is triggered that promotes bone loss, both by activating osteoclasts and by causing malabsorption of many bone-critical nutrients, including the fat-soluble vitamins, D, K, and A, plus amino acids, and many essential minerals.

The latest research papers are reporting that the classic symptoms associated with adult celiac disease (nutrient malabsorption, diarrhea and weight loss) are much less common than more subtle indicators of celiac disease, such as unexplained iron deficiency anemia, unexplained gastro-intestinal symptoms, fatigue, asymptomatic iron deficiency, bone loss, neurologic disease, dyspepsia (indigestion), non-specific abdominal symptoms, dermatitis herpetiformis, and malignancies.[454]

In a study conducted in the UK, less than half of the patients found to have celiac disease had any of its classical symptoms. Osteoporosis was the most common complication related to celiac disease. Among the patients in this study, 28% were found to have osteoporosis (T score <-2.5), and another 31% to have osteopenia (T score <-1.0.) One woman had developed hyperparathyroidism as a result of wheat intolerance. Thyroid disorders, particularly hypothyroidism, were also found to be commonly related to celiac disease, but the most common symptom in these patients was anemia, which was present in 66%.

In other words, just because you do not have the "classical symptoms" of celiac disease, this does not mean your bones are not being damaged by your body's reactions to gluten, the key protein in wheat. The average age at which the women in the aforementioned study learned that wheat was causing their bone loss, anemia and/or hypothyroidism was 53.2 years; some were in their 40s, others in their 60s. The good news is that a gluten-free diet has been shown to increase BMD in persons who are gluten intolerant.

A number of blood (serological) tests, available at many labs,[455] can be run to try to confirm whether wheat is a cause of your bone loss:

- *anti-IgE antibodies* indicate wheat allergy.

- *IgA autoantibodies to anti-tissue transglutaminase/anti-endomysium/anti-gliadin antibodies* (abbreviated as tTG/EMA/dAGA), indicates an auto-immune reaction to gluten. One caveat here: many people with celiac disease have an IgA deficiency, so relying on the presence of autoantibodies to IgA won't work for them. Recently, deamidated gliadin peptides (DGP) antibodies (especially of the IgG class) have been introduced with sensitivity and specificity comparable to anti-tTG and anti-EMA, but with more accurate performance in people who are IgA-deficient.

- *Human Leukocyte Antigen (HLA)-DQ2 and/or HLA-DQ8 haplotypes*—a haplotype is a combination of alleles (DNA sequences) at adjacent locations (loci) on a chromosome that are transmitted together. The haplotypes HLA-DQ2 and HLA-DQ8 are part of many people's genetic inheritance. They are cell surface receptor proteins found on white blood cells that serve as "antigen presenting cells." These are special immune cells that present antigens to T cells, which are then activated. (T cells are key players in our adaptive immune system, the part of our immune system that remembers formerly seen threats, so can quickly develop defenses that specifically target them.)

The problem is that, even if none of these blood tests come back positive, you could still be among the estimated 10% of the population who have an adverse (pro-inflammatory and potentially bone-damaging) reaction to gluten.[456] This leads us to one more, potentially more sensitive test:

The SIgA Stool Test

Why run a stool test to identify gluten/gliadin sensitivity? Because the blood tests for antigliadin and antiendomysial/antitissue transglutaminase antibodies are only routinely positive after damage to the intestinal villi (the finger-like projections on the inner surface of our intestines, which increase our ability to absorb digested nutrients 30- to 60-fold) is extensive. Only if you have full blown, untreated celiac disease will you certainly have IgA antibodies to gliadin in your blood as well as inside your intestines, where the gliadin/gluten containing foods are digested.

Evidence of an immune reaction to gluten in gluten-sensitive individuals who do not have villous atrophy (the vast majority) will only be revealed in a test that checks for antigliadin IgA antibodies where gluten/gliadin containing foods are first encountered: inside your intestinal tract, not in your blood.

This makes sense. The immune system in your intestines is going to do everything it can to keep something it sees as a noxious invader inside your intestines and neutralize it there, preventing it from penetrating into your bloodstream. To do so, your intestinal immune system will mount a defense with T cells and lymphocytes on and within the lining of your intestines (intestinal epithelium), and with secretory IgA (SIgA), a special form of IgA containing a component that enables it to be secreted from the lining right into your intestines.

The SIgA Stool Test, offered by EnteroLab, checks for antigliadin IgA antibodies excreted naturally in the stool. They combine the test for antigliadin IgA antibodies with a malabsorption test (also using the same stool specimen) and HLA gene testing, for which the sample is derived from a cotton-tipped swab rubbed inside your mouth. In Dr. Wright's clinical experience with hundreds of patients, he has found this form of testing to be more accurate than any other lab test for "hidden" gliadin/gluten sensitivity.[457]

The Very Best Test—Eliminate Wheat from Your Diet and See How YOU Feel

Especially if the cost of testing is an issue, why not just eliminate wheat and other gluten-containing grains from your diet and see how you respond? It's surprisingly easy as a wide variety of great-tasting gluten-free foods are now readily available. Ultimately, going gluten-free for a few months is the only absolutely certain way to know whether YOU are gluten-sensitive. If you feel healthier, if various symptoms (headache, fatigue, digestive disturbances, arthritic and skin complaints, etc.), lessen or go away, then you can be sure wheat is not your bones' friend. And more to the point regarding our main concern here, within 4–6 weeks of following a completely gluten-free diet, running one of the bone resorption tests described above should confirm your bone loss has slowed or halted.

APPENDIX B

Vitamin and Mineral Essentials for Healthy Bones

F OR OPTIMAL BONE HEALTH, your diet—plus supplements, including a high quality multiple vitamin and mineral supplement, which is highly recommended for everyone—must provide the following vitamins and minerals. Preferred forms, "average" dosage requirements and key special considerations are noted for each.

The daily doses recommended are necessarily "average" because each of us is unique, so our needs for certain nutrients, such as vitamin D_3 for example, may vary considerably. This list will give you the basics. Consider it a good place to *begin* determining YOUR optimal bone-building vitamin and mineral requirements.

BONE-BUILDING MINERALS

Calcium

For individuals aged 31–50 years, 1,000 milligrams/day; for those aged 51 and older, 1,200 milligrams/day. Calcium citrate and calcium derived from sea-algae are preferable to calcium carbonate.*

Magnesium

250 milligrams twice daily (in one of its chelated forms, e.g., as magnesium citrate, malate or aspartate). If you develop loose stools, try taking each dose of magnesium with 25 milligrams of pyridoxal-5-phosphate. P5P is the activated form of B_6 and is the form in which B_6 is responsible for getting magnesium inside your cells (see pages 224–232). If you still continue to experience "gastrointestinal hurry," which leads to nutrient malabsorption, reduce your supplemental magnesium dose to 200 milligrams daily, in divided doses if possible.

Boron

3 milligrams/day, some of which may be already provided by your multiple vitamin and mineral supplement.[†]

Zinc

15–20 milligrams/day, preferably in the form of zinc picolinate. Although the current recommended daily intake for zinc is just 8 milligrams/day in women and 11

---

* See pages 209–222.

† See pages 223–224.

milligrams/day in men, 35–45% of Americans aged 60 and older are not consuming this much zinc, unless they are taking zinc in a supplement. The amount of supplemental zinc associated with increases in BMD in postmenopausal women is 15 milligrams/day.[458] Zinc's special relationship with copper requires that you also get at least 1 milligram/day of copper from food and supplements when consuming 15 milligrams of zinc/day. Your multiple vitamin and mineral may provide these amounts of zinc and copper.*

Copper

1–3 milligrams/day. In addition to its special relationship with zinc,[†] copper is a cofactor for lysyl oxidase, the enzyme required to initiate cross-linking of collagen and elastin, a key step in new bone formation.[459]

Manganese

As manganese citrate, 5 milligrams/day. Manganese is needed for the biosynthesis of mucopolysaccharides (an important component of connective tissue and also used in bone matrix formation), and is a required cofactor for several enzymes in bone tissue. Without manganese, these enzymes cannot function. Manganese deficiency has also been shown in animal studies to significantly lower—by 66%—levels of IGF-1 (insulin-like growth factor-1), which is essential for bone growth.[460]

In a two-year study involving healthy older postmenopausal women (average age 66 years), when manganese (5 milligrams/day) was provided, in combination with

* See pages 232–239.

† See page 238.

calcium (calcium citrate malate, 1,000 mg elemental Ca/day), copper (2.5 mg/day), and zinc (15 mg/day), the result was a significantly greater gain in BMD than when calcium alone was given. In the women receiving only calcium, spinal BMD dropped (-1.25); in contrast, the women given calcium and trace minerals had a +1.48 gain in their spinal BMD.[461]

Molybdenum

As molybdenum amino acid chelate, 50 micrograms. Molybdenum is a major cofactor for the enzymes our bodies produce to metabolize sulfur compounds. These enzymes include sulfite oxidase. Sulfite oxidase is required to metabolize the sulfur-containing essential amino acids cysteine and methionine in foods. Cysteine, in turn, is required for the production of the body's most important internally produced antioxidant: glutathione. When our glutathione levels drop, we are unable to neutralize free radicals and other pro-inflammatory compounds. Our inflammation levels skyrocket—and among numerous other unpleasant results, osteoclasts' activity increases.

If you are sensitive to sulfite preservatives (in wines, dried fruits, salad bars), this may indicate a molybdenum insufficiency. Also, burning coal to produce energy produces the pollutant, sulfur dioxide, which our bodies detoxify using sulfite oxidase. If you live in an area where coal is mined and used as an energy source, having enough molybdenum on board may help protect not only your bones from osteoporosis, but your lungs from asthma.[462]

Silicon

As silicon amino acid chelate, 10 milligrams/day. Silicon is a common component of the diet found mainly in plant-based foods (cereal grains and some fruits and vegetables), drinking water (especially mineral water) and some alcoholic beverages, notably beer. In studies using human osteoblast precursor cells, silicon (which, for the technically inclined, is absorbed from water and digested food as orthosilicic acid, its soluble form) has been shown to stimulate collagen type 1 synthesis in human osteoblast-like cells and to enhance the development of osteoblasts.[463]

Recent studies suggest silicon may be more helpful for women who are premenopausal or on bio-identical hormone replacement and for men since it appears to interact with estrogen to impact bone health. Men do produce a little estrogen, which plays a very important role in maintaining their bones.[*464]

Selenium

As seleno L-methionine, 50 micrograms/day. Selenium is a cofactor for several enzymes essential for keeping inflammation in check. These include the antioxidant enzymes glutathione peroxidase and thioredoxin reductase, and also three of the four known types of thyroid hormone deiodinases, whose job is to activate and then deactivate various thyroid hormones. As discussed above in relation to molybdenum, glutathione is crucial for keeping inflammation under control.[†]

---

* See pages 128–129.

† The ways in which dysfunctional thyroid hormone production or activity contribute to bone loss are discussed on pages 114–117.

Strontium Citrate

680 milligrams/day of elemental strontium until initial improvement is seen then reduce to the 200–400 milligram/day range. Take strontium citrate several hours before or after consuming dietary or supplemental calcium. These two minerals compete for absorption. Calcium will win. Thus, to receive maximum benefit from your strontium citrate supplement, take it several hours before or after consuming calcium.*

BONE-BUILDING VITAMINS

Vitamin D₃

2,000—5,000 IU per day—or more depending upon genetic issues (e.g., vitamin D receptor SNPs that result in poorly formed cell receptors for vitamin D), latitude at which you reside (the further north or south of the Earth's equator, the fewer months during the year during which sun exposure will produce vitamin D in your skin), digestive function (impaired digestion results in lowered absorption of nutrients as does gastric bypass surgery,[†] your weight (being obese increases your vitamin D requirements) plus a number of other factors.[‡] Since 2,000 IU/day is very infrequently enough to achieve the "tropical optimum" blood levels of 60–100 ng/mL, we suggest starting with 4,000–5,000 IU/day, checking your blood levels of 25(OH)D after 3 months, then adjusting until "tropical optimum" levels are attained. Vitamin D₃ is the preferred form since it has

---

* See page 255.

† See pages 110–113.

‡ See pages 168–172.

been shown to be 87% better at increasing and maintaining blood levels of 25(OH)D than vitamin D_2.[*][465]

Vitamin K₂

If in the form of MK-7, 100 micrograms/day; if in the form of MK-4, 15 milligrams taken 3 times daily (ideally, every 6–8 hours) for a total of 45 milligrams/day.[†] MK-7 and MK-4 are handled differently by our bodies. MK-4 is cleared by the liver within a matter of hours, while MK-7 remains active for several days, and therefore accumulates when taken daily, providing a constant reserve of available K_2. For the vast majority of individuals, this is beneficial, but a few women have written us to say they felt MK-7 caused them to have trouble sleeping. Research has just been published indicating that common single nucleotide polymorphisms or SNPs (variations in our genetic inheritance) in certain key genes implicated in vitamin K metabolism (e.g., APOE, VKOR, CYP4F2) affect our nutritional requirements for vitamin K. Some of these SNPs cause us to eliminate vitamin K more quickly, increasing our needs for vitamin K, while others, found in a very small percentage of people, enable them to keep vitamin K around much longer.[466] In the unlikely event that you are among the few who retain vitamin K far longer than the "average" person, and you find MK-7 does not agree with you, just supplement with MK-4 instead.

---

* See pages 168–172.

† See pages 172–199.

Vitamin B₆

50 milligrams/day. Some B_6, also called pyridoxine, should be provided by your multiple vitamin and mineral supplement. Ideally, it will be in its activated form, which is called pyridoxal-5-phosphate, since approximately 25% of Americans have inherited a slow enzyme for the conversion of B_6 to P5P.[*]

Vitamin B₁₂

500 micrograms/day. Some B_{12}, also called cobalamin, should be provided by your multiple vitamin and mineral supplement. Ideally, it will be in its activated form, methylcobalamin.[†]

Folate

1,000–2,000 micrograms/day in its natural form of folinic acid or even better, 5-methyltetrahydrofolate, the "ready for action" form of folate. What you do not want is "folic acid," a synthetic and less expensive version of folate used in fortified foods and cheaper supplements. Folic acid has been linked to adverse effects including insomnia, intestinal dysfunction,[‡] and, most recently, increased risk for cancer, particularly prostate cancer.[467] The reason for this is that, as noted, folic acid is a synthetic compound. When ingested, it is supposed to be converted (by the enzyme, dihydrofolate reductase to the dihydrofolate and then to the tetrahydrofolate form of folate, for the technically inclined) to compounds iden-

---

[*] See page 232.

[†] See pages 99–105.

[‡] See page 201.

tical to those that would arise from consuming natural folate. However, large oral doses of folic acid, which is present in fortified foods as well as many supplements, can overwhelm this process, so folic acid does not get converted to reduced folate; instead, folic acid accumulates in the bloodstream. This does not occur after consumption of naturally occurring folate. Very little is known about how our bodies handle unmetabolized folic acid or its biological effects.[468] Stick with natural folate.*

Having a genetic inheritance that includes a slow enzyme [methyltetrahydrafolate reductase (MTHFR), for the technically inclined] for the conversion of folate into its methylated form, 5-methyltetrahydrofolate, is surprisingly common; at least two frequently seen single nucleotide polymorphisms (SNPs) result in a slow MTHFR. For this reason, either make sure your diet consistently includes lots of folate–rich foods, like leafy greens, or consider supplementing with 5-methyltetrahydrofolate.[469]

Riboflavin

25 milligrams/day. Riboflavin plays important roles in mitochondrial energy production and is also the cofactor for MTHFR, the enzyme that converts folate into its active form. Along with vitamins B_6, B_{12}, and folate, riboflavin is needed to keep your levels of highly inflammatory (and therefore osteoclast-activating) homocysteine down. Particularly if you have high blood pressure (which promotes inflammation) and are among those with a slow MTHFR, riboflavin may help you lower your blood pressure, lower your homocysteine levels, and protect your bones.[470]

---

* See page 199.

Vitamin C

1,000–2,000 milligrams per day (or more depending on diet, lifestyle.*) If you develop loose stools, try taking buffered vitamin C and/or taking smaller doses, e.g., 250–500 milligrams, several times over the course of your day.

Vitamin E

400 IU/day of mixed tocopherols and tocotrienols. Research has now documented a link between increased "oxidative stress" and bone loss in humans. "Oxidative stress" is "medspeak" for situations in which so many free radicals are being produced that our bodies can't neutralize them quickly enough to prevent damage. Damage = inflammation, and inflammation promotes the activation of osteoclasts. Real Vitamin E (mixed tocopherols and tocotrienols) can help turn the tide.

What's essential to know here is that vitamin E is not just alpha-tocopherol, the form of vitamin E provided by most supplements. Real vitamin E is a family of eight protective compounds that includes four tocopherols (alpha, beta, delta, and gamma tocopherol) and four tocotrienols (alpha, beta, delta, and gamma tocotrienol). It turns out that not only is alpha-tocopherol not the best vitamin E fraction for our bones (or our cardiovascular systems), but if taken by itself, alpha-tocopherol can, in fact, increase inflammation—a big NO NO where our bone (and cardiovascular) health is concerned.

---

* Consumption of refined grains, sugars, and smoking, including second hand smoking, greatly increase vitamin C needs, as do viral infections, such as colds or flu. See pages 201–204.

This is why studies using supplemental vitamin E (actually only alpha-tocopherol) have had mixed results, while studies looking at people eating diets rich in vitamin E have had only positive results. Gamma-tocopherol, which is the form of vitamin E highest in foods (and thus the vitamin E fraction we get in largest amounts when we eat these foods or take a supplement providing "mixed tocopherols and tocotrienols") is better for our bones. Numerous recent studies have shown that supplements providing only alpha-tocopherol suppress serum gamma-tocopherol levels by as much as 60%—which obviously leads to negative effects on bone.

Gamma-tocopherol has many anti-inflammatory actions, helps balance and protect alpha-tocopherol to make the most of its beneficial effects, and has been shown to lessen bone turnover, resulting in more bone formation than resorption. Plus the tocotrienols have numerous anti-inflammatory, bone-protective actions and also play important roles in normal bone calcification.[471]

Omega-3 Fatty Acids

1,000 milligrams of omega-3s per day (180 milligrams as EPA and 120 milligrams as DHA).

Alpha-linolenic acid, the omega-3 fat found in walnuts and flaxseed, has been shown to promote bone health by helping to prevent excessive bone turnover—when consumption of foods rich in this omega-3 fat results in a lower ratio of omega-6 to omega-3 fats in the diet.

Other studies have shown that diets rich in the omega-3s from fish (DHA and EPA), which also naturally result in a lowered ratio of omega-6 to omega-3 fats, reduce bone loss. Researchers think this is most likely because omega-6 fats are converted into pro-inflammatory prostaglandins, while omega-3 fats are metabolized into anti-inflammatory prostaglandins. (Prostaglandins are hormone-like substances made in our bodies from fatty acids.)

A study that compared the effects of diets containing a similar amount of fat, but very different ratios of omega 6: omega 3 fats, illustrates the beneficial effect of alpha-linolenic acid, the omega-3 fat concentrated in plant foods, specifically, in flaxseed and walnuts. In this study, 23 participants (20 men and 3 postmenopausal women) ate each of 3 diets for a 6-week period with a 3 week washout period in between diets.[472]

- Diet 1 provided 34% total fat with omega-6 and omega-3 fats in amounts typically seen in the standard American diet: 9% polyunsaturated fats (PUFAs) of which 7.7% were omega-6 and only 0.8% omega-3 fats, resulting in a pro-inflammatory ratio of 9.6:1.

- Diet 2, an omega-6-rich diet, provided 37% total fat containing 16% PUFAs of which 12% were omega-6 and 3.6% omega-3, a better but still pro-inflammatory ratio of 3.3:1.

- Diet 3, which provided 38% in total fats, was an omega-3-rich diet, containing 17% PUFAs, of which 10.5% were omega-6 and 6.5% omega-3 (in the form of alpha linolenic acid, an omega-3 fat richly supplied by flax seeds and walnuts), resulting in an anti-inflammatory ratio of 1.6:1.

After each diet, subjects' blood levels of N-telopeptides, a marker of bone breakdown,* were measured,

---

* See pages 158–160.

and were found to be 15.3% lower following Diet 3, the omega-3-rich diet, than either of the other two.

The level of N-telopeptides seen with each diet also correlated with that of a key marker of inflammation called tumor necrosis factor-alpha (TNF-alpha). Diets 1 and 2, which both had a significantly higher ratio of omega-6 to omega-3 fats, resulted in much higher levels of pro-inflammatory TNF-alpha than the diet high in omega-3 fats from walnuts and flaxseed.

Another recent study shows that combining omega-3s with exercise significantly lowers inflammation and boosts BMD in older women. In this study, 79 postmenopausal women were randomly divided into four groups. The first group acted as controls and received neither the exercise plan (walking and jogging three times a week) nor supplemental omega-3s. Group 2 only exercised. Group 3 were given omega-3 supplements only (containing 180 mg EPA and 120 mg DHA, to supply a total of 1000 mg/day). Group 4 got the whole enchilada—exercise and omega-3s. Six months later, women in the omega-3s + exercise group had increases in BMD of 15% in the lower back and 19% in the neck of the femur (thigh bone) at the hip (where many hip fractures occur). In the women taking omega-3s and exercising, levels of pro-inflammatory cytokines, IL-6 and TNF-alpha dropped by 40% and 80%, respectively. No increases in BMD or decreases in inflammatory markers were seen in the other three groups.[473]

The take-away here: in addition to frequently including omega-3-rich flaxseed and walnuts, as well as cold water fish, in your bone-building diet, supplement with omega-3s (180 mg EPA and 120 mg DHA, to supply approximately a total of 1000 mg/day) and exercise at least three times a week.

SOME COMBINATION SUPPLEMENT OPTIONS

To help make getting adequate amounts of all these minerals, plus vitamin D_3, vitamin K_1 and vitamin K_2 (as MK-7), easier, Dr. Wright formulated the Osteo-Mins® AM and PM supplements. They are intended to be used along with a multi-vitamin supplying the B vitamins, vitamin C, and vitamin E.[474]

Since the calcium in AlgaeCal Plus® is provided within the full matrix of minerals the sea-algae absorbed and utilized to build its bone-like structure, this supplement also provides a wide range of trace minerals, plus boron, magnesium, vitamin D_3, vitamin K_2 (as MK-7) and vitamin C.[475]

A variety of other bone support combination supplements are available. We've provided links for you to a number of others.[476] In addition, we suggest you run a Google search to see if any new bone support products have become available. Compare ingredients, dosages and cost—then choose the bone support product you feel will best meet YOUR needs.

Resources

Where Can I Find an "Integrative" Doctor Who Will Help Me Build and Keep My Bones Strong, Naturally?

To find an integrative doctor in your area, check with the organizations listed below.

- **THE ALLIANCE FOR NATURAL HEALTH USA**
  www.anh-usa.org
  6931 Arlington Road, Suite 304
  Bethesda, MD 20814
  800-230-2762
  office@anh-usa.org

- **AMERICAN ASSOCIATION OF NATUROPATHIC PHYSICIANS**
  www.Naturopathic.org
  4435 Wisconsin Avenue, NW, Suite 403
  Washington, DC 20016
  202-237-8150

142455759756858555

- **AMERICAN HOLISTIC MEDICAL ASSOCIATION**
  www.HolisticMedicine.org
  27629 Chagrin Blvd., Suite 213
  Woodmere, OH 44122
  216-292-6644

- **AMERICAN COLLEGE FOR ADVANCEMENT IN MEDICINE**
  www.acam.org
  8001 Irvine Center Drive, Suite 825
  Irvine, CA 92618
  949-309-3520

- **AMERICAN ACADEMY OF ENVIRONMENTAL MEDICINE**
  www.aaemonline.org
  6505 E. Central Avenue, # 296
  Wichita, KS 67207
  316-684-5500

- **INTERNATIONAL COLLEGE OF INTEGRATIVE MEDICINE**
  www.icimed.com
  Box 271
  Bluffton, OH 45817
  419-358-0273

- **THE INSTITUTE FOR FUNCTIONAL MEDICINE**
  www.FunctionalMedicine.org
  505 S. 336th Street, Suite 500
  Federal Way, WA 98003
  253-661-3010; 253-661-8310 (Fax)

Additional Helpful Resources

- Wright, J. and Lenard, L. *Stay Young and Sexy with Bio-Identical Hormone Replacement* (Petaluma, CA: Smart Publications, 2010).

- For more information on a bone-building diet and quick, delicious recipes, visit The World's Healthiest Foods at www.whfoods.org.

More Information on STOTT PILATES® for Osteoporosis

NANCY BROSE, BSF, MLA, STOTT PILATES® ADVANCED LEVEL INSTRUCTOR

Nancy earned her BS in Forest Resources at University of Washington and MA in Landscape Architecture at UC Berkeley before devoting herself to Pilates. Her knowledge of patterns, design and growth in nature has given her unique perspective and insight into the stress and growth response patterns of the human body. A STOTT PILATES® advanced level certified teacher and a Yamuna Body Rolling Practitioner, Nancy has been practicing and teaching Pilates since 2001 and is the owner of Inner Strength Pilates, located in Sammamish, WA (www.innerstrength-pilates.biz).

Nancy opened Inner Strength Pilates in 2004 and developed bone strengthening exercise programs specifically for osteoporosis and osteopenia. She has seen her clients improve their balance, avoid debilitating fractures during falls, and increase their bone density enough to successfully move out of the Osteoporosis T score range. In 2008, wanting to share her successes and the information she had learned to help others, she developed the Pilates for Osteoporosis I and II Teacher Training Program. In addition to working with private clients at Inner Strength Pilates, Nancy teaches Pilates for Osteoporosis and Pilates for Asymmetry at Body Center Studios in Seattle, WA.

KRISTI QUINN, MA, LMP, LEAD STOTT PILATES® INSTRUCTOR TRAINER

Born and raised in Wyoming, Kristi received her MA in Dance at American University in Washington, DC, in 1997, with core competencies in teaching, kinesiology and choreography. She danced professionally throughout the US and across Europe before moving to Seattle in 1998. Soon after landing in Seattle, she helped establish BodyCenter Studios (http://bodycenterstudios.com/).

Kristi's in-depth understanding of the body's biomechanics and correct movement patterns contributes to her deep insight into the specific needs of each of her many clients, including those seeking rehabilitation from injuries as well as those living with chronic conditions such as fibromyalgia, chronic fatigue, MS, and osteoporosis. As a Lead STOTT PILATES® Instructor Trainer, Kristi is helping to create the next generation of qualified instructors through her technically demanding courses such as "Injury and Special Populations" and her Osteoporosis Protocols Workshop with Nancy Brose.

Nancy and Kristi have worked together for several years and have combined their talents and resources to create the Osteoporosis and Asymmetry courses as an offering that meets the requirements for STOTT

PILATES® certified continuing education. Thanks to their efforts, Pilates for Osteoporosis certification for STOTT instructors is now being offered at Body-Center Studios.

ORGANIZATIONS OFFERING PILATES FOR OSTEOPOROSIS TRAINING:

- **Body Center Studios, Seattle, WA**
  www.bodycenterstudios.com
- **Inner Strength Pilates, Seattle, WA**
  www.innerstrengthpilates.biz
- **STOTT PILATES®**
  www.stottpilates.com
- **Polestar**
  www.polestarpilates.com
- **Physical Mind**
  www.themethodpilates.com
- **The Pilates Method Alliance**
  www.pilatesmethodalliance.orgappendix

Contact Lara Pizzorno

You can contact Lara Pizzorno, MA, LMT via Praktikos Books at www.praktikosinstitute.org/your-bones-from-the-author, or via her page at the website of her husband, Dr. Joe Pizzorno, ND: www.drpizzorno.com.

Glossary

akaline phosphatase: An enzyme that is a marker for the formation of the bone-building osteoblasts.

amenorrhea: Complete loss of menstrual periods.

androgens: Male hormones.

andropause: Male menopause. Testosterone levels drop with age, resulting in insufficient production of estrogen to maintain bone.

apoptosis: Cell suicide by means of a programmed sequence of self-destruct events. Apoptosis plays a crucial role in developing and maintaining health by eliminating old cells, unnecessary cells, and unhealthy cells.

aromatase: An enzyme responsible for a key step in the biosynthesis of estrogens; in particular, the aromatization of androgens into estrogens.

atrial fibrillation: Irregular heartbeat.

bronchospasm: When the bands of muscle around the airways tighten uncontrollably, as in asthma.

calcaneus: Anklebone.

calcium carbonate: A rock-derived form of calcium that is not as well absorbed as calcium citrate since it requires adequate stomach acid, calcium carbonate is the least expensive form of calcium and thus the form most commonly used in supplements.

calcium citrate: A more bioavailable form of calcium, which is absorbed even when stomach acid production is below normal.

corpus luteum: Formed from the remains of the follicle after ovulation and secretes progesterone, which prepares the uterine lining for implantation of the egg, if fertilized, and is required for activation of osteoblasts.

creatinine: A breakdown product of creatine phosphate in muscle tissue. Higher levels indicate a decrease in kidney function and ability to excrete waste products.

C-telopeptide: A serum bio-marker of bone breakdown.

DXA: The gold standard x-ray procedure used to evaluate bone density.

DRESS syndrome: Stands for "drug reaction with eosinophilia and systemic symptoms syndrome" and is also known as "drug hypersensitivity syndrome."

estradiol: The most potent form of estrogen.

first-degree relatives: The parents, brothers, sisters, or children.

flavin adenine dinucleotide or FAD: A coenzyme whose co-factor is riboflavin, FAD is required for the production of the activated forms of B6 and folate, and also in energy metabolism, in which it acts as an electron carrier during the production of the energy currency of the body, ATP.

fragility fracture: A fracture that occurs during normal daily activities as a result of having weak, thin bones.

gastric achlorhydria: Too little stomach acid to be able to properly digest food, also called hypochlorhydria.

gastric banding: An alternative surgical procedure for morbid obesity—alternative to the Roux-en-Y gastric bypass which has not been shown to produce as much bone loss as the Roux-en-Y procedure. In gastric banding, an inflatable silicone device is placed around the top portion of the stomach to create a small pouch at the top of the stomach.

gastric bypass: Surgical procedure used to treat morbid obesity, referred to in medical terminology as the Roux-en-Y procedure, greatly decreases one's ability to absorb nutrients and promotes osteoporosis.

Helicobacter pylori (H.pylori): A pathogenic bacterium that causes peptic ulcers.

hirsutism: Excessive hairiness in atypical areas, e.g., a mustache on a woman.

homocysteine: A highly inflammatory compound, homocysteine is produced as an intermediate product of a normal and important cellular process called the methylation cycle, which takes place constantly within our cells. Normally, as soon as homocysteine is produced from the amino acid, methionine in the methylation cycle, it is immediately converted into back into methionine (via the actions of enzymes that require folate and B_{12}) or into cysteine (via the action of a B6-dependent enzyme). When levels of

B_6, B_{12} and folate are inadequate, however, the methylation cycle stops mid-way at homocysteine, which builds up, flows out of cells into the bloodstream, and causes damage wherever it goes. High levels of homocysteine are associated with not only osteoporosis, but cardiovascular diseases, diabetes, rheumatoid arthritis and Alzheimer's disease.

hydroxyapatite: The complex of minerals in which calcium is joined with phosphorus forming calcium phosphate, hydroxyapatite is the principal bone storage form of calcium in bone and provides its structure and strength.

hypercalcemia: Elevated blood levels of calcium.

hyperparathyroidism: Overactivity of the parathyroid glands (hyper = excessive, above normal), resulting in excessive production of parathyroid hormone.

hyperthyroidism: An "hyperactive" thyroid.

ionized: Made to have fewer electrons.

low-energy thighbone fractures: Fractures occurring during normal daily activities. Their likelihood is increased by the bisphosphonates and denosumab.

menaquinone: Vitamin K_2, the form in which vitamin K activates osteocalcin, which pulls calcium into bone, and matrix-Gla protein, which prevents calcium from depositing in arteries.

mesenchymal stem cells: Undifferentiated cells that may develop into any one of several different types of cells, including osteoblasts, chondrocytes (cells that produce cartilage) or adipocytes (fat cells).

metformin: A patent medicine that lowers blood sugar levels and is prescribed for people with type 2 diabetes.

methionine: An essential amino acid that serves as a methyl donor in the methylation cycle (see also cysteine and homocysteine).

methylation: A cellular process involving the addition of a methyl group to a molecule, which jump starts and stops many vital processes in the body, including regulation of gene expression and protein function.

microbial biofilms: Supersized bacterial colonies that cause chronic infections, are involved in numerous diseases, and are highly resistant to antibiotics. Their likelihood of their development in the mouth, where they promote osteonecrosis of the jawbone, is increased by bisphosphonates and denosumab.

myalgia: Severe muscle pain.

non-alcoholic fatty liver disease or NAFLD: Rapidly increasing liver disease, caused by insulin resistance and type 2 diabetes.

N-telopeptide: Cross-linked N-telopeptides of type I collagen (NTX or NTx), a breakdown product of the type-I collagen in bone cartilage.

osteoblasts: The bone-forming cells that pull calcium, magnesium, and phosphorous from the blood to build new bone.

osteocalcin: A protein secreted by osteoblasts that plays a key role in the bone formation process.

osteoclasts: Specialized bone cells that remove worn out or dead bone to make room for new bone.

osteocytes: What osteoblasts turn into after they begin secreting the bone matrix.

osteoid: A cartilage-like material into which the osteoblasts deposit calcium; also required for the cross-linking of collagen fibrils in bone, which helps to form a strong bone matrix.

osteomalacia: Bone pain.

osteonecrosis of the jaw: Jaw bone death, osteo = bone, necrosis = death.

osteopenia: Bone thinning. Accelerated bone loss, an early warning signal for developing osteoporosis.

osteoporosis: Porous bone (osteo = bone, porosis = porous)—is a progressive loss of bone that results in bone thinning and increased vulnerability to fracture.

osteoporotic fractures: Also called fragility fractures because they happen in thinned out, fragile bone.

ovulation: The release of an egg from a follicle in the ovaries.

perimenopause: The years immediately preceding menopause when levels of estrogen and progesterone begin to decline (peri=around).

periodontal ligament: The ligament that attaches the tooth to its socket in the jawbone.

phylloquinone: Vitamin K_1—type of vitamin K found in plants.

primary hyperparathyroidism: An overactive parathyroid gland whose over-activity is not caused by vitamin D deficiency.

pyridoxal-5-phosphate (P-5-P): The activated form of vitamin B_6.

resorbed: To dissolve and re-absorb.

Roux-en-Y procedure: Gastric bypass surgery in which the stomach is made smaller and part of the small intestine where many minerals and vitamins are primarily absorbed is bypassed. This causes weight loss, but also nutrient deficiencies that greatly increase risk for osteoporosis and other health problems.

sarcopenia: Loss of skeletal muscle mass, typically with aging. Sarco= flesh or muscle; penia=loss.

soluble: Able to be dissolved.

standard deviation: A statistic used as a measure of how tightly all the various participants are clustered around the mean (midline or average) in a set of data. In relation to bone loss, it signifies how much the bone mass of a specific woman differs from that of the "average" healthy 20 year old woman, the time in a woman's life when her bone mass is highest.

subtrochanter of the femur: Below the trochanter but in the upper part of the body of the thigh bone.

symptomatic hypocalcemia: A serious condition in which too little calcium is in circulation, which may result in cardiovascular collapse, very low blood pressure unresponsive to fluids and vasopressors (patent medicines that cause blood vessel constriction), and dysrhythmias (abnormal cardiac rhythms).

transverse: Crosswise.

upper tolerable intake levels (ULs): How much of a nutrient we can take daily without risk of toxicity.

venous thromboembolism: Blood clot formation inside a blood vessel. Deep venous thrombosis can cause pulminary embolism, a blockage of the main artery of the lung.

Endnotes

1. http://en.wikipedia.org/wiki/Osteoporosis.

2. Riggs, B. L., L. J. Melton 3rd, R. A. Robb, et al. 2004. Population-based study of age and sex differences in bone volumetric density, size, geometry, and structure at different skeletal sites. *J Bone Miner Res* 19:1945–54. PMID: 15537436.

3. Bilezikian, J. P. 1999. Osteoporosis in men. *J Clin Endocrinol Metab* Oct.; 84(10):3431–4. PMID: 10522975.

4. Nochowitz, B. 2009. An update on osteoporosis. *Am J Ther* Sept-Oct;16(5):437–445. PMID: 19262365.

5. Binkley, N. 2006. Osteoporosis in men. *Arq Bras Endocrinol Metab* 50/4:764–774. PMID: 17117301.

   Stock, H., A. Schneider, and E. Strauss. 2004. Osteoporosis: a disease in men. *Clin Orthop Relat Res* Aug; (425):143–51. PMID: 15292799.

6. Center, J. R., T. V. Nguyen, D. Schneider, et al. 1999. Mortality after all major types of osteoporotic

fracture in men and women: an observational study. *Lancet* 353:878–82. PMID: 10093980.

Pande, I., D. L. Scott, T. W. O'Neill, et al. 2006. Quality of life, morbidity, and mortality after low trauma hip fracture in men. *Ann Rheum Dis* 65:87–92. PMID: 16079173.

7. Null, G., D. Rasio, and C. Dean. *Death by Medicine* (Mt. Jackson, VA: Praktikos Books, 2010).

8. American Association of Poison Control Centers. 2008 Report, http://www.aapcc.org/dnn/Portals/0/2008annualreport.pdf (accessed 6-2-2010).

9. http://www.fda.gov/cder/drug/infopage/bisphosphonates/default.htm.

10. Odvina, C.V., J. E. Zerwekh, D. S. Rao, et al. 2005. Severely suppressed bone turnover: a potential complication of alendronate therapy. *J Clin Endocrinol Metab* Mar;90(3):1294–301. PMID: 15598694.

11. http://www.mayoclinic.com/health/fosamax/AN01379.

12. http://www.ashcraftandgerel.com/practiceareas/dangerous-drugs-and-medical-products/fosamax-bisphosphonate-drugs-recall/?gclid=CJCZx5yp-LMCFQhyQgod730A1A.

13. Document #4, Judge Daubert ruling. "Opinion and 6 Order", from Judge John F Keenan, United States District Court, Southern District of New York, Case 1:06-md-01789-JFK-JCF. Document 750 filed 07/27/2009: pages 21, 36, 45.

14. Favia, G., G. P. Pilolli, E. Maiorano. 2009. Osteonecrosis of the jaw correlated to bisphosphonate therapy in non-oncologic patients: clinicopathological features of 24 patients. *J Rheumatol* Dec;36(12):2780–7. PMID: 19884275.

15. Lo, J. C., F. S. O'Ryan, N. P. Gordon, et al. 2009. Prevalence of osteonecrosis of the jaw in patients with oral bisphosphonate exposure. *J Oral Maxillofac Surg* Jun 30. PMID: 19772941.

16. Favia, G., G. P. Pilolli, and E. Maiorano. 2009. Osteonecrosis of the jaw correlated to bisphosphonate therapy in non-oncologic patients: clinicopathological features of 24 patients. *J Rheumatol* Dec;36(12):2780–7. PMID: 19884275.

   Palaska, P. K., V. Cartsos, and A. I. Zavras. 2009. Bisphosphonates and time to osteonecrosis development. *Oncologist* Nov;14(11):1154–66. PMID: 19897878.

   Marx, R. E. 2008. Bisphosphonate-induced osteonecrosis of the jaws: a challenge, a responsibility, and an opportunity. *Int J Periodontics Restorative Dent* Feb;28(1):5–6. PMID: 18351197.

   Rogers, S., N. Rahman, and D. Ryan. 2010. Guidelines for treating patients taking bisphosphonates prior to dental extractions. *J Ir Dent Assoc* Feb-Mar;56(1):40. PMID: 20337145.

   Dello Russo, N. M., M. K. Jeffcoat, R. E. Marx, et al. 2007. Osteonecrosis in the jaws of patients who are using oral biphosphonates to treat osteoporosis. *Int J Oral Maxillofac Implants* Jan-Feb;22(1):146–53. PMID: 17340909.

   Lee, J. 2009. Complication related to bisphosphonate therapy: osteonecrosis of the jaw. *J Infus Nurs* Nov-Dec;32(6):330–5. PMID: 19918142.

   Lo, J. C., F. S. O'Ryan, N. P. Gordon, et al. 2010. Prevalence of osteonecrosis of the jaw in patients with oral bisphosphonate exposure. *J Oral Maxillofac Surg* Feb;68(2):243–53. PMID: 19772941.

   Longo, R., M. A. Castellana, and G. Gasparini. 2009. Bisphosphonate-related osteonecrosis of the jaw and left thumb. *J Clin Oncol* Dec 10;27(35):e242–3. PMID: 19858386.

Kyrgidis, A. and E. Verrou. 2010. Fatigue in bone: a novel phenomenon attributable to bisphosphonate use. *Bone* Feb;46(2):556; author reply 557–8. Epub 2009 Sep 29. PMID: 19796720.

Vassiliou, V., N. Tselis, and D. Kardamakis. 2010. Osteonecrosis of the Jaws: Clinicopathologic and Radiologic Characteristics, Preventive and Therapeutic Strategies. *Strahlenther Onkol* Apr 26. [Epub ahead of print] PMID: 20437019.

Kyrgidis, A. and K. Vahtsevanos. 2010. Bisphosphonate-related osteonecrosis of the jaws: A review of 34 cases and evaluation of risk. *J Craniomaxillofac Surg* Apr 29. [Epub ahead of print] PMID: 20434920.

Assael, L. A. 2009. Oral bisphosphonates as a cause of bisphosphonate-related osteonecrosis of the jaws: clinical findings, assessment of risks, and preventive strategies. *J Oral Maxillofac Surg* May;67(5 Suppl):35–43. PMID: 19371813.

Migliorati, C. A., K. Mattos, and M. J. Palazzolo. 2010. How patients' lack of knowledge about oral bisphosphonates can interfere with medical and dental care. *J Am Dent Assoc* May;141(5):562–6. PMID: 20436104.

Filleul, O., E. Crompot and S. Saussez. 2010. Bisphosphonate-induced osteonecrosis of the jaw: a review of 2,400 patient cases. *J Cancer Res Clin Oncol* Aug;136(8):1117–24. Epub 2010 May 28. PMID: 20508948.

Sarin, J., S. S. DeRossi and S. O. Akintoye. 2008. Updates on bisphosphonates and potential pathobiology of bisphosphonate-induced jaw osteonecrosis. *Oral Dis* Apr;14(3):277–85. PMID: 18336375.

17. Favia, G., G. P. Pilolli, and E. Maiorano. 2009. Histologic and histomorphometric features of bisphosphonate-related osteonecrosis of the jaws:

an analysis of 31 cases with confocal laser scanning microscopy. *Bone* Sep;45(3):406–13. Epub 2009 May 18. PMID: 19450715.

Stepan, J. J., D. B. Burr, I. Pavo, et al. 2007. Low bone mineral density is associated with bone microdamage accumulation in postmenopausal women with osteoporosis. *Bone* Sep;41(3):378–85. PMID: 17597017.

18. Sedghizadeh, P. P., K. Stanley, M. Caligiuri, S. Hofkes, B. Lowry, and C. F. Shuler. 2009. Oral bisphosphonate use and the prevalence of osteonecrosis of the jaw: An institutional inquiry. *J Am Dent Assoc* 40:61–66. PMID: 19119168.

Sedghizadeh, P. P., S. K. Kumar, A. Gorur, et al. 2008. Identification of microbial biofilms in osteonecrosis of the jaws secondary to bisphosphonate therapy. *J Oral Maxillofac Surg* Apr;66(4):767–75. PMID: 18355603.

19. Pazianas, M., P. Miller, W. A. Blumentals, et al. 2007. A review of the literature on osteonecrosis of the jaw in patients with osteoporosis treated with oral bisphosphonates: prevalence, risk factors, and clinical characteristics. *Clin Ther* Aug;29(8):1548–58. PMID: 17919538.

20. Edwards, B. J., J. W. Hellstein, P. L. Jacobsen, et al. 2008. Updated recommendations for managing the care of patients receiving oral bisphosphonate therapy: an advisory statement from the American Dental Association Council on Scientific Affairs. *J Am Dent Assoc* Dec;139(12):1674–7. PMID: 19047674.http://www.ada.org/prof/resources/topics/osteonecrosis.asp.

21. Hellstein, J. W., R. A. Adler, B. Edwards, P. L. Jacobsen, J. R. Kalmar, S. Koka, C. A. Migliorati, and H. Ristic. "Managing the Care of Patients Receiving Antiresorptive Therapy for Prevention and Treatment of Osteoporosis: Executive Summary

of Recommendations from the American Dental Association Council on Scientific Affairs." [In eng]. J Am Dent Assoc 142, no. 11 (Nov 2011): 1243-51.

22.　Parker Waichman Alonso LLP. Breaking News. Osteo-necrosis of the Jaw, http://www.yourlawyer.com/topics/overview/osteonecrosis_of_the_jaw_onj/.

Arrain, Y. and T. Masud. 2009. Bisphosphonates and osteonecrosis of the jaw—current thoughts. *Dent Update* Sep;36(7):415–9. PMID: 19810397.

23.　Estefanía Fresco, R., R. Ponte Fernández, J. M. Aguirre Urizar. 2006. Bisphosphonates and oral pathology II. Osteonecrosis of the jaws: review of the literature before 2005. *Med Oral Patol Oral Cir Bucal* Nov 1;11(6):E456–61. PMID: 17072246.

24.　Kumar, S. K., M. Meru, and P. Sedghizadeh. 2008. Osteonecrosis of the jaws secondary to bisphos-phonate therapy: a case series. *J Contemp Dent Pract* Jan 1;9(1):63–9. PMID: 18176650.

25.　Sedghizadeh, P. P., S. K. Kumar, A. Gorur, et al. 2008. Identification of microbial biofilms in osteo-necrosis of the jaws secondary to bisphosphonate therapy. *J Oral Maxillofac* Surg Apr;66(4):767–75. PMID: 18355603.

26.　Mak, A., M. W. Cheung, R. C. Ho, et al. 2009. Bisphosphonates and atrial fibrillation: Bayesian meta-analyses of randomized controlled trials and observational studies. *BMC Musculoskelet Disord* Sep 21;10:113. PMID: 19772579.

Bhuriya, R., M. Singh, J. Molnar, et al. 2010. Bisphosphonate use in women and the risk of atrial fibrillation: A systematic review and meta-analysis. *Int J Cardiol* Jan 3. [Epub ahead of print] PMID: 20051297.

27.　Naccarelli. G., A. Capucci, C. Lau, and O. Oseroff. Identifying atrial fibrillation-preventing stroke. On-line medical seminar. November 13, 2010, http://www.theheart.org/article/1020235.do.

Lopes, R. D., J. P. Piccini, E. M. Hylek, et al. 2008. Antithrombotic therapy in atrial fibrillation: guidelines translated for the clinician. *J Thromb Thrombolysis* Dec;26(3):167–74. PMID: 18807225.

28. Cummings, S. R., A. V. Schwartz, et al. 2007. Alendronate and atrial fibrillation. *N Engl J Med* May 3;356(18):1895–6. PMID: 17476024.

29. Huang, W. F., Y. W. Tsai, Y. W. Wen, et al. 2009. Osteoporosis treatment and atrial fibrillation: alendronate versus raloxifene. *Menopause* Aug 12. [Epub ahead of print] PMID: 19680161.

30. Heckbert, S. R., G. Li, S. R. Cummings, et al. 2008. Use of alendronate and risk of incident atrial fibrillation in women. *Arch Intern Med* Apr 28;168(8):826–31. PMID: 18443257.

31. Papapetrou, P. D. 2009. Bisphosphonate-associated adverse events. *Hormones* (Athens) Apr-Jun;8(2):96–110. PMID: 19570737.

32. Woo, C., G. Gao, S. Wade, et al. 2010. Gastrointestinal side effects in postmenopausal women using osteoporosis therapy: 1-year findings in the POSSIBLE US study. *Curr Med Res Opin* Apr;26(4):1003–9. PMID: 20201623.

33. Green, J., G. Czanner, G. Reeves, et al. 2010. Oral bisphosphonates and risk of cancer of oesophagus, stomach, and colorectum: case-control analysis within a UK primary care cohort. *BMJ* Sep 1;341:c4444. doi: 10.1136/bmj.c4444. PMID: 20813820.

34. Body, J. J. 2001. Dosing regimens and main adverse events of bisphosphonates. *Semin Oncol* Aug;28(4 Suppl 11):49–53. PMID: 11544576.

35. Merck Sharp & Dohme (New Zealand). Limited. Fosamax (alendronate) data sheet, 17 October 2005, http://www.medsafe.govt.nz/profs/Datasheet/f/Fosamaxtab.htm.

36. Mazj, S. and S. M. Lichtman. 2004. Renal dysfunction associated with bisphosphonate use: Retrospective analysis of 293 patients with respect to age and other clinical characteristics. *Journal of Clinical Oncology* ASCO Annual Meeting Proceedings (Post-Meeting Edition). Vol 22, No 14S (July 15 Supplement), 8039, available at http://meeting.ascopubs.org/cgi/content/abstract/22/14_suppl/8039 (accessed 6-18-10).

Diel, I. J., R. Weide, H. Köppler, et al. 2009. Risk of renal impairment after treatment with ibandronate versus zoledronic acid: a retrospective medical records review. *Support Care Cancer* Jun;17(6):719–25. Epub 2008 Dec 17. PMID: 19089462.

37. Perman, M. J., A. W. Lucky, J. E. Heubi, et al. 2009. Severe symptomatic hypocalcemia in a patient with RDEB treated with intravenous zoledronic acid. *Arch Dermatol* Jan;145(1):95–6. PMID: 19153360.

Mishra, A. 2008. Symptomatic hypocalcemia following intravenous administration of zoledronic acid in a breast cancer patient. *J Postgrad Med* Jul-Sep;54(3):237. PMID: 18626181.

Chennuru, S., J. Koduri, M. A. Baumann. 2008. Risk factors for symptomatic hypocalcaemia complicating treatment with zoledronic acid. *Intern Med J* Aug;38(8):635–7. Epub 2008 Feb 17. PMID: 18284458.

Aksoy, S., H. Abali, M. Dinçer, et al. 2004. Hypocalcemic effect of zoledronic acid or other bisphosphonates may contribute to their antiangiogenic properties. *Med Hypotheses* 62(6):942–4. PMID: 15142653.

Tanvetyanon, T. and A. M. Choudhury. 2004. Hypocalcemia and azotemia associated with zoledronic acid and interferon alfa. *Ann Pharmacother* Mar;38(3):418–21. PMID: 14970365.

38. Kyrgidis, A. and E. Verrou. 2009. Fatigue in bone: A novel phenomenon attributable to bisphosphonate use. *Bone* Sep 29.PMID: 19796720.

39. Odvina, C.V., J. E. Zerwekh, D. S. Rao, et al. 2005. Severely suppressed bone turnover: a potential complication of alendronate therapy. *J Clin Endocrinol Metab* Mar;90(3):1294–301. PMID: 15598694.

40. Goh, S. K., K.Y. Yang, J. S. Koh, et al. 2007. Subtrochanteric insufficiency fractures in patients on alendronate therapy: a caution. *J Bone Joint Surg Br* 89(3):349–353. PMID: 17356148.

41. Nevasier, A.S., J. M. Lane, B. A. Lenart, et al. 2008. Low-energy femoral shaft fractures associated with alendronate use. *J Orthop Trauma* 22(5):346–350. PMID: 18448990.

42. Stepan, J. J., D. B. Burr, I. Pavo, et al. 2007. Low bone mineral density is associated with bone microdamage accumulation in postmenopausal women with osteoporosis. *Bone* Sep;41(3):378–85. PMID: 17597017.

43. Ing-Lorenzini, K., J. Desmeules, O. Plachta, et al. 2009. Low-energy femoral fractures associated with the long-term use of bisphosphonates: a case series from a Swiss university hospital. *Drug Saf* 32(9):775–85. PMID: 19670917.

44. Watters, C. 2010. Bisphosphonate Therapy for Osteoporosis: A Potential Risk for Subtrochanteric Fractures. *Orthopaedic Nursing* 29(3):210–213, May/June doi: 10.1097/NOR.ob013e3181db5485.

   Bamrungsong, T. and C. Pongchaiyakul. 2010. Bilateral atypical femoral fractures after long-term alendronate therapy: a case report. *J Med Assoc Thai* May;93(5):620–4. PMID: 20524451.

   Abrahamsen, B. 2010. Adverse effects of bisphosphonates. *Calcif Tissue Int* Jun;86(6):421–35. Epub 2010 Apr 21. PMID: 20407762.

Giusti, A., N. A. Hamdy and S. E. Papapoulos. 2010. Atypical fractures of the femur and bisphosphonate therapy: A systematic review of case/case series studies. *Bone* Aug;47(2):169–80. Epub 2010 May 20. PMID: 20493982.

Girgis, C. M. and M. J. Seibel. 2010. Atypical femur fractures: a complication of prolonged bisphosphonate therapy? *Med J Aust* Aug 16;193(4):196–8. PMID: 20712536.

45. Benhamou, C. L. 2007. Effects of osteoporosis medications on bone quality. *Joint Bone Spine* Jan;74(1):39–47. PMID: 17196423.

Capeci, C. M. and N. C. Tejwani. 2009. Bilateral low-energy simultaneous or sequential femoral fractures in patients on long-term alendronate therapy. *J Bone Joint Surg Am* Nov;91(11):2556–61. PMID: 19884427.

Schneider, J. P. 2009. Bisphosphonates and low-impact femoral fractures: current evidence on alendronate-fracture risk. *Geriatrics* Jan;64(1):18–23. PMID: 19256578.

Bunning, R.D., R. J. Rentfro and J. S. Jelinek. 2010. Low-energy femoral fractures associated with long-term bisphosphonate use in a rehabilitation setting: a case series. *PM R* Jan;2(1):76–80. PMID: 20129517.

Schilcher, J. and P. Aspenberg. 2009. Incidence of stress fractures of the femoral shaft in women treated with bisphosphonate. *Acta Orthop* Aug;80(4):413–5. PMID: 19568963.

Lenart, B. A., A. S. Neviaser, S. Lyman, et al. 2009. Association of low-energy femoral fractures with prolonged bisphosphonate use: a case control study. *Osteoporos Int* Aug;20(8):1353–62. Epub 2008 Dec 9. PMID: 19066707.

Goddard, M. S., K. R. Reid, J. C. Johnston, et al. 2009. Atraumatic bilateral femur fracture in long-term bisphosphonate use. *Orthopedics* Aug;32(8). PMID: 19708622.

Capeci, C. M. and N. C. Tejwani. 2009. Bilateral low-energy simultaneous or sequential femoral fractures in patients on long-term alendronate therapy. *J Bone Joint Surg Am* Nov;91(11):2556–61. PMID: 19884427.

46. Yamaguchi, T. and T. Sugimoto. 2009. [New development in bisphosphonate treatment. When and how long should patients take bisphosphonates for osteoporosis?] *Clin Calcium* Jan;19(1):38–43. PMID: 19122263.

47. Romo, C. and L. Salahi. Fosamax: Is Long Term Use of Bone Strengthening Drug Linked to Fractures? ABC News, March 8, 2010, http://abcnews.go.com/WN/WorldNews/osteoporosis-drugs-fosamax-increase-risk-broken-bones-women/story?id=10044066.

Romo, C., L. Salahi and D. Childs. FDA to Investigate Possible Osteoporosis Drug-Femur Fracture Link After ABC News Report. ABC News, March 10, 2010, http://abcnews.go.com/WN/WellnessNews/fda-consult-experts-fracture-risk-bone-drugs/story?id=10065341.

FDA Drug Safety Communication: Ongoing safety review of oral bisphosphonates and atypical subtrochanteric femur fractures. http://www.fda.gov/Drugs/DrugSafety/PostmarketDrugSafetyInformationforPatientsandProviders/ucm203891.htm.

48. FDA Drug Safety Communication. http://www.fda.gov/Drugs/DrugSafety/ucm229009.htm.

FDA Consumer Update. http://www.fda.gov/ForConsumers/ConsumerUpdates/ucm229127.htm.

49. Solomon, D.H., M. C. Hochberg, H. Mogun, et al. 2009. The relation between bisphosphonate use and non-union of fractures of the humerus in

older adults. *Osteoporos Int* Jun;20(6):895–901. Epub 2008 Oct 9. PMID: 18843515.

50. Knight, R. J., C. Reddy, M. A. Rtshiladze, et al. 2010. Bisphosphonate-related osteonecrosis of the jaw: tip of the iceberg. *J Craniofac Surg* Jan;21(1):25–32. Review. PMID: 20072026.

51. Prommer, E. E. 2009. Toxicity of bisphosphonates. *J Palliat Med* Nov;12(11):1061–5. PMID: 19922007.

Kyrgidis, A., S. Triaridis, K. Vahtsevanos, et al. 2009. Osteonecrosis of the jaw and bisphosphonate use in breast cancer patients. *Expert Rev Anticancer Ther* Aug;9(8):1125–34. PMID: 19671032.

Gebara, S. N. and H. Moubayed. 2009. Risk of osteonecrosis of the jaw in cancer patients taking bisphosphonates. *Am J Health Syst Pharm* Sep 1;66(17):1541–7. PMID: 19710437.

52. Ferran, L. and K. McKarthy. New Weapon in Breast Cancer Battle? Experts Cautious. Dec. 11, 2009, http://abcnews.go.com/.

53. Body, J. J. 2008. [Update on treatment of postmenopausal osteoporosis] *Rev Med Brux* Sep;29(4):301–9. PMID: 18949981.

Valverde, P. 2008. Pharmacotherapies to manage bone loss-associated diseases: a quest for the perfect benefit-to-risk ratio. *Curr Med Chem* 15(3):284–304. Review. PMID: 18288984.

Uebelhart, D., D. Frey, P. Frey-Rindova, et al. 2003. [Therapy of osteoporosis: bisphosphonates, SERM's, teriparatide and strontium] *Z Rheumatol* Dec;62(6):512–7. Review. PMID: 14685711.

O'Donnell, S., A. Cranney, G. A. Wells, et al. 2006. Strontium ranelate for preventing and treating postmenopausal osteoporosis. *Cochrane Database Syst Rev* Oct 18;(4):CD005326. PMID: 17054253.

Stevenson, M., S. Davis, M. Lloyd-Jones, et al. 2007. The clinical effectiveness and cost-effectiveness of strontium ranelate for the prevention of osteoporotic fragility fractures in postmenopausal women. *Health Technol Assess* Feb;11(4):1–134. PMID: 17280622.

Reginster, J. Y., R. Deroisy and I. Jupsin. 2003. Strontium ranelate: a new paradigm in the treatment of osteoporosis. *Drugs Today* (Barc) Feb;39(2):89–101. PMID: 12698204.

54. Coleman, R. E., H. Marshall, D. Cameron, D. Dodwell, R. Burkinshaw, M. Keane, M. Gil, *et al.* "Breast-Cancer Adjuvant Therapy with Zoledronic Acid." [In eng]. *N Engl J Med* 365, no. 15 (Oct 13 2011): 1396–405.

55. Frost, M. L., M. Siddique, G. M. Blake, A. E. Moore, P. K. Marsden, P. J. Schleyer, R. Eastell, and I. Fogelman. "Regional Bone Metabolism at the Lumbar Spine and Hip Following Discontinuation of Alendronate and Risedronate Treatment in Postmenopausal Women." [In Eng]. *Osteoporos Int* (Oct 8 2011).

56. Reclast (zoledronic acid): Patent medicine Safety Communication - New Contraindication and Updated Warning on Kidney Impairment, posted 9-1-2011, available at http://www.fda.gov/Safety/MedWatch/SafetyInformation/SafetyAlerts-forHumanMedicalProducts/ucm270464.htm. This url is so long, I am also including a bitly version for you here: http://1.usa.gov/IUwi99.

57. Ayus, J. C., and A. I. Arieff. "Abnormalities of Water Metabolism in the Elderly." [In eng]. *Semin Nephrol* 16, no. 4 (Jul 1996): 277–88.

Faes, M. C., M. G. Spigt. Olde Rikkert MGM. "Dehydration in Geriatrics." *Geriatrics and Aging.* 2007;10(9):590–596. Posted 12-26-2007 @ http://www.medscape.com/viewarticle/567678FDA.

58. Ho, J. W. "Bisphosphonate Stimulation of Osteo-blasts and Osteoblastic Metastasis as a Mecha-nism of Hypocalcaemia." [In eng]. *Med Hypotheses* 78, no. 3 (Mar 2012): 377–9.

59. Green, J., G. Czanner, G. Reeves, J. Watson, L. Wise, and V. Beral. "Oral Bisphosphonates and Risk of Cancer of Oesophagus, Stomach, and Colorectum: Case-Control Analysis within a Uk Primary Care Cohort." [In eng]. *BMJ* 341 (2010): c4444.

60. McKague, M., D. Jorgenson, and K. A. Buxton. "Ocular Side Effects of Bisphosphonates: A Case Report and Literature Review." [In eng]. *Can Fam Physician* 56, no. 10 (Oct 2010): 1015–7.

61. Etminan, M., F. Forooghian, and D. Maberley. "Inflammatory Ocular Adverse Events with the Use of Oral Bisphosphonates: A Retrospective Cohort Study." [In eng]. *CMAJ* 184, no. 8 (May 15 2012): E431–4.

62. Vestergaard, P., K. Schwartz, L. Rejnmark, L. Mosekilde, and E. M. Pinholt. "Oral Bisphospho-nate Use Increases the Risk for Inflammatory Jaw Disease: A Cohort Study." [In eng]. *J Oral Maxillo-fac Surg* 70, no. 4 (Apr 2012): 821–9.

63. Puhaindran, M. E., A. Farooki, M. R. Steensma, M. Hameed, J. H. Healey, and P. J. Boland. "Atypi-cal Subtrochanteric Femoral Fractures in Patients with Skeletal Malignant Involvement Treated with Intravenous Bisphosphonates." [In eng]. *J Bone Joint Surg Am* 93, no. 13 (Jul 6 2011): 1235–42.

Hussein, W., C. Cunningham, H. Logan, C. Fallon, and S. Murphy. "Atypical Fractures on Long-Term Bisphosphonates Therapy." [In eng]. *Ir Med J* 104, no. 10 (Nov-Dec 2011): 308, 10.

Depasquale, R., R. Jones and A. Hunt. "Bisphos-phonate-related bilateral atypical femoral frac-tures - Be aware and beware." *Malta Med. J.* Vol 23, Issue 2, available at http://www.um.edu.mt/umms/mmj/showpdf.php?article=322.

Sellmeyer, D. E. "Atypical Fractures as a Potential Complication of Long-Term Bisphosphonate Therapy." [In eng]. *JAMA* 304, no. 13 (Oct 6 2010): 1480–4.

64. Perre, M. C. "Subtrochanteric fractures in patients on long term bisphosphonate therapy." *J Surg Radiol.* 2011 Jul 2(3): 207–326. http://www.surgisphere.com/SurgRad/issues/volume-2/1-july-2011--pages-207-326.html.

65. Ng, Y. H., P. D. Gino, K. Lingaraj, and S. Das De. "Femoral Shaft Fractures in the Elderly—Role of Prior Bisphosphonate Therapy." [In eng]. *Injury* 42, no. 7 (Jul 2011): 702–6.

66. Nieves, J. W., and F. Cosman. "Atypical Subtrochanteric and Femoral Shaft Fractures and Possible Association with Bisphosphonates." [In eng]. *Curr Osteoporos Rep* 8, no. 1 (Mar 2010): 34–9.

67. Reddy, S. V., and S. K. Gupta. "Atypical Femoral Shaft Fracture in a Patient with Non-Metastatic Prostate Cancer on Zoledronic Acid Therapy: Effect of Therapy or Coincidence?" [In eng]. *Singapore Med J* 53, no. 3 (Mar 2012): e52–4.

68. Shin, D. Y., C. R. Ku, K. M. Kim, H. S. Choi, Y. Rhee, E. J. Lee, and S. K. Lim. "Spontaneous Non-Traumatic Stress Fractures in Bilateral Femoral Shafts in a Patient Treated with Bisphosphonates." [In eng]. *Korean J Intern Med* 27, no. 1 (Mar 2012): 98–102.

Murphy, C. G., S. O'Flanagan, P. Keogh, and P. Kenny. "Subtrochanteric Stress Fractures in Patients on Oral Bisphosphonate Therapy: An Emerging Problem." [In eng]. *Acta Orthop Belg* 77, no. 5 (Oct 2011): 632–7.

69. Zhang, J., K. G. Saag, and J. R. Curtis. "Long-Term Safety Concerns of Antiresorptive Therapy." [In eng]. *Rheum Dis Clin North Am* 37, no. 3 (Aug 2011): 387–400, vi.

Hollick, R. J., and D. M. Reid. "Role of Bisphosphonates in the Management of Postmenopausal Osteoporosis: An Update on Recent Safety Anxieties." [In eng]. *Menopause Int* 17, no. 2 (Jun 2011): 66–72.

Lewiecki, E. M. "Safety of Long-Term Bisphosphonate Therapy for the Management of Osteoporosis." [In eng]. *Drugs* 71, no. 6 (Apr 16 2011): 791–814.

Howard, P. A., B. J. Barnes, J. L. Vacek, W. Chen, and S. M. Lai. "Impact of Bisphosphonates on the Risk of Atrial Fibrillation." [In eng]. *Am J Cardiovasc Drugs* 10, no. 6 (2010): 359–67.

Mortimer, J. E., and S. K. Pal. "Safety Considerations for Use of Bone-Targeted Agents in Patients with Cancer." [In eng]. *Semin Oncol* 37 Suppl 1 (Jun 2010): S66–72.

Vassiliou, V., N. Tselis and D. Kardamakis. "Osteonecrosis of the Jaws: Clinicopathologic and Radiologic Characteristics, Preventive and Therapeutic Strategies." [In eng]. *Strahlenther Onkol* 186, no. 7 (Jul 2010): 367–73.

Abrahamsen, B. "Adverse Effects of Bisphosphonates." [In eng]. *Calcif Tissue Int* 86, no. 6 (Jun 2010): 421–35.

John, Camm A. "Review of the cardiovascular safety of zoledronic acid and other bisphosphonates for the treatment of osteoporosis." *Clin Ther* (Mar 2010):32(3):426–36.

Bhuriya, R., M. Singh, J. Molnar, R. Arora, and S. Khosla. "Bisphosphonate Use in Women and the Risk of Atrial Fibrillation: A Systematic Review and Meta-Analysis." [In eng]. *Int J Cardiol* 142, no. 3 (Jul 23 2010): 213–7.

Papapetrou, P. D. "Bisphosphonate-Associated Adverse Events." [In eng]. *Hormones (Athens)* 8, no. 2 (Apr-Jun 2009): 96–110.

Shannon, J., S. Modelevsky, and A. A. Grippo. "Bisphosphonates and Osteonecrosis of the Jaw." [In eng]. *J Am Geriatr Soc* 59, no. 12 (Dec 2011): 2350–5.

70. Barasch, A., J. Cunha-Cruz, F. A. Curro, P. Hujoel, A. H. Sung, D. Vena, A. E. Voinea-Griffin, *et al.* "Risk Factors for Osteonecrosis of the Jaws: A Case-Control Study from the Condor Dental Pbrn." [In eng]. *J Dent Res* 90, no. 4 (Apr 2011): 439–44.

71. Shannon, J., S. Modelevsky, and A. A. Grippo. "Bisphosphonates and Osteonecrosis of the Jaw." [In eng]. *J Am Geriatr Soc* 59, no. 12 (Dec 2011): 2350–5.

Nicoletti, P., V. M. Cartsos, P. K. Palaska, Y. Shen, A. Floratos, and A. I. Zavras. "Genomewide Pharmacogenetics of Bisphosphonate-Induced Osteonecrosis of the Jaw: The Role of Rbms3." [In eng]. *Oncologist* 17, no. 2 (2012): 279–87.

Marx, R. E., and R. Tursun. "Suppurative Osteomyelitis, Bisphosphonate Induced Osteonecrosis, Osteoradionecrosis: A Blinded Histopathologic Comparison and Its Implications for the Mechanism of Each Disease." [In eng]. *Int J Oral Maxillofac Surg* 41, no. 3 (Mar 2012): 283–9.

Stockmann, P., F. Wehrhan, S. Schwarz-Furlan, F. Stelzle, S. Trabert, F. W. Neukam, and E. Nkenke. "Increased Human Defensine Levels Hint at an Inflammatory Etiology of Bisphosphonate-Associated Osteonecrosis of the Jaw: An Immunohistological Study." [In eng]. *J Transl Med* 9 (2011): 135.

Filleul, O., E. Crompot, and S. Saussez. "Bisphosphonate-Induced Osteonecrosis of the Jaw: A Review of 2,400 Patient Cases." [In eng]. *J Cancer Res Clin Oncol* 136, no. 8 (Aug 2010): 1117–24.

Vestergaard, P., K. Schwartz, L. Rejnmark, L. Mosekilde, and E. M. Pinholt. "Oral Bisphosphonate Use Increases the Risk for Inflammatory Jaw Disease: A Cohort Study." [In eng]. *J Oral Maxillofac Surg* 70, no. 4 (Apr 2012): 821–9.

72. Lai, P. S., S. S. Chua, and S. P. Chan. "Pharmaceutical Care Issues Encountered by Post-Menopausal Osteoporotic Women Prescribed Bisphosphonates." [In Eng]. *J Clin Pharm Ther* (Mar 1 2012).

73. Rizzoli, R., K. Akesson, M. Bouxsein, J. A. Kanis, N. Napoli, S. Papapoulos, J. Y. Reginster, and C. Cooper. "Subtrochanteric Fractures after Long-Term Treatment with Bisphosphonates: A European Society on Clinical and Economic Aspects of Osteoporosis and Osteoarthritis, and International Osteoporosis Foundation Working Group Report." [In eng]. *Osteoporos Int* 22, no. 2 (Feb 2011): 373–90.

74. Vestergaard, P., F. Schwartz, L. Rejnmark, and L. Mosekilde. "Risk of Femoral Shaft and Subtrochanteric Fractures among Users of Bisphosphonates and Raloxifene." [In eng]. *Osteoporos Int* 22, no. 3 (Mar 2011): 993–1001.

75. La Rocca Vieira, R., Z. S. Rosenberg, M. B. Allison, S. A. Im, J. Babb, and V. Peck. "Frequency of Incomplete Atypical Femoral Fractures in Asymptomatic Patients on Long-Term Bisphosphonate Therapy." [In eng]. *AJR Am J Roentgenol* 198, no. 5 (May 2012): 1144–51.

76. Walker, E. FDA Panel Waffles on Limiting Duration of Bisphosphonae Use, available at http://www.medpagetoday.com/Endocrinology/Osteoporosis/28442?utm_content=&utm_medium=email&utm_campaign=DailyHeadlines&utm_source=WC&eun=g320126dor&userid=320126.

77. Bauer, J. S., N. Beck, J. Kiefer, P. Stockmann, M. Wichmann, and S. Eitner. "Awareness and Education of Patients Receiving Bisphosphonates." [In eng]. *J Craniomaxillofac Surg* 40, no. 3 (Apr 2012): 277–82.

78. Genuis, S. J., and T. P. Bouchard. "Combination of Micronutrients for Bone (Comb) Study: Bone Den-

sity after Micronutrient Intervention." [In eng]. *J Environ Public Health* 2012 (2012): 354151.

79. Prolia® is the trade name given to denosumab marketed to women at risk of osteoporosis; Xgeva® is the trade name given to the patent medicine when used for the prevention of skeletal-related events in patients with bone metastases from solid tumors.

80. Reid, I. R. and J. Cornish. 2012. Epidemiology and pathogenesis of osteonecrosis of the jaw. *Nat Rev Rheumatol* Feb;8(2):90–96. http://www.nature.com/nrrheum/journal/v8/n2/full/nrrheum.2011.181.html.

http://www.genengnews.com/gen-news-highlights/amgen-s-denosumab-cleared-by-fda-for-second-indication/81244270/.

81. Reid, I. R. and J. Cornish. 2012. Epidemiology and pathogenesis of osteonecrosis of the jaw. *Nat Rev Rheumatol* Feb;8(2):90–96. http://www.nature.com/nrrheum/journal/v8/n2/full/nrrheum.2011.181.html.

82. Ibid.

83. Fattore, A. D., and A. Teti. "The Tight Relationship between Osteoclasts and the Immune System." [In eng]. *Inflamm Allergy Drug Targets* 11, no. 3 (Jun 1 2012): 181–7.

84. Khosla, S. "Increasing Options for the Treatment of Osteoporosis." [In eng]. *N Engl J Med* 361, no. 8 (Aug 20 2009): 818–20.

85. McClung, M. R., E. M. Lewiecki, S. B. Cohen, M. A. Bolognese, G. C. Woodson, A. H. Moffett, M. Peacock, *et al.* "Denosumab in Postmenopausal Women with Low Bone Mineral Density." [In eng]. *N Engl J Med* 354, no. 8 (Feb 23 2006): 821–31.

86. Godinez-Puig, V. and B. Nardone, West, D.P., et al. 2012. Denosumab is associated with dermatologic toxicity in the FDA-AERS database. *J Investigative*

Dermatology, Vol. 132, Suppl. 1, May, 75th, May 9–12, 2012. http://www.nature.com/jid/journal/v132/n1s/full/jid201286a.html.

87. Reid, I. R. and J. Cornish. 2012. Epidemiology and pathogenesis of osteonecrosis of the jaw. *Nat Rev Rheumatol* Feb;8(2):90–96. http://www.nature.com/nrrheum/journal/v8/n2/full/nrrheum.2011.181.html.

88. Bridgeman, M. B., and R. Pathak. "Denosumab for the Reduction of Bone Loss in Postmenopausal Osteoporosis: A Review." [In eng]. *Clin Ther* 33, no. 11 (Nov 2011): 1547–59.

89. Haberfeld, H, ed. (2009) (in German). Austria-Codex (2009/2010 ed.). (Vienna: Österreichischer Apothekerverlag). ISBN 3-85200-196-X.

90. Watts, N. B., C. Roux, J. F. Modlin, J. P. Brown, A. Daniels, S. Jackson, S. Smith, *et al.* "Infections in Postmenopausal Women with Osteoporosis Treated with Denosumab or Placebo: Coincidence or Causal Association?" [In eng]. *Osteoporos Int* 23, no. 1 (Jan 2012): 327–37.

91. Walker, Emily P. 2012. "Benefit of Bone Patent medicine in Prostate Cancer in Doubt". *MedPage Today* Feb 7, http://www.medpagetoday.com/HematologyOncology/ProstateCancer/31039.

92. Dore, R. K. "Data from Extension Trials: Denosumab and Zoledronic Acid." [In eng]. *Curr Osteoporos Rep* 10, no. 1 (Mar 2012): 16–21.

93. Body, J. J., P. Bergmann, S. Boonen, J. P. Devogelaer, E. Gielen, S. Goemaere, J. M. Kaufman, S. Rozenberg, and J. Y. Reginster. "Extraskeletal Benefits and Risks of Calcium, Vitamin D and Anti-Osteoporosis Medications." [In eng]. *Osteoporos Int* 23 Suppl 1 (Feb 2012): S1–23.

94. http://blogs.wsj.com/health/2009/08/14/analysts-react-to-fda-panel-it-wasnt-a-perfect-day-for-amgen/.

95. Marcus, R. "Present at the Beginning: A Personal Reminiscence on the History of Teriparatide." [In eng]. *Osteoporos Int* 22, no. 8 (Aug 2011): 2241–8.

96. Subbiah, V., V. S. Madsen, A. K. Raymond, R. S. Benjamin, and J. A. Ludwig. "Of Mice and Men: Divergent Risks of Teriparatide-Induced Osteosarcoma." [In eng]. *Osteoporos Int* 21, no. 6 (Jun 2010): 1041–5.

   Tastekin, N., and C. Zateri. "Probable Osteosarcoma Risk after Prolonged Teriparatide Treatment: Comment on the Article by Saag Et Al." [In eng]. *Arthritis Rheum* 62, no. 6 (Jun 2010): 1837; author reply 37–8.

97. Ibid.

98. Forteo Trial on Idiopathic Osteoporosis in Premenopausal Women, accessed 4-18-2012 at http://clinicaltrials.gov/ct2/show/NCT01440803.

99. Miller, P. D. "Safety of Parathyroid Hormone for the Treatment of Osteoporosis." [In eng]. *Curr Osteoporos Rep* 6, no. 1 (Mar 2008): 12–6.

100. Bunyaratavej, N. "Experience of Application: Blood Screening and Bone Turnover Markers for Prevention of Unwanted Effects and Early Outcomes of Teriparatide." [In eng]. *J Med Assoc Thai* 94 Suppl 5 (Oct 2011): S31–4.

101. Cumali. K., K. Kadir, K. Hanifi, et al. Severe hypercalcemia due to teriparatide. *Indian J Pharmacol* [serial online] 2012 [cited 2012 Apr 19]; 44:270-1. Available from: http://www.ijp-online.com/text.asp?2012/44/2/270/93869.

102. Lasco, A., A. Catalano, N. Morabito, A. Gaudio, G. Basile, A. Trifiletti, and M. Atteritano. "Adrenal Effects of Teriparatide in the Treatment of Severe Postmenopausal Osteoporosis." [In eng]. *Osteoporos Int* 22, no. 1 (Jan 2011): 299–303.

103. Morelli, V., B. Masserini, A. S. Salcuni, C. Eller-Vainicher, C. Savoca, R. Viti, F. Coletti, *et al.* "Subclinical Hypercortisolism: Correlation between Biochemical Diagnostic Criteria and Clinical Aspects." [In eng]. *Clin Endocrinol (Oxf)* 73, no. 2 (Aug 2010): 161–6.

104. Lasco, A., A. Catalano, N. Morabito, A. Gaudio, G. Basile, A. Trifiletti, and M. Atteritano. "Adrenal Effects of Teriparatide in the Treatment of Severe Postmenopausal Osteoporosis." [In eng]. *Osteoporos Int* 22, no. 1 (Jan 2011): 299–303.

105. Braverman, E. R., T. J. Chen, A. L. Chen, V. Arcuri, M. M. Kerner, A. Bajaj, J. Carbajal, *et al.* "Age-Related Increases in Parathyroid Hormone May Be Antecedent to Both Osteoporosis and Dementia." [In eng]. *BMC Endocr Disord* 9 (2009): 21.

106. Am Acad Orthopaedic Surgeons. 2012. Mtg: Abstract 190, (presented 2-8-12) http://bit.ly/wG9lAT.

107. Genuis, S. J., and T. P. Bouchard. "Combination of Micronutrients for Bone (Comb) Study: Bone Density after Micronutrient Intervention." [In eng]. *J Environ Public Health* 2012 (2012): 354151.

108. Lappe, J., I. Kunz, I. Bendik, K. Prudence, P. Weber, R. Recker, and R. P. Heaney. "Effect of a Combination of Genistein, Polyunsaturated Fatty Acids and Vitamins D3 and K1 on Bone Mineral Density in Postmenopausal Women: A Randomized, Placebo-Controlled, Double-Blind Pilot Study." [In Eng]. *Eur J Nutr* (Feb 3 2012).

109. Rizzoli, R., and J. Y. Reginster. "Adverse Drug Reactions to Osteoporosis Treatments." [In eng]. *Expert Rev Clin Pharmacol* 4, no. 5 (Sep 2011): 593–604.

110. Ma, J., R. A. Johns and R. S. Stafford. 2007. Americans are not meeting current calcium recommendations. *Am J Clin Nutr* May;85(5):1361–6. PMID: 17490974.

111. Hale, G.E. and H. G. Burger. 2009. Hormonal changes and biomarkers in late reproductive age, menopausal transition and menopause. *Best Pract Res Clin Obstet Gynaecol* Feb;23(1):7–23. PMID: 19046657.

112. Binkley, N. 2006. Osteoporosis in men. *Arq Bras Endocrinol Metabol* Aug;50(4):764–74. PMID: 17117301.

   Tuck, S. P. and R. M. Francis. 2009. Testosterone, bone and osteoporosis. *Front Horm Res* 37:123–32. PMID: 19011293.

113. Ross, R. W. and E. J. Small. 2002. Osteoporosis in men treated with androgen deprivation therapy for prostate cancer. *J Urol* May;167(5):1952–6. PMID: 11956415.

114. Grossman, M. I., J. B. Kirsner and I. E. Gillespie. 1963. Basal and histalog-stimulated gastric secretion in control subjects and in patients with peptic ulcer or gastric cancer. *Gastroenterology* Jul;45:14–26. PMID: 14046306.

115. Nicar, M. J. and C. Y. Pak. 1985. Calcium bioavailability from calcium carbonate and calcium citrate. *J Clin Endocrinol Metab* Aug;61(2):391–3. PMID: 4008614.

   Wood, R. J. and C. Serfaty-Lacrosniere. 1992. Gastric acidity, atrophic gastritis, and calcium absorption. *Nutr Rev* Feb;50(2):33–40. PMID: 1570081.

116. Nicar, M. J. and C. Y. Pak. 1985. Calcium bioavailability from calcium carbonate and calcium citrate. *J Clin Endocrinol Metab* Aug;61(2):391–3. PMID: 4008614.

   Wood, R. J. and C. Serfaty-Lacrosniere. 1992. Gastric acidity, atrophic gastritis, and calcium absorption. *Nutr Rev* Feb;50(2):33–40. PMID: 1570081.

117. Hanzlik, R.P., S. C. Fowler and D. H. Fisher. 2005. Relative bioavailability of calcium from calcium

formate, calcium citrate, and calcium carbonate. *J Pharmacol Exp Ther* Jun;313(3):1217–22. PMID: 15734899.

Reinwald, S., C. M. Weaver and J. J. Kester. 2008. The health benefits of calcium citrate malate: a review of the supporting science. *Adv Food Nutr Res* 54:219–346. PMID: 18291308.

Tondapu, P., D. Provost, B. Adams-Huet, et al. 2009. Comparison of the absorption of calcium carbonate and calcium citrate after Roux-en-Y gastric bypass. *Obes Surg* Sep;19(9):1256–61. PMID: 19437082.

118. Straub, D. A. 2007. Calcium supplementation in clinical practice: a review of forms, doses, and indications. *Nutr Clin Pract* Jun;22(3):286–96. PMID: 17507729.

119. Licata, A. A., E. Bou, F. C. Bartter, et al. 1981. Acute effects of dietary protein on calcium metabolism in patients with osteoporosis. *J Gerontol* Jan;36(1):14–9. PMID: 7451829.

120. New, S. A. 2004. Do vegetarians have a normal bone mass? *Osteoporos Int* Sep;15(9):679–88. PMID: 15258721.

Marsh, A. G., T. V. Sanchez, F. L. Chaffee, et al. 1983. Bone mineral mass in adult lacto-ovo-vegetarian and omnivorous males. *Am J Clin Nutr* Mar;37(3):453–6. PMID: 6687507.

Cooper, C., E. J. Atkinson, D. D. Hensrud, et al. 1996. Dietary protein intake and bone mass in women. *Calcif Tissue Int* May;58(5):320–5. PMID: 8661965.

121. Fulgoni, V. L. 3rd. 2008. Current protein intake in America: analysis of the National Health and Nutrition Examination Survey, 2003–2004. *Am J Clin Nutr* May;87(5):1554S-1557S. PMID: 18469286.

122. Kerstetter, J. E., K. O. O'Brien and K. L. Insogna. 2003. Low protein intake: the impact on calcium and bone

homeostasis in humans. *J Nutr* Mar;133(3):855S-861S. PMID: 12612169.

123. Kerstetter, J. E., K. O. O'Brien and K. L. Insogna. 2003. Dietary protein, calcium metabolism, and skeletal homeostasis revisited. *Am J Clin Nutr* Sep;78(3 Suppl):584S-592S. PMID: 12936953.

124. Pizzorno, J. E. and M. T. Murray eds. *Textbook of Natural Medicine*, 3rd Ed. Vol. 2, (St Louis, MO: Elsevier, 2006), p. 1982.

   Gross, L. S., L. Li, E. S. Ford and S. Liu. 2004. Increased consumption of refined carbohydrates and the epidemic of type 2 diabetes in the United States: an ecologic assessment. *Am J Clin Nutr* May;79(5):774-9. PMID: 15113714.

125. Olshansky, S. J., D. J. Passaro, R. C. Hershow, et al. 2005. A potential decline in life expectancy in the United States in the 21st century. *N Engl J Med* Mar 17;352(11):1138-45. PMID: 15784668.

126. Pizzorno, J. E. and M. T. Murray eds. *Textbook of Natural Medicine*, 3rd Ed. Vol. 2, (St Louis, MO: Elsevier, 2006), p. 1982.

127. Byers, T. 1993. Dietary trends in the United States. Relevance to cancer prevention. *Cancer* Aug 1;72(3 Suppl):1015-8. PMID: 8334652.

128. Block, G. 1991. Dietary guidelines and the results of food consumption surveys. *Am J Clin Nutr* Jan;53(1 Suppl):356S-357S. PMID: 1985410.

129. Saito, M. 2009. [Biochemical markers of bone turnover. New aspect. Bone collagen metabolism: new biological markers for estimation of bone quality] *Clin Calcium* Aug;19(8):1110-7. PMID: 19638694.

   Petramala, L., M. Acca, C. M. Francucci, et al. 2009. Hyperhomocysteinemia: a biochemical link between bone and cardiovascular system diseases? *J Endocrinol Invest* 32(4 Suppl):10-4. PMID: 19724160.

Yilmaz, N. and E. Eren. 2009. Homocysteine oxidative stress and relation to bone mineral density in postmenopausal osteoporosis. *Aging Clin Exp Res* Aug-Oct;21(4–5):353–7. PMID: 19959926.

Haliloglu, B., F. B. Aksungar, E. Ilter, et al. 2010. Relationship between bone mineral density, bone turnover markers and homocysteine, folate and vitamin B12 levels in postmenopausal women. *Arch Gynecol Obstet* Apr;281(4):663–8. Epub 2009 Nov 28. PMID: 19946695.

Leboff, M. S., R. Narweker, A. LaCroix, et al. 2009. *J Clin Endocrinol Metab* Apr;94(4):1207–13. PMID: 19174498.

130. Andreotti, F., F. Burzotta, A. Manzoli, et al. 2000. Homocysteine and risk of cardiovascular disease. *J Thromb Thrombolysis* Jan;9(1):13–21. PMID: 10590184.

131. Stanger, O., B. Fowler, K. Piertzik, et al. 2009. Homocysteine, folate and vitamin B12 in neuropsychiatric diseases: review and treatment recommendations. *Expert Rev Neurother* Sep;9(9):1393–412. PMID: 19769453.

132. Ferechide, D. and D. Radulescu. 2009. Hyperhomocysteinemia in renal diseases. *J Med Life* Jan-Mar;2(1):53–9. PMID: 20108491.

Zoccali, C. 2005. Biomarkers in chronic kidney disease: utility and issues towards better understanding. *Curr Opin Nephrol Hypertens* Nov;14(6):532–7. PMID: 16205471.

Ingrosso, D., A. F. Perna. 2009. Epigenetics in hyperhomocysteinemic states. A special focus on uremia. *Biochim Biophys Acta* Sep;1790(9):892–9. PMID: 19245874.

Righetti, M. 2009. Protective effect of vitamin B therapy on bone and cardiovascular disease. *Recent Pat Cardiovasc Drug Discov* Jan;4(1):37–44. PMID: 19149705.

Trimarchi, H., P. Young, M. L. Díaz, et al. 2005. [Hyperhomocysteinemia as a vascular risk factor in chronic hemodialysis patients] *Medicina* (B Aires) 65(6):513–7. PMID: 16433478.

133. Woolf, K., M. M. Manore. 2008. Elevated plasma homocysteine and low vitamin B-6 status in non-supplementing older women with rheumatoid arthritis. *J Am Diet Assoc* Mar;108(3):443–53; discussion 454. PMID: 18313425.

134. Wile, D. J. and C. Toth. 2010. Association of metformin, elevated homocysteine, and methylmalonic acid levels and clinically worsened diabetic peripheral neuropathy. *Diabetes Care.* 2010 Jan;33(1):156–61. Epub 2009 Oct 21. PMID: 19846797.

   Pflipsen, M. C., R. C. Oh, A. Saguil, et al. 2009. The prevalence of vitamin B(12) deficiency in patients with type 2 diabetes: a cross-sectional study. *J Am Board Fam Med* Sep-Oct;22(5):528–34. PMID: 19734399.

135. Shah, S., R. J. Bell, S. R. Davis. 2006. Homocysteine, estrogen and cognitive decline. *Climacteric* Apr;9(2):77–87. PMID: 16698655.

   Sultan, N., M. A. Khan and S. Malik. 2007. Effect of folic acid supplementation on homocysteine level in postmenopausal women. *J Ayub Med Coll Abbottabad* Oct-Dec;19(4):78–81. PMID: 18693605.

136. McLean, R. R., P. F. Jacques, J. Selhub, et al. 2008. Plasma B vitamins, homocysteine, and their relation with bone loss and hip fracture in elderly men and women. *J Clin Endocrinol Metab* Jun;93(6):2206–12. PMID: 18364381.

137. Lussana, F., M. L. Zighetti, P. Bucciarelli, et al. 2003. Blood levels of homocysteine, folate, vitamin B_6 and B12 in women using oral contraceptives compared to non-users. *Thromb Res* 112(1–2):37–41. PMID: 15013271.

138. Pfeiffer, C. M., S. P. Caudill, E. W. Gunter, et al. 2005. Biochemical indicators of B vitamin status in the US population after folic acid fortification: results from the National Health and Nutrition Examination Survey 1999–2000. *Am J Clin Nutr* Aug;82(2):442–50. PMID: 16087991.

139. Pennypacker, L. C., R. H. Allen, et al. 1992. High prevalence of cobalamin deficiency in elderly outpatients. *J Am Geriatr Soc* Dec;40(12):1197–204. PMID: 1447433.

140. Allen, L. H. 2009. How common is vitamin B-12 deficiency? *Am J Clin Nutr* Feb;89(2):693S-6S. Epub 2008 Dec 30. PMID: 19116323.

141. Pflipsen, M. C., R. C. Oh, A. Saguil, et al. 2009. The prevalence of vitamin B(12) deficiency in patients with type 2 diabetes: a cross-sectional study. *J Am Board Fam Med* Sep-Oct;22(5):528–34. PMID: 19734399.

142. Fain, O. 2005. Musculoskeletal manifestations of scurvy. *Joint Bone Spine* Mar;72(2):124–8. PMID: 15797491.

    Hall, S. L. and G. A. Greendale. 1998. The relation of dietary vitamin C intake to bone mineral density: results from the PEPI study. *Calcif Tissue Int* Sep;63(3):183–9. PMID: 9701620.

143. Sahni, S., M. T. Hannan, D. Gagnon, et al. 2009. Protective effect of total and supplemental vitamin C intake on the risk of hip fracture—a 17-year follow-up from the Framingham Osteoporosis Study. *Osteoporos Int* Nov;20(11):1853–61. PMID: 19347239.

144. Martínez-Ramírez, M. J., S. Palma Pérez, A. D. Delgado-Martínez, et al. 2007. Vitamin C, vitamin B12, folate and the risk of osteoporotic fractures. A case-control study. *Int J Vitam Nutr Res* Nov;77(6):359–68. PMID: 18622945.

145. Pasco, J. A., M. J. Henry, L. K. Wilkinson, et al. 2006. Antioxidant vitamin supplements and markers of bone turnover in a community sample of nonsmoking women. *J Womens Health* (Larchmt) Apr;15(3):295–300. PMID: 16620188.

146. Schleicher, R. L., M. D. Carroll, E. S. Ford, et al. 2009. Serum vitamin C and the prevalence of vitamin C deficiency in the United States: 2003–2004 National Health and Nutrition Examination Survey (NHANES). *Am J Clin Nutr* Nov;90(5):1252–63 PMID: 19675106.

147. Palacios, C. 2006. The role of nutrients in bone health, from A to Z. *Crit Rev Food Sci Nutr* 46(8):621–8. PMID: 17092827.

Morton, D. J., E. L. Barrett-Connor and D. L. Schneider. 2001. Vitamin C supplement use and bone mineral density in postmenopausal women. *J Bone Miner Res* Jan;16(1):135–40. PMID: 11149477.

148. Pizzorno, J. E. *Total Wellness* (Rocklin, CA: Prima Publishing, 1996), p. 44–45, 62.

149. Schleicher, R. L., M. D. Carroll, E. S. Ford, et al. 2009. Serum vitamin C and the prevalence of vitamin C deficiency in the United States: 2003–2004 National Health and Nutrition Examination Survey (NHANES). *Am J Clin Nutr* Nov;90(5):1252–63 PMID: 19675106.

150. Lazcano-Ponce, E., J. Tamayo, R. Díaz, et al. 2009. Correlation trends for bone mineral density in Mexican women: evidence of familiar predisposition. *Salud Publica Mex* 51 Suppl 1:s93–9. PMID: 19287898.

151. Pizzorno, J. E. and M. T. Murray, "Osteoporosis", in *Textbook of Natural Medicine*, 3rd ed., (St. Louis: Elsevier, 2006), Ch. 196, 2:1978.

152. Makovey, J., T. V. Nguyen, V. Naganathan, et al. 2007. Genetic effects on bone loss in peri- and postmenopausal women: a longitudinal twin

study. *J Bone Miner Res* Nov;22(11):1773–80. PMID: 17620052.

Sigurdsson, G., B. V. Halldorsson, U. Styrkarsdottir, et al. 2008. Impact of genetics on low bone mass in adults. *J Bone Miner Res* Oct;23(10):1584–90. PMID: 18505373.

Zhai, G., T. Andrew, B. S. Kato, et al. 2009. Genetic and environmental determinants on bone loss in postmenopausal Caucasian women: a 14-year longitudinal twin study. *Osteoporos Int* Jun;20(6):949–53. PMID: 18810303.

153. Valderas, J. P., S. Velasco, S. Solari, et al. 2009. Increase of bone resorption and the parathyroid hormone in postmenopausal women in the long-term after Roux-en-Y gastric bypass. *Obes Surg* Aug;19(8):1132–8. Epub 2009 Jun 11. PMID: 19517199.

De Prisco, C. and S. N. Levine. 2005. Metabolic bone disease after gastric bypass surgery for obesity. *Am J Med Sci* Feb;329(2):57–61. PMID: 15711420.

154. Tice, J. A., L. Karliner, J. Walsh, et al. 2008. Gastric banding or bypass? A systematic review comparing the two most popular bariatric procedures. *Am J Med* Oct;121(10):885–93. PMID: 18823860.

155. Wang, A. and A. Powell. 2009. The effects of obesity surgery on bone metabolism: what orthopedic surgeons need to know. *Am J Orthop* (Belle Mead NJ) Feb;38(2):77–9. PMID: 19340369.

156. Goode, L. R., R. E. Brolin, H. A. Chowdhury, et al. 2004. Bone and gastric bypass surgery: effects of dietary calcium and vitamin D. *Obes Res* Jan;12(1):40–7. PMID: 14742841.

157. Nakchbandi, I. A., S. W. van der Merwe. 2009. Current understanding of osteoporosis associated with liver disease. *Nat Rev Gastroenterol Hepatol* Nov;6(11):660–70. PMID: 19881518.

Jean, G., J. C. Terrat, T. Vanel, et al. 2008. Daily oral 25-hydroxycholecalciferol supplementation for vitamin D deficiency in haemodialysis patients: effects on mineral metabolism and bone markers. *Nephrol Dial Transplant* Nov;23(11):3670–6. PMID: 18579534.

Jean, G., J. C. Terrat, T. Vanel, et al. 2008. Evidence for persistent vitamin D 1-alpha-hydroxylation in hemodialysis patients: evolution of serum 1,25-dihydroxycholecalciferol after 6 months of 25-hydroxycholecalciferol treatment. *Nephron Clin Pract* 110(1):c58–65. PMID: 18724068.

Frith, J. and J. L. Newton. 2009. Liver disease in older women. *Maturitas* Dec 2. [Epub ahead of print] PMID: 19962256.

158. Levey, A. S., L. A. Stevens, C. H. Schmid, et al. 2009. A new equation to estimate glomerular filtration rate. *Ann Intern Med* May 5;150(9):604–12. PMID: 19414839.

159. Frith, J., D. Jones and J. L. Newton. 2009. Chronic liver disease in an ageing population. *Age Ageing* Jan;38(1):11–8. Epub 2008 Nov 22. PMID: 19029099.

160. George, J., H. K. Ganesh, S. Acharya, et al. 2009. Bone mineral density and disorders of mineral metabolism in chronic liver disease. *World J Gastroenterol* Jul 28;15(28):3516–22. PMID: 19630107.

Murlikiewicz, K., A. Zawiasa, M. Nowicki. 2009. [Vitamin D—a panacea in nephrology and beyond] *Pol Merkur Lekarski* Nov;27(161):437–41. PMID: 19999813.

Moe, S. M., T. Drüeke, N. Lameire, et al. 2007. Chronic kidney disease-mineral-bone disorder: a new paradigm. *Adv Chronic Kidney Dis* Jan;14(1):3–12. PMID: 17200038.

Spasovski , G. B. 2007. Bone health and vascular calcification relationships in chronic kidney disease. *Int Urol Nephrol* 39(4):1209–16. Epub 2007 Sep 26. PMID: 17899431.

Jean, G., B. Charra and C. Chazot. 2008. Vitamin D deficiency and associated factors in hemodialysis patients. *J Ren Nutr* Sep;18(5):395–9. PMID: 18721733.

161. Braverman, E. R., T. J. Chen, A. L. Chen, et al. 2009. Age-related increases in parathyroid hormone may be antecedent to both osteoporosis and dementia. *BMC Endocr Disord* Oct 13;9:21. PMID: 19825157.

162. Bonjour, J. P., V. Benoit, O. Pourchaire , et al. 2009. Inhibition of markers of bone resorption by consumption of vitamin D and calcium-fortified soft plain cheese by institutionalised elderly women. *Br J Nutr* Oct;102(7):962–6. PMID: 19519975.

163. Braverman, E. R., T. J. Chen, A. L. Chen, et al. 2009. Age-related increases in parathyroid hormone may be antecedent to both osteoporosis and dementia. *BMC Endocr Disord* Oct 13;9:21. PMID: 19825157.

164. Williams, G. R. 2009. Actions of thyroid hormones in bone. *Endokrynol Pol* Sep-Oct;60(5):380–8. PMID: 19885809.

Zaidi, M., T. F. Davies, A. Zallone, H. C. Blair, et al. 2009. Thyroid-stimulating hormone, thyroid hormones, and bone loss. *Curr Osteoporos Rep* Jul;7(2):47–52. PMID: 19631028.

165. Suominen, H. 2006. Muscle training for bone strength. *Aging Clin Exp Res* Apr;18(2):85–93. PMID: 16702776.

166. Schmitt, N. M., J. Schmitt, M. Dören. 2009. The role of physical activity in the prevention of osteoporosis in postmenopausal women-An update.

Maturitas May 20;63(1):34–8. Epub 2009 Apr 7. PMID: 19356867.

167. de Matos, O., D. J. Lopes da Silva, et al. 2009. Effect of specific exercise training on bone mineral density in women with postmenopausal osteopenia or osteoporosis. *Gynecol Endocrinol* Sep;25(9):616–20. PMID: 19533480.

168. Iwamoto, J., Y. Sato, T. Takeda, et al. 2009. Effectiveness of exercise in the treatment of lumbar spinal stenosis, knee osteoarthritis, and osteoporosis. *Aging Clin Exp Res* Nov 6. [Epub ahead of print] PMID: 19920410.

169. Brooke-Wavell. K., P. R. Jones, A. E. Hardman, et al. 2001. Commencing, continuing, and stopping brisk walking: effects on bone mineral density, quantitative ultrasound of bone and markers of bone metabolism in postmenopausal women. *Osteoporos Int* 12(7):581–7. PMID: 11527057.

170. Angin, E. and Z. Erden. 2009. [The effect of group exercise on postmenopausal osteoporosis and osteopenia] *Acta Orthop Traumatol Turc* Aug-Oct;43(4):343–50. PMID: 19809232.

171. Pizzorno, L. and J. Pizzorno. 2005. Clinical Pearls from the 12th Annual International Symposium on Functional Medicine, The Immune System Under Seige: New Clinical Approaches to Immunological Imbalances in the 21st Century, held May 26–28, 2005, Palm Springs, CA. Presentation by Michael Holick, How Vitamin D Modulates Immune and Inflammatory Processes. *IMCJ* Oct;4(5):30–33.

172. Guzel, R., E. Kozanoglu, F. Guler-Uysal, et al. 2001. Vitamin D status and bone mineral density of veiled and unveiled Turkish women. *J Womens Health Gend Based Med* Oct;10(8):765–70. PMID: 11703889.

Gannagé-Yared, M. H., G. Maalouf, S. Khalife, et al. 2009. Prevalence and predictors of vitamin

D inadequacy amongst Lebanese osteoporotic women. *Br J Nutr* Feb;101(4):487–91.PMID: 18631414.

173. Binkley, N., R. Novotny, D. Krueger, et al. 2007. Low vitamin D status despite abundant sun exposure. *J Clin Endocrinol Metab* 92:2130–5. PMID: 17426097.

174. Gannagé-Yared, M. H., G. Maalouf, S. Khalife, et al. 2009. Prevalence and predictors of vitamin D inadequacy amongst Lebanese osteoporotic women. *Br J Nutr* Feb;101(4):487–91.PMID: 18631414.

175. Chapuy, M. C., M. E. Arlot, P. D. Delmas, et al. 1994. Effect of calcium and cholecalciferol treatment for three years on hip fractures in elderly women. *BMJ* Apr 23;308(6936):1081–2. PMID: 8173430.

176. Chapuy, M. C., M. E. Arlot, F. Duboeuf , et al. 1992. Vitamin D3 and calcium to prevent hip fractures in the elderly women. *N Engl J Med* Dec 3;327(23):1637–42. PMID: 1331788.

   Meunier, P. J., M. C. Chapuy, M. E. Arlot, et al. 1994. Can we stop bone loss and prevent hip fractures in the elderly? *Osteoporos Int* 4 Suppl 1:71–6. PMID: 8081065.

177. Chapuy, M. C., R. Pamphile, E. Paris, et al. 2002. Combined calcium and vitamin D3 supplementation in elderly women: confirmation of reversal of secondary hyperparathyroidism and hip fracture risk: the Decalyos II study. *Osteoporos Int* Mar;13(3):257–64. PMID: 11991447.

178. http://www.vitamindcouncil.org.

179. Legroux-Gérot, I., J. Vignau, M. D'Herbomez, et al. 2007. Evaluation of bone loss and its mechanisms in anorexia nervosa. *Calcif Tissue Int* Sep;81(3):174–82. PMID: 17668143.

   Legroux-Gérot, I., J. Vignau, E. Biver, et al. 2010. Anorexia nervosa, osteoporosis and circulating leptin: the missing link. *Osteoporos Int* Jan 6. [Epub ahead of print] PMID: 20052458.

180. Perez-Lopez, F. R., M. Brincat, C. T. Erel, F. Tremollieres, M. Gambacciani, I. Lambrinoudaki, M. H. Moen, *et al.* "Emas Position Statement: Vitamin D and Postmenopausal Health." [In eng]. *Maturitas* 71, no. 1 (Jan 2012): 83–8.

181. http://en.wikipedia.org/wiki/List_of_benzodiazepines.

182. Luz Rentero, M., C. Carbonell, M. Casillas, M. Gonzalez Bejar, and R. Berenguer. "Risk Factors for Osteoporosis and Fractures in Postmenopausal Women between 50 and 65 Years of Age in a Primary Care Setting in Spain: A Questionnaire." [In eng]. *Open Rheumatol J* 2 (2008): 58–63.

183. http://en.wikipedia.org/wiki/List_of_benzodiazepines.

184. A more complete listing can be found at http://en.wikipedia.org/wiki/SSRI#List_of_agents.

185. http://en.wikipedia.org/wiki/Atypical_antipsychotics#List_of_atypical_antipsychotics.

186. Bolton, J. M., L. E. Targownik, S. Leung, J. Sareen, and W. D. Leslie. "Risk of Low Bone Mineral Density Associated with Psychotropic Medications and Mental Disorders in Postmenopausal Women." [In eng]. *J Clin Psychopharmacol* 31, no. 1 (Feb 2011): 56–60.

187. Bolton, J. M., C. Metge, L. Lix, H. Prior, J. Sareen, and W. D. Leslie. "Fracture Risk from Psychotropic Medications: A Population-Based Analysis." [In eng]. *J Clin Psychopharmacol* 28, no. 4 (Aug 2008): 384–91.

188. Damsa, C., A. Bumb, F. Bianchi-Demicheli, P. Vidailhet, R. Sterck, A. Andreoli, and S. Beyenburg. ""Dopamine-Dependent" Side Effects of Selective Serotonin Reuptake Inhibitors: A Clinical Review." [In eng]. *J Clin Psychiatry* 65, no. 8 (Aug 2004): 1064–8.

189. O'Keane, V. "Antipsychotic-Induced Hyperprolactinaemia, Hypogonadism and Osteoporosis in the Treatment of Schizophrenia." [In eng]. *J Psychopharmacol* 22, no. 2 Suppl (Mar 2008): 70–5.

O'Keane, V., and A. M. Meaney. "Antipsychotic Drugs: A New Risk Factor for Osteoporosis in Young Women with Schizophrenia?" [In eng]. *J Clin Psychopharmacol* 25, no. 1 (Feb 2005): 26–31.

190. http://en.wikipedia.org/wiki/List_of_benzodiazepines.

191. http://en.wikipedia.org/wiki/Atypical_antipsychotics# List_of_atypical_antipsychotics.

192. Loke, Y. K., S. Singh, and C. D. Furberg. "Long-Term Use of Thiazolidinediones and Fractures in Type 2 Diabetes: A Meta-Analysis." [In eng]. *CMAJ* 180, no. 1 (Jan 6 2009): 32–9.

Dormuth, C. R., G. Carney, B. Carleton, K. Bassett, and J. M. Wright. "Thiazolidinediones and Fractures in Men and Women." [In eng]. *Arch Intern Med* 169, no. 15 (Aug 10 2009): 1395–402.

Douglas, I. J., S. J. Evans, S. Pocock, and L. Smeeth. "The Risk of Fractures Associated with Thiazolidinediones: A Self-Controlled Case-Series Study." [In eng]. *PLoS Med* 6, no. 9 (Sep 2009): e1000154.

Aubert, R. E., V. Herrera, W. Chen, S. M. Haffner, and M. Pendergrass. "Rosiglitazone and Pioglitazone Increase Fracture Risk in Women and Men with Type 2 Diabetes." [In eng]. *Diabetes Obes Metab* 12, no. 8 (Aug 2010): 716–21.

Bodmer, M., C. Meier, M. E. Kraenzlin, and C. R. Meier. "Risk of Fractures with Glitazones: A Critical Review of the Evidence to Date." [In eng]. *Drug Saf* 32, no. 7 (2009): 539–47.

Douglas, I. J., S. J. Evans, S. Pocock, and L. Smeeth. "The Risk of Fractures Associated with Thiazolidinediones: A Self-Controlled Case-Series Study." [In eng]. *PLoS Med* 6, no. 9 (Sep 2009): e1000154.

193. Bruedigam, C., M. Eijken, M. Koedam, J. van de Peppel, K. Drabek, H. Chiba, and J. P. van Leeuwen. "A New Concept Underlying Stem Cell Lineage Skewing That Explains the Detrimental Effects of Thiazolidinediones on Bone." [In eng]. *Stem Cells* 28, no. 5 (May 2010): 916–27.

194. Daniell, H. W. "Opioid Endocrinopathy in Women Consuming Prescribed Sustained-Action Opioids for Control of Nonmalignant Pain." [In eng]. *J Pain* 9, no. 1 (Jan 2008): 28–36.

195. Rhodin, A., M. Stridsberg, and T. Gordh. "Opioid Endocrinopathy: A Clinical Problem in Patients with Chronic Pain and Long-Term Oral Opioid Treatment." [In eng]. *Clin J Pain* 26, no. 5 (Jun 2010): 374–80.

196. Pizorno, J. E. and M. T. Murray., "Osteoporosis," in the *Textbook of Natural Medicine*, 3rd ed.,: (St Louis, MO: Churchill Livingstone, 2006), chap 146.

National Institutes of Health. 2000. Osteoporosis prevention, diagnosis, and therapy. *NIH Consensus Statement* Mar 27–29;17(1):1–45.

Xu, L., P. McElduff, C. D'Este and J. Attia. 2004. Does dietary calcium have a protective effect on bone fractures in women? A meta-analysis of observational studies. *Br J Nutr* 91:625–634. PMID: 15035690.

Reid, I. R., R. W. Ames, M. C. Evans, et al. 1995. Long-term effects of calcium supplementation on bone loss and fractures in postmenopausal women: a randomized controlled trial. *Am J Med* 98:331–335. PMID: 7709944.

Devine, A., I. M. Dick, S. J. Heal, et al. 1997. A 4-year follow-up study of the effects of calcium supplementation on bone density in elderly postmenopausal women. *Osteoporos Int* 7:23–28. PMID: 9102058.

Elders, P. J., P. Lips, J. C. Netelenbos, et al. 1994. Long-term effect of calcium supplementation on bone loss in perimenopausal women. *J Bone Miner Res* 9:963–970. PMID: 7942164.

Shea, B., G. Wells, A. Cranney, et al. 2007. WITH-DRAWN: Calcium supplementation on bone loss in postmenopausal women. *Cochrane Database Syst Rev* Jul 18;(1):CD004526. PMID: 17636765.

Bourgoin, B. P., D. R. Evans, J. R. Cornett, et al. 1993. Lead content in 70 brands of dietary calcium supplements. *Am J Public Health* 83:1155–1160. PMID: 8342726.

Scelfo, G. M. and A. R. Flegal. 2000. Lead in calcium supplements. *Environ Health Perspect* Apr;108(4):309–19. PMID: 10753088.

Pizzorno, L. U., J. E. Pizzorno and M. T. Murray. "Osteoporosis," in *Natural Medicine Instructions for Patients*, (Churchill Livingstone/Elsevier, 2002), p. 251–9.

Pounder, R. E. and D. Ng. The prevalence of Helicobacter pylori infection in different countries. *Aliment Pharmacol Ther* 9 Suppl 2:33–9. PMID: 8547526.

197. Colameco, S. Opioid-induced endocrinopathy: diagnosis and screening. *J Pain Palliat Care Pharmacother*. 2012;26(1):73–5.

Elliott, J. A., E. Horton, and E. E. Fibuch. "The Endocrine Effects of Long-Term Oral Opioid Therapy: A Case Report and Review of the Literature." [In eng]. *J Opioid Manag* 7, no. 2 (Mar-Apr 2011): 145–54.

198. Straub, D. A. 2007. Calcium supplementation in clinical practice: a review of forms, doses, and indications. *Nutr Clin Pract* Jun;22(3):286–96. PMID: 17507729.

World's Healthiest Foods, Calcium, http://www.whfoods.org/genpage.php?tname=nutrient&dbid=45 (accessed 5-16-2010).

Linus Pauling Institute, Calcium, http://lpi.oregonstate. edu/infocenter/minerals/calcium/ (accessed 5-16-2010).

Castelo-Branco, C., M. Ciria-Recasens, M. J. Cancelo-Hidalgo, et al. 2009. Efficacy of ossein-hydroxyapatite complex compared with calcium carbonate to prevent bone loss: a meta-analysis. *Menopause* Sep-Oct;16(5):984–91. PMID: 19407667.

199. Adler, R. A., J. R. Curtis, K. Saag, et al. Glucocorticoid-induced osteoporosis. In: Marcus, R., D. Feldman, D. A. Nelsen, C. J. Rosen, eds. *Osteoporosis.* 3rd ed. (San Diego, CA: Elsevier-Academic Press, 2008), 1135–66.

Van Staa, T. P., R. F. Laan, I. P. Barton, S. Cohen, D. M. Reid, and C. Cooper. "Bone Density Threshold and Other Predictors of Vertebral Fracture in Patients Receiving Oral Glucocorticoid Therapy." [In eng]. *Arthritis Rheum* 48, no. 11 (Nov 2003): 3224–9.

Steinbuch, M., T. E. Youket, and S. Cohen. "Oral Glucocorticoid Use Is Associated with an Increased Risk of Fracture." [In eng]. *Osteoporos Int* 15, no. 4 (Apr 2004): 323–8.

200. Weinstein, R. S. "Clinical Practice. Glucocorticoid-Induced Bone Disease." [In eng]. *N Engl J Med* 365, no. 1 (Jul 7 2011): 62–70.

201. Weinstein, R. S. Glucocorticoid-induced osteoporosis. In: Rosen, C., ed. *The ASBMR primer on the metabolic bone diseases and disorders of mineral metabolism.* 7th ed. (Washington, DC: ASBMR, 2008), 267–72.

202. Wright, J. V., L. Lenard. *Why Stomach Acid is Good for You, Natural Relief from Heartburn, Indigestion, Reflux & GERD.* (Lanham, Maryland:,M. Evans, 2001), 25–28.

203. Mackay, J. D. and P. T. Bladon. "Hypomagnesaemia Due to Proton-Pump Inhibitor Therapy: A Clinical Case Series." [In eng]. *QJM* 103, no. 6 (Jun 2010): 387–95.

204. O'Keane, V. "Antipsychotic-Induced Hyperprolactinaemia, Hypogonadism and Osteoporosis in the Treatment of Schizophrenia." [In eng]. *J Psychopharmacol* 22, no. 2 Suppl (Mar 2008): 70–5.

O'Keane, V., and A. M. Meaney. "Antipsychotic Drugs: A New Risk Factor for Osteoporosis in Young Women with Schizophrenia?" [In eng]. *J Clin Psychopharmacol* 25, no. 1 (Feb 2005): 26–31.

205. Slemenda, C.W., S. L. Hui, C. Longcope and C. C. Johnston, Jr. 1989. Cigarette smoking, obesity, and bone mass. *J Bone Miner Res* Oct;4(5):737–41. PMID: 2816518.

Krall, E. A. and B. Dawson-Hughes. 1991. Smoking and bone loss among postmenopausal women. *J Bone Miner Res* Apr;6(4):331–8. PMID: 1858519.

Vestergaard, P. and L. Mosekilde. 2003. Fracture risk associated with smoking: a meta-analysis. *J Intern Med* Dec;254(6):572–83. PMID: 14641798.

Ward, K. D. and R. C. Klesges. 2001. A meta-analysis of the effects of cigarette smoking on bone mineral density. *Calcif Tissue Int* May;68(5):259–70. PMID: 11683532.

206. Høidrup, S., E. Prescott, T. I. Sørensen, et al. 2000. Tobacco smoking and risk of hip fracture in men and women. *Int J Epidemiol* Apr;29(2):253–9. PMID: 10817121.

207. Seeman, E., L. J. Melton, 3rd, W. M. O'Fallon, et al. 1983. Risk factors for spinal osteoporosis in men. *Am J Med* Dec;75(6):977–83. PMID: 6650552.

208. Kazantzis, G. 2004. Cadmium, osteoporosis, and calcium metabolism. *Biometals* Oct;17(5):493–8. PMID: 15688852.

209. Friberg, L. 1983. Cadmium. *Annu Rev Public Health* 4:367–73. PMID: 6860444.

210. Apeti, D. A., G. G. Lauenstein and G. F. Riedel. 2009. Cadmium distribution in coastal sediments and mollusks of the US. *Mar Pollut Bull* Jul;58(7):1016–24. PMID: 19342067.

211. Wilkinson, J. M., J. Hill and C. J. Phillips. 2003. The accumulation of potentially toxic metals by grazing ruminants. *Proc Nutr Soc* May;62(2):267–77. PMID: 14506874.

212. Akesson, A., P. Bjellerup, T. Lundh, et al. 2006. Cadmium-induced effects on bone in a population-based study of women. *Environ Health Perspect* Jun;114(6):830–4. PMID: 16759980.

 McElroy, J. A., M. M. Shafer, J. M. Hampton, et al. 2007. Predictors of urinary cadmium levels in adult females. *Sci Total Environ* Sep 1;382(2–3):214–23. PMID: 17544058.

213. Hogervorst, J., M. Plusquin, J. Vangronsveld, et al. 2007. House dust as possible route of environmental exposure to cadmium and lead in the adult general population. *Environ Res* Jan;103(1):30–7. PMID: 16843453.

214. "US Agency Goes After Cadmium in Children's Jewelry," http://abcnews.go.com/Health/WellnessNews/wireStory?id=9527916 (accessed 3-2-10).

 "Cadmium: The New Made-in-China Scare," http://www.businessweek.com/globalbiz/blog/eyeonasia/archives/2010/01/cadmium_the_new.html.

 "U.S. to Develop Safety Standards for Toxic Metals," (Update 2), http://www.businessweek.com/news/2010-01-12/u-s-to-develop-safety-standards-for-toxic-metals-update1-.html.

215. Andujar, P., L. Bensefa-Colas, A. Descatha. 2009. [Acute and chronic cadmium poisoning.] *Rev*

Med Interne Aug 24. [Epub ahead of print] PMID: 19709784.

Järup, L., A. Akesson. 2009. Current status of cadmium as an environmental health problem. *Toxicol Appl Pharmacol* Aug 1;238(3):201–8. Epub 2009 May 3. PMID: 19409405.

216. Gallagher, C. M., J. S. Kovach, J. R. Meliker. 2008. Urinary cadmium and osteoporosis in U.S. Women >or= 50 years of age: NHANES 1988–1994 and 1999–2004. *Environ Health Perspect* Oct;116(10):1338–43. PMID: 18941575.

217. Laroche, M., Y. Lasne, A. Felez, L. Moulinier, et al. 1994. [Osteocalcin and smoking] *Rev Rhum Ed Fr* Jun;61(6):433–6. PMID: 7833868.

218. Lee, N. K., H. Sowa, E. Hinoi, et al. 2007. Endocrine regulation of energy metabolism by the skeleton. *Cell* Aug 10;130(3):456–69. PMID: 17693256.

Wolf, G. 2008. Energy regulation by the skeleton. *Nutr Rev* Apr;66(4):229–33. PMID: 18366536.

219. Rothem, D. E., L. Rothem, M. Soudry, et al. 2009. Nicotine modulates bone metabolism-associated gene expression in osteoblast cells. *J Bone Miner Metab* 27(5):555–61. PMID: 19436947.

Kamer, A. R., N. El-Ghorab, N. Marzec, et al. 2006. Nicotine induced proliferation and cytokine release in osteoblastic cells. *Int J Mol Med* Jan;17(1):121–7. PMID: 16328020.

220. Mueck, A. O., H. Seeger. 2005. Smoking, estradiol metabolism, and hormone replacement therapy. *Curr Med Chem Cardiovasc Hematol Agents* Jan;3(1):45–54. PMID: 15638743.

221. Benson, B. W. and J. D. Shulman. 2005. Inclusion of tobacco exposure as a predictive factor for decreased bone mineral content. *Nicotine Tob Res* Oct;7(5):719–24. PMID: 16191742.

222. Oncken, C., K. Prestwood, A. Kleppinger, et al. 2006. Impact of smoking cessation on bone mineral density in postmenopausal women. *J Womens Health* (Larchmt) Dec;15(10):1141–50. PMID: 17199455.

223. Chakkalakal, D. A. 2005. Alcohol-induced bone loss and deficient bone repair. *Alcohol Clin Exp Res* Dec;29(12):2077–90. PMID: 16385177.

Broulik, P. D., J. Rosenkrancová, P. Růžička, et al. 2009. The effect of chronic alcohol administration on bone mineral content and bone strength in male rats. *Physiol Res* Nov 20. [Epub ahead of print] PMID: 19929136.

224. Wosje, K. S. and H. J. Kalkwarf. 2007. Bone density in relation to alcohol intake among men and women in the United States. *Osteoporos Int* Mar;18(3):391–400. PMID: 17091218.

225. Kanis, J. A., H. Johansson, O. Johnell, et al. 2005. Alcohol intake as a risk factor for fracture. *Osteoporos Int* Jul;16(7):737–42. PMID: 15455194.

226. Pedrera-Zamorano, J. D., J. M. Lavado-Garcia, R. Roncero-Martin, et al. 2009. Effect of beer drinking on ultrasound bone mass in women. *Nutrition* Oct;25(10):1057–63. Epub 2009 Jun 13. PMID: 19527924.

227. Tucker, K. L., 2009. Jugdaohsingh R, Powell JJ, et al. Effects of beer, wine, and liquor intakes on bone mineral density in older men and women. *Am J Clin Nutr* Apr;89(4):1188–96. Epub 2009 Feb 25. PMID: 19244365.

Liu, Z. P., W. X. Li, B. Yu, et al. 2005. Effects of trans-resveratrol from Polygonum cuspidatum on bone loss using the ovariectomized rat model. *J Med Food Spring* 8(1):14–9. PMID: 15857203.

King, R. E., J. A. Bomser and D. B. Min. Bioactivity of resveratrol. Compr Rev Food Sci Food Saf 5:65–70.

DOI 10.1111/j.1541-4337.2006.00001.x, http://www3.interscience.wiley.com/journal/118607162/abstract.

228. Jha, S. K., V. K. Mishra, D. K. Sharma, and T. Damodaran. "Fluoride in the Environment and Its Metabolism in Humans." [In eng]. *Rev Environ Contam Toxicol* 211 (2011): 121–42.

Everett, E. T. "Fluoride's Effects on the Formation of Teeth and Bones, and the Influence of Genetics." [In eng]. *J Dent Res* 90, no. 5 (May 2011): 552–60.

229. Ibid.

230. Whitford, G. M. "Intake and Metabolism of Fluoride." [In eng]. *Adv Dent Res* 8, no. 1 (Jun 1994): 5–14.

231. Bergandi, L., V. Aina, G. Malavasi, C. Morterra, and D. Ghigo. "The Toxic Effect of Fluoride on Mg-63 Osteoblast Cells Is Also Dependent on the Production of Nitric Oxide." [In eng]. *Chem Biol Interact* 190, no. 2-3 (Apr 25 2011): 179–86.

Bergandi, L., V. Aina, S. Garetto, G. Malavasi, E. Aldieri, E. Laurenti, L. Matera, C. Morterra, and D. Ghigo. "Fluoride-Containing Bioactive Glasses Inhibit Pentose Phosphate Oxidative Pathway and Glucose 6-Phosphate Dehydrogenase Activity in Human Osteoblasts." [In eng]. *Chem Biol Interact* 183, no. 3 (Feb 12 2010): 405–15.

232. Song, Y. E., H. Tan, K. J. Liu, Y. Z. Zhang, Y. Liu, C. R. Lu, D. L. Yu, J. Tu, and C. Y. Cui. "Effect of Fluoride Exposure on Bone Metabolism Indicators Alp, Balp, and Bgp." [In eng]. *Environ Health Prev Med* 16, no. 3 (May 2011): 158–63.

233. Everett, E. T. "Fluoride's Effects on the Formation of Teeth and Bones, and the Influence of Genetics." [In eng]. *J Dent Res* 90, no. 5 (May 2011): 552–60.

234. DePaula, C. A., Y. Pan, and N. Guzelsu. "Uniform Partial Dissolution of Bone Mineral by Using Fluoride

and Phosphate Ions Combination." [In eng]. *Connect Tissue Res* 49, no. 5 (2008): 328–42.

235. Everett, E. T. "Fluoride's Effects on the Formation of Teeth and Bones, and the Influence of Genetics." [In eng]. *J Dent Res* 90, no. 5 (May 2011): 552–60.

236. Jha, S. K., V. K. Mishra, D. K. Sharma, and T. Damodaran. "Fluoride in the Environment and Its Metabolism in Humans." [In eng]. *Rev Environ Contam Toxicol* 211 (2011): 121–42.

237. Wright, J. V. Fight tooth decay and dramatically slash or even eliminate dental cavities for a lifetime! Nutrition & Healing. Vol. 19, Issue 3, May 2012.

238. Binkley, N. 2009. A perspective on male osteoporosis. *Best Pract Res Clin Rheumatol* Dec;23(6):755–68. PMID: 19945687.

239. Binkley, N. 2006. Osteoporosis in men. *Arq Bras Endocrinol Metabol* Aug;50(4):764–74. PMID: 17117301.

240. Orwoll, E., C. M. Nielson, L. M. Marshall, et al. 2009. Vitamin D deficiency in older men. *J Clin Endocrinol Metab* Apr;94(4):1214–22. PMID: 19174492.

241. van Hogezand, R. A., N. A. Hamdy. 2006. Skeletal morbidity in inflammatory bowel disease. *Scand J Gastroenterol Suppl* May;(243):59–64. PMID: 16782623.

242. Orlic, Z. C., T. Turk, B. M. Sincic, et al. 2010. How activity of inflammatory bowel disease influences bone loss. *J Clin Densitom* Jan-Mar;13(1):36–42. PMID: 20171567.

243. Liu, G., M. Peacock, O. Eilam, et al. 1997. Effect of osteoarthritis in the lumbar spine and hip on bone mineral density and diagnosis of osteoporosis in elderly men and women. *Osteoporos Int* 7(6):564–9. PMID: 9604053.

244. Khosla, S., S. Amin, E. Orwoll. 2008. Osteoporosis in men. *Endocr Rev* Jun;29(4):441–64. PMID: 18451258 Clarke BL, Khosla S. Androgens and bone. *Steroids*. 2009 Mar;74(3):296–305. PMID: 18992761.

245. Binkley, N. 2006. Osteoporosis in men. *Arq Bras Endocrinol Metabol* Aug;50(4):764–74. PMID: 17117301.

246. Shahinian, V. B., Y. F. Kuo, J. L. Freeman, et al. 2005. Risk of fracture after androgen deprivation for prostate cancer. *N Engl J Med* Jan 13;352(2):154–64. PMID: 15647578.

247. *Assessment of Fracture Risk and Its Application to Screening for Postmenopausal Osteoporosis.* (Geneva: WHO, 1994).

248. Ahuja, J., D. Rhodes, D. Goldman, et al. Intakes and sources of vitamin D in the US population. http://www.fasebj.org/cgi/content/meeting_abstract/24/1_MeetingAbstracts/917.6?maxtoshow=&hits=20&RESULTFORMAT=&searchid=1&FIRSTINDEX=0&displaysectionid=Calcium%2C+Phosphorus%2C+Magnesium%2C+and+Vitamin+D&volume=24&issue=1_MeetingAbstracts&resourcetype=HWCIT (accessed 5-11-2010).

249. Bischoff-Ferrari, H. A. 2008. Optimal serum 25-hydroxyvitamin D levels for multiple health outcomes. *Adv Exp Med Biol* 624:55–71. PMID: 18348447.

250. Mistretta, V. I., P. Delanaye, J. P. Chapelle JP, et al. 2008. [Vitamin D2 or vitamin D3?] *Rev Med Interne* Oct;29(10):815–20. PMID: 18406498.

251. Vieth, R. 2007. Vitamin D toxicity, policy, and science. *J Bone Miner Res* Dec;22 Suppl 2:V64–8. PMID: 18290725.

252. Mundy, G. R. 2007. Osteoporosis and inflammation. *Nutr Rev* Dec;65(12 Pt 2):S147–51. PMID: 18240539.

Shea, M. K., S. L. Booth, J. M. Massaro, et al. 2008. Vitamin K and vitamin D status: associations with inflammatory markers in the Framingham Offspring Study. *Am J Epidemiol* Feb 1;167(3):313–20. PMID: 18006902.

253. Pizzorno, L. Vitamin K, *Longevity Medicine Review*, 2009, http://www.lmreview.com/articles/view/vitamin-k/.

Pizzorno, L. Vitamin K2, but not vitamin K1, is helpful for bone density. *Longevity Medicine Review* 2009, http://www.lmreview.com/articles/view/vitamin-k2-but-not-vitamin-k1-is-helpful-for-bone-density/.

Pizzorno, L. Vitamin D and Vitamin K team up to lower CVD risk: Part I, *Longevity Medicine Review* 2009, http://www.lmreview.com/articles/view/vitamin-d-and-vitamin-k-team-up-to-lower-cvd-risk-part-1/.

Pizzorno, L. Vitamin D and Vitamin K team up to lower CVD risk: Part 2, Longevity Medicine Review 2009, http://www.lmreview.com/articles/view/vitamin-d-and-vitamin-k-team-up-to-lower-cvd-risk-part-2/.

254. Hart, J. P., A. Catterall, R. A. Dodds, et al. 1984. Circulating vitamin K1 levels in fractured neck of femur. *Lancet* Aug 4;2(8397):283. PMID: 6146829.

Hodges, S. J., M. J. Pilkington, T. C. Stamp, et al. 1991. Depressed levels of circulating menaquinones in patients with osteoporotic fractures of the spine and femoral neck. *Bone* 12(6):387–9. PMID: 1797053.

255. Booth, S. L., K. L. Tucker, H. Chen, et al. 2000. Dietary vitamin K intakes are associated with hip fracture but not with bone mineral density in elderly men and women. *Am J Clin Nutr* May;71(5):1201–8. PMID: 10799384.

256. Iinuma, N. 2005. [Vitamin K2 (menatetrenone) and bone quality] *Clin Calcium* Jun;15(6):1034–9. PMID: 15930719.

257. Plaza, S. M., D. W. Lamson. 2005. Vitamin K2 in bone metabolism and osteoporosis. *Altern Med Rev* Mar;10(1):24–35. PMID: 15771560.

258. Cockayne, S., J. Adamson, S. Lanham-New, et al. 2006. Vitamin K and the prevention of fractures: systematic review and meta-analysis of randomized controlled trials. *Arch Intern Med* Jun 26;166(12):1256–61. PMID: 16801507.

259. Pizzorno, L. 2008. Vitamin K: beyond coagulation to uses in bone, vascular and anti-cancer metabolism, *IMCJ* Apr; 7(2): 24–30.

260. Source: Food Processor Version 7.60, *ESHA Research*, Salem, OR, December 2000.

261. Kanellakis, S., G. Moschonis, R. Tenta, A. Schaafsma, E. G. van den Heuvel, N. Papaioannou, G. Lyritis, and Y. Manios. "Changes in Parameters of Bone Metabolism in Postmenopausal Women Following a 12-Month Intervention Period Using Dairy Products Enriched with Calcium, Vitamin D, and Phylloquinone (Vitamin K(1)) or Menaquinone-7 (Vitamin K (2)): The Postmenopausal Health Study Ii." [In eng]. *Calcif Tissue Int* 90, no. 4 (Apr 2012): 251–62.

262. Marini, H., L. Minutoli, F. Polito, A. Bitto, D. Altavilla, M. Atteritano, A. Gaudio, *et al.* "Opg and Srankl Serum Concentrations in Osteopenic, Postmenopausal Women after 2-Year Genistein Administration." [In eng]. *J Bone Miner Res* 23, no. 5 (May 2008): 715–20.

263. Iwamoto, J., T. Takeda and S. Ichimura. 2000. Effect of combined administration of vitamin D3 and vitamin K2 on bone mineral density of the lumbar spine in postmenopausal women with osteoporosis. *J Orthop Sci* 5(6):546–51. PMID: 11180916.

264. Ushiroyama, T., A. Ikeda and M. Ueki. 2002. Effect of continuous combined therapy with vitamin K(2) and vitamin D(3) on bone mineral density and coagulofibrinolysis function in postmenopausal women. *Maturitas* Mar 25;41(3): 211–21. PMID: 11886767.

265. McCann, J. C. and B. N. Ames. 2009. Vitamin K, an example of triage theory: is micronutrient inadequacy linked to diseases of aging? *Am J Clin Nutr* Oct;90(4):889–907. PMID: 19692494.

266. Pizzorno, L. 2008. Vitamin K: beyond coagulation to uses in bone, vascular and anti-cancer metabolism, *IMCJ* Apr; 7(2): 24–30.

267. Natto, http://en.wikipedia.org/wiki/Natt%C5%8D (accessed 5-13-10).

268. Schurgers, L. J., J. M. Geleijnse, D. E. Grobbee, et al. "Nutritional intake of vitamins K1 (phylloquinone) and K2 (menaquinone) in the Netherlands: . J,Nutr. Environ. Med. (June 1999): 9(2):115–122. DOI: 10.1080/13590849961717 accessed at Ingentaconnect 7-15-11 @ http://www.ingentaconnect.com/content/routledg/cjne/1999/00000009/00000002/art00004.

269. Forli, L., J. Bollerslev, S. Simonsen, et al. 2010. Dietary vitamin K2 supplement improves bone status after lung and heart transplantation. *Transplantation*. 2010 Feb 27;89(4):458–64. PMID: 20177349.

270. Yamaguchi, M. 2006. Regulatory mechanism of food factors in bone metabolism and prevention of osteoporosis. *Yakugaku Zasshi*. 2006 Nov; 126(11): 1117–37. PMID: 17077614.

271. Food and Nutrition Board, Institute of Medicine. Vitamin K. Dietary Reference Intakes for Vitamin A, Vitamin K, Arsenic, Boron, Chromium, Copper, Iodine, Iron, Manganese, Molybdenum, Nickel, Silicon, Vanadium, and Zinc. Washington, D.C.

National Academy Press 2001:162–196, http://www.nap.edu/openbook.php?isbn=0309072794.

272. Schurgers, L. J., K. J. Teunissen and K. Hamulyák. 2007. Vitamin K-containing dietary supplements: comparison of synthetic vitamin K1 and natto-derived menaquinone-7. *Blood Apr* 15;109(8):3279–83. PMID: 17158229.

   Schurgers, L. J. Vitamin K2 as MenaQ7, Improve bone health and inhibit arterial calcification. Monograph published April 2007, *NattoPharma*, ASA, Norway, http://www.menaq7.com/index.php?s=Research.

273. Tanko, L. B., C. Christiansen, D. A. Cox, M. J. Geiger, M. A. McNabb, and S. R. Cummings. "Relationship between Osteoporosis and Cardiovascular Disease in Postmenopausal Women." [In eng]. *J Bone Miner Res* 20, no. 11 (Nov 2005): 1912–20.

274. Gerber, Y., L. J. Melton, 3rd, S. A. Weston, and V. L. Roger. "Association between Myocardial Infarction and Fractures: An Emerging Phenomenon." [In eng]. *Circulation* 124, no. 3 (Jul 19 2011): 297–303.

275. Gast, G. C., N. M. de Roos, I. Sluijs, M. L. Bots, J. W. Beulens, J. M. Geleijnse, J. C. Witteman, *et al.* "A High Menaquinone Intake Reduces the Incidence of Coronary Heart Disease." [In eng]. *Nutr Metab Cardiovasc Dis* 19, no. 7 (Sep 2009): 504–10.

276. Tigas, S. and A. Tsatsoulis. "Endocrine and metabolic manifestations in inflammatory bowel disease." *Annals of Gastroenterology, North America*, 25 (Feb 2012). Available at: <http://www.annalsgastro.gr/index.php/annalsgastro/article/view/1020>. Date accessed: 15 Apr. 2012.)

277. Geleijnse, J. M., C. Vermeer, D. E. Grobbee, L. J. Schurgers, M. H. Knapen, I. M. van der Meer, A. Hofman, and J. C. Witteman. "Dietary Intake of Menaquinone Is Associated with a Reduced Risk

of Coronary Heart Disease: The Rotterdam Study."
[In eng]. *J Nutr* 134, no. 11 (Nov 2004): 3100–5.

278. Beulens, J. W., M. L. Bots, F. Atsma, M. L. Bartelink, M. Prokop, J. M. Geleijnse, J. C. Witteman, D. E. Grobbee, and Y. T. van der Schouw. "High Dietary Menaquinone Intake Is Associated with Reduced Coronary Calcification." [In eng]. *Atherosclerosis* 203, no. 2 (Apr 2009): 489–93.

279. Erkkila, A. T., S. L. Booth, F. B. Hu, P. F. Jacques, J. E. Manson, K. M. Rexrode, M. J. Stampfer, and A. H. Lichtenstein. "Phylloquinone Intake as a Marker for Coronary Heart Disease Risk but Not Stroke in Women." [In eng]. *Eur J Clin Nutr* 59, no. 2 (Feb 2005): 196–204.

Erkkila, A. T., S. L. Booth, F. B. Hu, P. F. Jacques, and A. H. Lichtenstein. "Phylloquinone Intake and Risk of Cardiovascular Diseases in Men." [In eng]. *Nutr Metab Cardiovasc Dis* 17, no. 1 (Jan 2007): 58–62.

280. Shearer, M. J., X. Fu, and S. L. Booth. "Vitamin K Nutrition, Metabolism, and Requirements: Current Concepts and Future Research." [In eng]. Adv Nutr 3, no. 2 (Mar 2012): 182-95.

281. Ibid.

282. Bhalerao, S., and T. R. Clandinin. "Cell Biology. Vitamin K2 Takes Charge." [In eng]. Science 336, no. 6086 (Jun 8 2012): 1241-2.

Vos, M., G. Esposito, J. N. Edirisinghe, S. Vilain, D. M. Haddad, J. R. Slabbaert, S. Van Meensel, et al. "Vitamin K2 Is a Mitochondrial Electron Carrier That Rescues Pink1 Deficiency." [In eng]. Science 336, no. 6086 (Jun 8 2012): 1306-10.

283. IOM Report: Dietary Reference Intakes for Vitamin A, Vitamin K, Arsenic, Boron, Chromium, Copper, Iodine, Iron, Manganese, Molybdenum, Nickel, Silicon, Vanadium, and Zinc, http://www.iom.edu/~/media/Files/Activity%20Files/Nutrition/DRIs/DRI_Vitamins.ashx.

284. Aspirin similar to warfarin in stroke prevention, article available at http://news.nurse.com/article/20120205/NATIONAL02/102130013.

285. Schurgers, L. J., K. J. Teunissen, K. Hamulyak, M. H. Knapen, H. Vik, and C. Vermeer. "Vitamin K-Containing Dietary Supplements: Comparison of Synthetic Vitamin K1 and Natto-Derived Menaquinone-7." [In eng]. *Blood* 109, no. 8 (Apr 15 2007): 3279–83.

286. McCormick, R. K. 2007. Osteoporosis: integrating biomarkers and other diagnostic correlates into the management of bone fragility. *Altern Med Rev* Jun;12(2):113–45. PMID: 17604458.

287. Koh, J. M., Y. S. Lee, Y. S. Kim, et al. 2006. Homocysteine enhances bone resorption by stimulation of osteoclast formation and activity through increased intracellular ROS generation. *J Bone Miner Res* Jul;21(7):1003–11. PMID: 16813521.

Kim, D. J., J. M. Koh, O. Lee, et al. 2006. Homocysteine enhances apoptosis in human bone marrow stromal cells. *Bone* Sep 39(3):582–90. PMID: 16644300.

288. Lee, N. K., Y. G. Choi, J. Y. Baik, et al. 2005. A crucial role for reactive oxygen species in RANKL-induced osteoclast differentiation, *Blood* 106, pp. 852–859. PMID: 15817678.

Ginaldi, L., M. C. Di Benedetto, M. De Martinis. 2005. Osteoporosis, inflammation and ageing. *Immun Ageing* 2:14. PMID: 16271143.

289. Choi, K. M., Y. K. Seo, H. H. Yoon, et al. 2008. Effect of ascorbic acid on bone marrow-derived mesenchymal stem cell proliferation and differentiation. *J Biosci Bioeng* Jun;105(6):586–94. PMID: 18640597.

Sahni, S., M. T. Hannan, D. Gagnon, et al. 2008. High vitamin C intake is associated with lower 4-year bone loss in elderly men. *J Nutr* Oct;138(10):1931–8. PMID: 18806103.

290. Ibid.

291. Rowe, D. J., S. Ko, X. M. Tom, et al. 1999. Enhanced production of mineralized nodules and collagenous proteins in vitro by calcium ascorbate supplemented with vitamin C metabolites. *J Periodontol* Sep;70(9):992–9. PMID: 10505801.

292. Prevalence and Incidence of Iron deficiency anemia, http://www.wrongdiagnosis.com/i/iron_deficiency_anemia/prevalence.htm#incidence_intro (accessed 5-13-10).

293. National Osteoporosis Foundation, What You Should Know About Calcium, http://www.nof.org/prevention/calcium2.htm (accessed 5-13-10).

294. Pizorno, J. E. and M. T. Murray., "Osteoporosis," in the *Textbook of Natural Medicine*, 3rd ed.,: (St Louis, MO: Churchill Livingstone, 2006), chap 146.

National Institutes of Health. 2000. Osteoporosis prevention, diagnosis, and therapy. *NIH Consensus Statement* Mar 27–29;17(1):1–45.

Xu, L., P. McElduff, C. D'Este and J. Attia. 2004. Does dietary calcium have a protective effect on bone fractures in women? A meta-analysis of observational studies. *Br J Nutr* 91:625–634. PMID: 15035690.

Reid, I. R., R. W. Ames, M. C. Evans, et al. 1995. Long-term effects of calcium supplementation on bone loss and fractures in postmenopausal women: a randomized controlled trial. *Am J Med* 98:331–335. PMID: 7709944.

Devine, A., I. M. Dick, S. J. Heal, et al. 1997. A 4-year follow-up study of the effects of calcium supplementation on bone density in elderly postmenopausal women. *Osteoporos Int* 7:23–28. PMID: 9102058.

Elders, P. J., P. Lips, J. C. Netelenbos, et al. 1994. Long-term effect of calcium supplementation on bone loss in perimenopausal women. *J Bone Miner Res* 9:963–970. PMID: 7942164.

295. Shea, B., G. Wells, A. Cranney, et al. 2007. WITH-DRAWN: Calcium supplementation on bone loss in postmenopausal women. *Cochrane Database Syst Rev* Jul 18;(1):CD004526. PMID: 17636765.

296. Bourgoin, B. P., D. R. Evans, J. R. Cornett, et al. 1993. Lead content in 70 brands of dietary calcium supplements. *Am J Public Health* 83:1155–1160. PMID: 8342726.

Scelfo, G. M. and A. R. Flegal. 2000. Lead in calcium supplements. *Environ Health Perspect* Apr;108(4):309–19. PMID: 10753088.

297. Pizzorno, L. U., J. E. Pizzorno and M. T. Murray. "Osteoporosis", in *Natural Medicine Instructions for Patients*, (Churchill Livingstone/Elsevier, 2002), p. 251–9.

298. World's Healthiest Foods, Calcium, http://www.whfoods.org/genpage.php?tname=nutrient&dbid=45 (accessed 5-16-2010).

Linus Pauling Institute, Calcium, http://lpi.oregonstate.edu/infocenter/minerals/calcium/ (accessed 5-16-2010).

299. Pounder, R. E. and D. Ng. The prevalence of Helicobacter pylori infection in different countries. *Aliment Pharmacol Ther* 9 Suppl 2:33–9. PMID: 8547526.

300. Straub, D. A. 2007. Calcium supplementation in clinical practice: a review of forms, doses, and indications. *Nutr Clin Pract* Jun;22(3):286–96. PMID: 17507729.

301. Castelo-Branco, C., M. Ciria-Recasens, M. J. Cancelo-Hidalgo, et al. 2009. Efficacy of ossein-hydroxyapatite complex compared with calcium carbonate to prevent bone loss: a meta-analysis. *Menopause* Sep-Oct;16(5):984–91. PMID: 19407667.

302. Pines, A., H. Raafat, A. H. Lynn and J.Whittington J. 1984. Clinical trial of microcrystalline hydroxyapatite compound ('Ossopan') in the prevention of osteoporosis due to corticosteroid therapy. *Curr Med Res Opin* 8(10):734–42. PMID: 6373153.

Stellon, A., A. Davies, A. Webb and R. Williams. 1985. Microcrystalline hydroxyapatite compound in prevention of bone loss in corticosteroid-treated patients with chronic active hepatitis. *Postgrad Med J* Sep;61(719):791–6. PMID: 2997764.

303. Adluri, R. S., L. Zhan, M. Bagchi, N. Maulik, and G. Maulik. "Comparative Effects of a Novel Plant-Based Calcium Supplement with Two Common Calcium Salts on Proliferation and Mineralization in Human Osteoblast Cells." [In eng]. *Mol Cell Biochem* 340, no. 1-2 (Jul 2010): 73–80.

304. Michalek, J. E., H. G. Preuss, H. A. Croft, P. L. Keith, S. C. Keith, M. Dapilmoto, N. V. Perricone, R. B. Leckie, and G. R. Kaats. "Changes in Total Body Bone Mineral Density Following a Common Bone Health Plan with Two Versions of a Unique Bone Health Supplement: A Comparative Effectiveness Research Study." [In eng]. *Nutr J* 10 (2011): 32.

305. Kaats, G. R., H. G. Preuss, H. A. Croft, S. C. Keith, and P. L. Keith. "A Comparative Effectiveness Study of Bone Density Changes in Women over 40 Following Three Bone Health Plans Containing Variations of the Same Novel Plant-Sourced Calcium." [In eng]. *Int J Med Sci* 8, no. 3 (2011): 180–91.

306. Kaats, G. R.: The Clicker, the Glycemic Index and the Glycemic Load, Estimating and Balancing Calories. In: *Restructuring Body Composition: How the Kind, Not the Amount, of Weight Loss Defines a Pathway to Optimal Health.* (Dallas: Taylor Publishing, 2008), 223–294.

307. Tang, B. M., G. D. Eslick, C. Nowson, et al. Use of calcium or calcium in combination with vitamin

D supplementation to prevent fractures and bone loss in people aged 50 years and older: a meta-analysis. *Lancet* (2007): 370:657–666.

308. Park, H. M., J. Heo, and Y. Park. "Calcium from Plant Sources Is Beneficial to Lowering the Risk of Osteoporosis in Postmenopausal Korean Women." [In eng]. *Nutr Res* 31, no. 1 (Jan 2011): 27–32.

309. Nieves, J. W. "Osteoporosis: The Role of Micronutrients." [In eng]. *Am J Clin Nutr* 81, no. 5 (May 2005): 1232S-39S.

310. Lanham-New, S. A. "Fruit and Vegetables: The Unexpected Natural Answer to the Question of Osteoporosis Prevention?" [In eng]. *Am J Clin Nutr* 83, no. 6 (Jun 2006): 1254–5.

311. Pizzorno, L. Beyond Tocopherol: A Review of Natural Vitamin E's Therapeutic Potential in Human Health and Disease, Part I, *Longevity Medicine Review* http://www.lmreview.com/articles/view/beyond-tocopherol-a-review-of-natural-vitamin-es-therapeutic-potential-in-human-health-and-disease-part-I/.

312. Bolland, M. J., A. Avenell, J. A. Baron, A. Grey, G. S. MacLennan, G. D. Gamble, and I. R. Reid. "Effect of Calcium Supplements on Risk of Myocardial Infarction and Cardiovascular Events: Meta-Analysis." [In eng]. *BMJ* 341 (2010): c3691.

Bolland, M. J., A. Grey, A. Avenell, G. D. Gamble, and I. R. Reid. "Calcium Supplements with or without Vitamin D and Risk of Cardiovascular Events: Reanalysis of the Women's Health Initiative Limited Access Dataset and Meta-Analysis." [In eng]. *BMJ* 342 (2011): d2040.

313. Wallace, R. B., J. Wactawski-Wende, M. J. O'Sullivan, J. C. Larson, B. Cochrane, M. Gass, and K. Masaki. "Urinary Tract Stone Occurrence in the Women's Health Initiative (Whi) Randomized Clinical Trial of Calcium and Vitamin D Supplements." [In eng]. *Am J Clin Nutr* 94, no. 1 (Jul 2011): 270–7.

314. Pizzorno, L. http://www.lmreview.com/articles/view/vitamin-d-and-vitamin-k-team-up-to-lower-cvd-risk-part-I/.

Pizzorno, L. http://www.lmreview.com/articles/view/Vitamin-K2-Essential-for-Prevention-of-Age-Associated-Chronic-Disease/.

315. Nielsen, F. H., B. J. Stoecker. 2009. *J Trace Elem Med Biol* 23(3):195–203. PMID: 19486829; And Nielsen F.H. 2008. Is boron nutritionally relevant? Nutr Rev Apr;66(4):183–91. PMID: 18366532.

Gorustovich, A. A., T. Steimetz, F. H. Nielsen, et al. 2008. Histomorphometric study of alveolar bone healing in rats fed a boron-deficient diet. *Anat Rec* (Hoboken) Apr;291(4):441–7. PMID: 18361451.

Nielsen, F. H. 2000. The emergence of boron as nutritionally important throughout the life cycle. *Nutrition* Jul-Aug;16(7–8):512–4. PMID: 10906539.

Nielsen, F. H. 2009. Micronutrients in parenteral nutrition: boron, silicon, and fluoride. *Gastroenterology* Nov;137(5 Suppl):S55–60. PMID: 19874950.

Nielsen, F. H. and B. J. Stoecker. 2009. Boron and fish oil have different beneficial effects on strength and trabecular microarchitecture of bone. *J Trace Elem Med Biol* 23(3):195–203. PMID: 19486829.

316. Samman, S., M. R. Naghii, Lyons Wall PM, et al. 1998. The nutritional and metabolic effects of boron in humans and animals. *Biol Trace Elem Res* Winter;66(1–3):227–35. PMID: 10050922.

Schaafsma, A., P. J. de Vries and W. H. Saris. 2001. Delay of natural bone loss by higher intakes of specific minerals and vitamins. *Crit Rev Food Sci Nutr* May;41(4):225–49. PMID: 11401244.

Nielsen, F. H. 1990. Studies on the relationship between boron and magnesium which possibly affects the formation and maintenance of bones. *Magnes Trace Elem* 9(2):61–9. PMID: 2222801.

317. Nielsen, F. H., C. D. Hunt, L. M. Mullen, et al. 1987. Effect of dietary boron on mineral, estrogen, and testosterone metabolism in postmenopausal women. *FASEB J* Nov;1(5):394–7. PMID: 3678698.

318. Dietary Reference Intakes for Vitamin A, Vitamin K, Arsenic, Boron, Chromium, Copper, Iodine, Iron, Manganese, Molybdenum, Nickel, Silicon, Vanadium, and Zinc. 2001. Food and Nutrition Board, Institute of Medicine, available at http://books.nap.edu/openbook.php?record_id=10026&page=1 (accessed 5-13-10).

319. Johnson, S. 2001. The multifaceted and widespread pathology of magnesium deficiency. *Med Hypotheses* Feb;56(2):163–70. PMID: 11425281.

320. Rude, R. K., F. R. Singer and H. E. Gruber. 2009. Skeletal and hormonal effects of magnesium deficiency. *J Am Coll Nutr* Apr;28(2):131–41. PMID: 19828898.

321. Rosanoff, A., C. M. Weaver, and R. K. Rude. "Suboptimal Magnesium Status in the United States: Are the Health Consequences Underestimated?" [In eng]. *Nutr Rev* 70, no. 3 (Mar 2012): 153–64.

322. World's Healthiest Foods, Magnisium, http://www.whfoods.org/genpage.php?tname=nutri-ent&dbid=75 (accessed 5-16-2010).

Magnesium, Eat Right Ontario, https://www.eatrightontario.ca/en/viewdocument.aspx?id=67 (accessed 5-16-2010).

323. Dhillon, K. S., J. Singh, and J. S. Lyall. "A New Horizon into the Pathobiology, Etiology and Treatment of Migraine." [In eng]. *Med Hypotheses* 77, no. 1 (Jul 2011): 147–51.

Dullo, P., and N. Vedi. "Changes in Serum Calcium, Magnesium and Inorganic Phosphorus Levels During Different Phases of the Menstrual Cycle." [In eng]. *J Hum Reprod Sci* 1, no. 2 (Jul 2008): 77–80.

324. Nielsen, F. H. "Magnesium, Inflammation, and Obesity in Chronic Disease." [In eng]. *Nutr Rev* 68, no. 6 (Jun 2010): 333–40.

Barbagallo, M., and L. J. Dominguez. "Magnesium and Aging." [In eng]. *Curr Pharm Des* 16, no. 7 (2010): 832–9.

325. Trenkwalder, C., W. A. Hening, P. Montagna, W. H. Oertel, R. P. Allen, A. S. Walters, J. Costa, K. Stiasny-Kolster, and C. Sampaio. "Treatment of Restless Legs Syndrome: An Evidence-Based Review and Implications for Clinical Practice." [In eng]. *Mov Disord* 23, no. 16 (Dec 15 2008): 2267–302.

Bartell, S., and S. Zallek. "Intravenous Magnesium Sulfate May Relieve Restless Legs Syndrome in Pregnancy." [In eng]. *J Clin Sleep Med* 2, no. 2 (Apr 15 2006): 187–8.

Popoviciu, L., B. Asgian, D. Delast-Popoviciu, A. Alexandrescu, S. Petrutiu, and I. Bagathal. "Clinical, Eeg, Electromyographic and Polysomnographic Studies in Restless Legs Syndrome Caused by Magnesium Deficiency." [In eng]. *Rom J Neurol Psychiatry* 31, no. 1 (Jan-Mar 1993): 55–61.

Fawcett, W. J. "Ketamine for Restless Legs Syndrome." [In eng]. *Anesth Analg* 96, no. 4 (Apr 2003): 1238; author reply 38–9.

Fawcett, W. J., E. J. Haxby, and D. A. Male. "Magnesium: Physiology and Pharmacology." [In eng]. *Br J Anaesth* 83, no. 2 (Aug 1999): 302–20.

Hornyak, M., U. Voderholzer, F. Hohagen, M. Berger, and D. Riemann. "Magnesium Therapy for Periodic Leg Movements-Related Insomnia and Restless Legs Syndrome: An Open Pilot Study." [In eng]. *Sleep* 21, no. 5 (Aug 1 1998): 501–5.

326. Rosanoff, A., C. M. Weaver, and R. K. Rude. "Suboptimal Magnesium Status in the United States: Are the Health Consequences Underestimated?" [In eng]. *Nutr Rev* 70, no. 3 (Mar 2012): 153–64.

327. IntraCellular Diagnostics, Inc.®, provides buccal smear testing, http://www.exatest.com/.

328. https://www.mymedlab.com/vitamin-levels/rbc-magnesium.

http://www.drmyhill.co.uk/wiki/Magnesium_test_-_red_cell.

http://www.privatemdlabs.com/lab_tests.php?view=search_results&show=1559&category=12&search=MAGNESIUM#1559.

329. Rude, R. K., J. S. Adams, E. Ryzen, et al. 1985. Low serum concentrations of 1,25-dihydroxyvitamin D in human magnesium deficiency. *J Clin Endocrinol Metab* Nov;61(5):933–40. PMID: 3840173.

330. Rude, R. K., F. R. Singer and H. E. Gruber. 2009. Skeletal and hormonal effects of magnesium deficiency. *J Am Coll Nutr* Apr;28(2):131–41. PMID: 19828898.

331. Cohen, L. and R. Kitzes. 1981. Infrared spectroscopy and magnesium content of bone mineral in osteoporotic women. Infrared spectroscopy and magnesium content of bone mineral in osteoporotic women. *Isr J Med Sci* Dec;17(12):1123–5. PMID: 7327911.

Cohen, L. 1988. Recent data on magnesium and osteoporosis. *Magnes Res* Jul;1(1–2):85–7. PMID: 3079205.

Launius, B.K., P. A. Brown, E. M. Cush, et al. 2004. Osteoporosis: The dynamic relationship between magnesium and bone mineral density in the heart transplant patient. *Crit Care Nurs Q* Jan-Mar;27(1):96–100. PMID: 14974529.

Takami, M. and S. Shinnichi. 2005. [Bone and magnesium] *Clin Calcium* Nov;15(11):91–6. PMID: 16272618.

332. Ryder, K. M., R. I. Shorr, A. J. Bush, S. B. Kritchevsky, T. Harris, K. Stone, J. Cauley, and F. A.

Tylavsky. "Magnesium Intake from Food and Supplements Is Associated with Bone Mineral Density in Healthy Older White Subjects." [In eng]. *J Am Geriatr Soc* 53, no. 11 (Nov 2005): 1875–80.

333. Musayev, F.N., M. L. Di Salvo, M. A. Saavedra, et al. 2009. Molecular basis of reduced pyridoxine 5'-phosphate oxidase catalytic activity in neonatal epileptic encephalopathy disorder. *J Biol Chem* Nov 6;284(45):30949–56. PMID: 19759001.

Khayat, M., S. H. Korman, P. Frankel, et al. 2008. PNPO deficiency: an under diagnosed inborn error of pyridoxine metabolism. *Mol Genet Metab* Aug;94(4):431–4. PMID: 18485777.

Hoey, L., H. McNulty and J. J. Strain. 2009. Studies of biomarker responses to intervention with riboflavin: a systematic review. *Am J Clin Nutr* Jun;89(6):1960S-1980S. PMID: 19403631.

334. Wong, C. P., and E. Ho. "Zinc and Its Role in Age-Related Inflammation and Immune Dysfunction." [In eng]. *Mol Nutr Food Res* 56, no. 1 (Jan 2012): 77–87.

335. Gurban, C. V., and O. Mederle. "The Opg/Rankl System and Zinc Ions Are Promoters of Bone Remodeling by Osteoblast Proliferation in Postmenopausal Osteoporosis." [In eng]. *Rom J Morphol Embryol* 52, no. 3 Suppl (2011): 1113–9.

336. Allen, L. H. "Zinc and Micronutrient Supplements for Children." [In eng]. *Am J Clin Nutr* 68, no. 2 Suppl (Aug 1998): 495S-98S.

337. Barrie, S. A., J. V. Wright, J. E. Pizzorno, E. Kutter, and P. C. Barron. "Comparative Absorption of Zinc Picolinate, Zinc Citrate and Zinc Gluconate in Humans." [In eng]. *Agents Actions* 21, no. 1-2 (Jun 1987): 223–8.

338. Ijuin, H. "Evaluation of Pancreatic Exocrine Function and Zinc Absorption in Alcoholism." [In eng]. *Kurume Med J* 45, no. 1 (1998): 1–5.

Sakai, F., S. Yoshida, S. Endo, and H. Tomita. "Double-Blind, Placebo-Controlled Trial of Zinc Picolinate for Taste Disorders." [In eng]. *Acta Otolaryngol Suppl*, no. 546 (2002): 129–33.

Heffernan, M. P., M. M. Nelson, and M. J. Anadkat. "A Pilot Study of the Safety and Efficacy of Picolinic Acid Gel in the Treatment of Acne Vulgaris." [In eng]. *Br J Dermatol* 156, no. 3 (Mar 2007): 548–52.

Kirkil, G., M. Hamdi Muz, D. Seckin, K. Sahin, and O. Kucuk. "Antioxidant Effect of Zinc Picolinate in Patients with Chronic Obstructive Pulmonary Disease." [In eng]. *Respir Med* 102, no. 6 (Jun 2008): 840–4.

339. Di Silvestro, R. and M. Swan. "Comparison of Four Commercially Available Zinc Supplements for Performance in a Zinc Tolerance Test." *The FASEB Journal*. 2008;22:693.3. http://www.fasebj.org/cgi/content/meeting_abstract/22/1_MeetingAbstracts/693.3?sid=f bcb3444-f9a0-461e-b851-e6aaf8a66b6f).

340. Reginster, J. Y., R. Deroisy, M. Dougados, et al. 2002. Prevention of early postmenopausal bone loss by strontium ranelate: the randomized, two-year, double-masked, dose-ranging, placebo-controlled PREVOS trial. *Osteoporos Int* Dec;13(12):925–31. PMID: 12459934.

341. Seeman, E., J. Devogelaer, R. Lorenc, et al. 2008. Strontium ranelate reduces the risk of vertebral fractures in patients with osteopenia. *J Bone Miner Res* Mar;23(3):433–8. PMID: 17997711.

342. Meunier, P., C. Roux, S. Ortolani, et al. 2009. Effects of long-term strontium ranelate treatment on vertebral fracture risk in postmenopausal women with osteoporosis. *Osteoporos Int* Oct;20(10):1663–73. PMID: 19153678.

Meunier, P., C. Roux, E. Seeman, et al. 2004. The effects of strontium ranelate on the risk of vertebral fracture in women with postmenopausal osteoporosis. *N Engl J Med* Jan 29;350(5):459–68. PMID: 14749454.

Reginster, J., E. Seeman, M. C. De Vernejoul, et al. 2005. Strontium ranelate reduces the risk of nonvertebral fractures in postmenopausal women with osteoporosis: Treatment of Peripheral Osteoporosis (TROPOS) study. *J Clin Endocrinol Metab* May;90(5):2816–22. Epub 2005 Feb 22. PMID: 15728210.

343. Arlot, M. E., Y. Jiang, H. K. Genant, et al. 2008. Histomorphometric and microCT analysis of bone biopsies from postmenopausal osteoporotic women treated with strontium ranelate. *J Bone Miner Res* Feb;23(2):215–22. PMID: 17922612.

344. Seeman, E., J. Devogelaer, R. Lorenc, et al. 2008. Strontium ranelate reduces the risk of vertebral fractures in patients with osteopenia. *J Bone Miner Res* Mar;23(3):433–8. PMID: 17997711.

345. Neuprez, A., J. Y. Reginster. 2008. Bone-forming agents in the management of osteoporosis. *Best Pract Res Clin Endocrinol Metab* Oct;22(5):869–83. PMID: 19028361.

346. Liu, J. M., A. Wai-Chee Kung, et al. 2009. Efficacy and safety of 2 g/day of strontium ranelate in Asian women with postmenopausal osteoporosis. *Bone* Sep;45(3):460–5. Epub 2009 May 21. PMID: 19464401.

347. Middleton, E. T., S. A. Steel, M. Aye, et al. 2010. The effect of prior bisphosphonate therapy on the subsequent BMD and bone turnover response to strontium ranelate. *J Bone Miner Res* Mar;25(3):455–62. PMID: 20201000.

348. Patnaik, P. *Handbook of Inorganic Chemicals* (McGraw-Hill, 2002), ISBN 0070494398.

349. Marie, P. J. 2006. Strontium ranelate: a dual mode of action rebalancing bone turnover in favour of bone formation. *Curr Opin Rheumatol* Jun;18 Suppl 1:S11–5. PMID: 16735840.

Marie, P. J. 2006. Strontium ranelate: a physiological approach for optimizing bone formation and resorption. *Bone* Feb;38(2 Suppl 1):S10–4. Epub 2006 Jan 24. PMID: 16439191.

Boivin, G. and P. J. Meunier. 2003. The mineralization of bone tissue: a forgotten dimension in osteoporosis research. *Osteoporos Int* 14 Suppl 3:S19–24. Epub 2003 Mar 18. Review. PMID: 12730799.

Boivin, G., D. Farlay, M. T. Khebbab, et al. 2010. In osteoporotic women treated with strontium ranelate, strontium is located in bone formed during treatment with a maintained degree of mineralization. *Osteoporos Int.* Apr;21(4):667–77. Epub 2009 Jul 14. PMID: 19597910.

Uebelhart, D., D. Frey, P. Frey-Rindova, et al. 2003. [Therapy of osteoporosis: bisphosphonates, SERM's, teriparatide and strontium] *Z Rheumatol* Dec;62(6):512–7. PMID: 14685711.

350. Deeks, E. D., S. Dhillon. 2010. Strontium ranelate: a review of its use in the treatment of postmenopausal osteoporosis. *Drugs* Apr 16;70(6):733–59. PMID: 20394457.

351. http://saveourbones.com/strontium-demistyfied/ (accessed 2-24-12).

352. Neufeld, E. B. and A. L. Boskey. "Strontium Alters the Complexed Acidic Phospholipid Content of Mineralizing Tissues." [In eng]. *Bone* 15, no. 4 (Jul-Aug 1994): 425–30.

353. Ozgur, S., H. Sumer, and G. Kocoglu. "Rickets and Soil Strontium." [In eng]. *Arch Dis Child* 75, no. 6 (Dec 1996): 524–6.

354. Centers for Disease Control's Agency for Toxic Substances and Disease Registry. Health Effects of Strontium report accessible @ http://www.atsdr. cdc.gov/ToxProfiles/tp159-c3.pdf.

355. Osborne, V., D. Layton, M. Perrio, L. Wilton, and S. A. Shakir. "Incidence of Venous Thromboembolism in Users of Strontium Ranelate: An Analysis of Data from a Prescription-Event Monitoring Study in England." [In eng]. *Drug Saf* 33, no. 7 (Jul 1 2010): 579–91.

Le Merlouette, M., H. Adamski, M. Dinulescu, F. Le Gall, F. Colin, H. Grimaud, and J. Chevrant-Breton. "[Strontium Ranelate-Induced Dress Syndrome]." [In fre]. *Ann Dermatol Venereol* 138, no. 2 (Feb 2011): 124–8.

356. Jonville-Bera, A. P., and E. Autret-Leca. "[Adverse Drug Reactions of Strontium Ranelate(Protelos((R)) in France]." [In fre]. *Presse Med* 40, no. 10 (Oct 2011): e453–62.

357. No authors listed. 2005. Strontium: new drug. Postmenopausal osteoporosis: too many unknowns. *Prescrire Int.* Dec;14(80):207–11. PMID: 16397977.

358. http://www.protelos.com/healthcare-professionals/osteoporosis/protelos.

359. Lehnerdt F. Zur Frage der Substitution des Calcium im Knochensystem durch Strontium, *Beitr Path Anat* 1909;46:468-585; *Beitr Path Anat* 1910;47:215–247.

360. Dr. Brunel's talk on strontium is available at: http://www.youtube.com/watch?v=fANeTg4Fwrc &feature=youtube.

361. No authors listed. 2012. Strontium ranelate: too many adverse effects (continued) Do not use. *Prescrire Int.* Mar;21(125):72. PMID: 22428195.

362. Pizzorno, J., L. A. Frassetto, and J. Katzinger. "Diet-Induced Acidosis: Is It Real and Clinically

Relevant?" [In eng]. *Br J Nutr* 103, no. 8 (Apr 2010): 1185–94.

363. Barenholdt, O., N. Kolthoff, and S. P. Nielsen. "Effect of Long-Term Treatment with Strontium Ranelate on Bone Strontium Content." [In eng]. *Bone* 45, no. 2 (Aug 2009): 200–6.

364. Belissa-Chatelain, P., I. Dupin-Roger, F. Cournarie, and Y. Tsouderos. "Re: "Effect of Long-Term Treatment with Strontium Ranelate on Bone Strontium Content" by Barenholdt Et Al. (Bone, 2009)." [In eng]. *Bone* 45, no. 5 (Nov 2009): 1024-5; author reply 26–7.

365. Siccardi, A. J., 3rd, S. Padgett-Vasquez, H. W. Garris, T. R. Nagy, L. R. D'Abramo, and S. A. Watts. "Dietary Strontium Increases Bone Mineral Density in Intact Zebrafish (Danio Rerio): A Potential Model System for Bone Research." [In eng]. *Zebrafish* 7, no. 3 (Sep 2010): 267–73.

Boivin, G., and P. J. Meunier. "The Mineralization of Bone Tissue: A Forgotten Dimension in Osteoporosis Research." [In eng]. *Osteoporos Int* 14 Suppl 3 (2003): S19–24.

Marie, P. J., P. Ammann, G. Boivin, and C. Rey. "Mechanisms of Action and Therapeutic Potential of Strontium in Bone." [In eng]. *Calcif Tissue Int* 69, no. 3 (Sep 2001): 121–9.

366. Pizzorno, J., L. A. Frassetto, and J. Katzinger. "Diet-Induced Acidosis: Is It Real and Clinically Relevant?" [In eng]. *Br J Nutr* 103, no. 8 (Apr 2010): 1185–94.

Barenholdt, O., N. Kolthoff, and S. P. Nielsen. "Effect of Long-Term Treatment with Strontium Ranelate on Bone Strontium Content." [In eng]. *Bone* 45, no. 2 (Aug 2009): 200–6.

Belissa-Chatelain, P., I. Dupin-Roger, F. Cournarie, and Y. Tsouderos. "Re: "Effect of Long-Term Treatment with Strontium Ranelate on Bone Strontium

Content" by Barenholdt Et Al. (Bone, 2009)." [In eng]. *Bone* 45, no. 5 (Nov 2009): 1024-5; author reply 26-7.

367. Reginster, J. Y., J. M. Kaufman, S. Goemaere, J. P. Devogelaer, C. L. Benhamou, D. Felsenberg, M. Diaz-Curiel, *et al.* "Maintenance of Antifracture Efficacy over 10 Years with Strontium Ranelate in Postmenopausal Osteoporosis." [In eng]. *Osteoporos Int* 23, no. 3 (Mar 2012): 1115-22.

368. Reginster, J. Y. "Strontium Ranelate in Osteoporosis." [In eng]. *Curr Pharm Des* 8, no. 21 (2002): 1907-16.

369. Bonnelye, E., A. Chabadel, F. Saltel, and P. Jurdic. "Dual Effect of Strontium Ranelate: Stimulation of Osteoblast Differentiation and Inhibition of Osteoclast Formation and Resorption in Vitro." [In eng]. *Bone* 42, no. 1 (Jan 2008): 129-38.

370. Chen, F. P., K. C. Wang and J. D. Huang. 2009. Effect of estrogen on the activity and growth of human osteoclasts in vitro. Taiwan *J Obstet Gynecol* Dec;48(4):350-5. PMID: 20045755.

Imai, Y., M. Y. Youn, S. Kondoh, et al. 2009. Estrogens maintain bone mass by regulating expression of genes controlling function and life span in mature osteoclasts. *Ann N Y Acad Sci* Sep;1173 Suppl 1:E31-9. PMID: 19751412.

McLean, R. R. 2009. Pro-inflammatory cytokines and osteoporosis. *Curr Osteoporos Rep* Dec;7(4):134-9. PMID: 19968917.

Boyce, B. F. and L. Xing. 2008. Functions of RANKL/RANK/OPG in bone modeling and remodeling. *Arch Biochem Biophys* May 15;473(2):139-46. Epub 2008 Mar 25. PMID: 18395508.

Mundy, G. R. 2007. Osteoporosis and inflammation. *Nutr Rev* Dec;65(12 Pt 2):S147-51. PMID: 18240539.

D'Amelio, P., A. Grimaldi, S. Di Bella, et al. 2008. Estrogen deficiency increases osteoclastogenesis up-regulating T cells activity: a key mechanism in osteoporosis. *Bone* Jul;43(1):92–100. Epub 2008 Mar 7. PMID: 18407820.

Pérez, A. V., G. Picotto, A. R. Carpentieri, et al. 2008. Mini-review on regulation of intestinal calcium absorption. Emphasis on molecular mechanisms of transcellular pathway. *Digestion* 77(1):22–34. Epub 2008 Feb 15. PMID: 18277073.

Dick, I. M., A. Devine, J. Beilby, et al. 2005. Effects of endogenous estrogen on renal calcium and phosphate handling in elderly women. *Am J Physiol Endocrinol Metab* Feb;288(2):E430–5. Epub 2004 Oct 5. PMID: 15466921.

Mauras, N., N. E. Vieira, A. L. Yergey. 1997. Estrogen therapy enhances calcium absorption and retention and diminishes bone turnover in young girls with Turner's syndrome: a calcium kinetic study. *Metabolism* Aug;46(8):908–13. PMID: 9258273.

Weaver, C. M. 1994. Age related calcium requirements due to changes in absorption and utilization. *J Nutr* Aug;124(8 Suppl):1418S-1425S. PMID: 8064395.

371. Wright, J. V. and L. Lenard. *Stay Young and Sexy with Bio-Identical Hormone Replacement*, Chapter 6, "Preventing and Reversing Osteoporosis," (Petaluma, CA: Smart Publications), 149.

Prior, J. C. 1990. Progesterone as a bone-trophic hormone. *Endocr Rev* May;11(2):386–98. PMID: 2194787.

Prior, J. C. 2005. Ovarian aging and the perimenopausal transition: the paradox of endogenous ovarian hyperstimulation. *Endocrine* Apr;26(3):297–300. PMID: 16034185.

372. Freeman, S. and L. P. Shulman. 2010. Considerations for the use of progestin-only contraceptives. *J Am Acad Nurse Pract* Feb;22(2):81–91. PMID: 20132366.

373. Quinkler, M., K. Kaur, M. Hewison, et al. 2008. Progesterone is extensively metabolized in osteoblasts: implications for progesterone action on bone. *Horm Metab Res* Oct;40(10):679–84. Epub 2008 Jun 6. PMID: 18537080.

Liang, M., E. Y. Liao, X. Xu, et al. 2003. Effects of progesterone and 18-methyl levonorgestrel on osteoblastic cells. *Endocr Res* Nov;29(4):483–501. PMID: 14682477.

Luo, X. H., E. Y. Liao, X. Su. 2002. Progesterone upregulates TGF-b isoforms (b1, b2, and b3) expression in normal human osteoblast-like cells. *Calcif Tissue Int* Oct;71(4):329–34. Epub 2002 Aug 6. PMID: 12154395.

MacNamara, P., C. O'Shaughnessy, P. Manduca, et al. 1995. Progesterone receptors are expressed in human osteoblast-like cell lines and in primary human osteoblast cultures. *Calcif Tissue Int* Dec;57(6):436–41. PMID: 8581876.

Kaunitz, A. M., R. Arias, M. McClung. 2008. Bone density recovery after depot medroxyprogesterone acetate injectable contraception use. *Contraception* Feb;77(2):67–76. PMID: 18226668.

374. Isley, M. M., and A. M. Kaunitz. "Update on Hormonal Contraception and Bone Density." [In eng]. *Rev Endocr Metab Disord* 12, no. 2 (Jun 2011): 93–106.

Seifert-Klauss, V., M. Schmidmayr, E. Hobmaier, and T. Wimmer. "Progesterone and Bone: A Closer Link Than Previously Realized." [In eng]. *Climacteric* 15 Suppl 1 (Apr 2012): 26–31.

Bahamondes, M. V., I. Monteiro, S. Castro, X. Espejo-Arce, and L. Bahamondes. "Prospective Study of the Forearm Bone Mineral Density of Long-Term Users of the Levonorgestrel-Releasing Intra-uterine System." [In eng]. *Hum Reprod* 25, no. 5 (May 2010): 1158–64.

375. Zhang, W. and H. Jia. 2007. Effect and mechanism of cadmium on the progesterone synthesis of ovaries. *Toxicology* Oct 8;239(3):204–12. Epub 2007 Jul 13. PMID: 17719163.

376. Prior, J. C., S. A. Kirkland, L. Joseph, et al. 2001. Oral con-traceptive use and bone mineral density in premenopausal women: cross-sectional, population-based data from the Ca-nadian Multicentre Osteoporosis Study. *CMAJ* Oct 16;165(8):1023–9. PMID: 11699697.

377. Hagen, J., N. Gott and D. R. Miller. 2003. Reliability of saliva hormone tests. *J Am Pharm Assoc* Nov-Dec;43(6):724–6. PMID: 14717270.

378. Wright, J. V. and L. Lenard. "Getting the Most Out of BHRT," in *Stay Young and Sexy with Bio-Identical Hormone Replacement*, (Petaluma, CA: Smart Publications), p. 301–308.

379. Rossouw, J. E., G. L. Anderson, R. L. Prentice, et al. 2002. Risks and benefits of estrogen plus progestin in healthy postmenopausal women: principal results From the Women's Health Initiative randomized controlled trial. *JAMA* Jul 17;288(3):321–33. PMID: 12117397.

380. Cauley, J. A., J. Robbins, Z. Chen, et al. 2003. Effects of estrogen plus progestin on risk of fracture and bone mineral density: the Women's Health Initiative randomized trial. *JAMA* Oct 1;290(13):1729–38. PMID: 14519707.

381. Coombs, N. J., K. A. Cronin, R. J. Taylor, et al. 2010. The impact of changes in hormone therapy on breast cancer incidence in the US population. *Cancer Causes Control* Jan;21(1):83–90. Epub 2009 Oct 1. PMID: 19795215.

382. Romieu, I., A. Fabre, A. Fournier, et al. 2010. Post-menopausal hormone therapy and asthma onset in the E3N cohort. *Thorax* Apr;65(4):292–7. Epub 2010 Feb 8. PMID: 20142267.

Nath, A. and R. Sitruk-Ware. 2009. Different cardiovascular effects of progestins according to structure and activity. *Climacteric* 12 Suppl 1:96–101. PMID: 19811251.

Canonico, M., A. Fournier, L. Carcaillon, et al. 2010. Postmenopausal hormone therapy and risk of idiopathic venous thromboembolism: results from the E3N cohort study. *Arterioscler Thromb Vasc Biol* Feb;30(2):340–5. Epub 2009 Oct 15. PMID: 19834106.

Razavi, P., M. C. Pike, P. L. Horn-Ross, et al. 2010. Long-term postmenopausal hormone therapy and endometrial cancer. *Cancer Epidemiol Biomarkers Prev* Feb;19(2):475–83. Epub 2010 Jan 19. PMID: 20086105.

Shapiro, S. 2007. Recent epidemiological evidence relevant to the clinical management of the menopause. *Climacteric* Oct;10 Suppl 2:2–15. PMID: 17882666.

Pike, M.C., A. H. Wu, D. V. Spicer, et al. 2007. Estrogens, progestins, and risk of breast cancer. *Ernst Schering Found Symp Proc* (1):127–50. PMID: 18540571.

383. Sitruk-Ware, R. 2004. New progestogens: a review of their effects in perimenopausal and postmenopausal women. *Drugs Aging* 21(13):865–83. PMID: 15493951.

384. Puel, C., V. Coxam, M. J. Davicco. 2007. [Mediterranean diet and osteoporosis prevention] *Med Sci* (Paris) Aug-Sep;23(8–9):756–60. PMID: 17875296.

385. Pollan, M. In Defense of Food (New York: Penguin Press, 2008), p.1.

386. Dai, Z., Y. Li, L. D. Quarles, T. Song, et al. 2007. Resveratrol enhances proliferation and osteoblastic differentiation in human mesenchymal stem cells via ER-dependent ERK1/2 activation. *Phytomedicine* Dec;14(12):806–14. PMID: 17689939.

Habold, C., I. Momken, A. Ouadi, et al. 2010. Effect of prior treatment with resveratrol on density and structure of rat long bones under tail-suspension. *J Bone Miner Metab* May 11. PMID: 20458604.

Boissy, P., T. L. Andersen, B. M. Abdallah, et al. 2005. Resveratrol inhibits myeloma cell growth, prevents osteoclast formation, and promotes osteoblast differentiation. *Cancer Res* Nov 1;65(21):9943–52. PMID: 16267019.

Zhou, H., L. Shang, X. Li, et al. 2009. Resveratrol augments the canonical Wnt signaling pathway in promoting osteoblastic differentiation of multipotent mesenchymal cells. *Exp Cell Res* Oct 15;315(17):2953–62. Epub 2009 Aug 6. PMID: 19665018.

Liu, Z. P., W. X. Li, B. Yu, et al. 2005. Effects of trans-resveratrol from Polygonum cuspidatum on bone loss using the ovariectomized rat model. *J Med Food Spring* 8(1):14–9. PMID: 15857203.

387. Worthington, V. 1998. Effect of agricultural methods on nutritional quality: a comparison of organic with conventional crops. *Altern Ther Health Med* Jan;4(1):58–69. PMID: 9439021.

388. The Organic Center. Nutrient Decline Linked to the "Dilution" Effect. September 2005 report, http://www.organic-center.org/science.hot.php?action=view&report_id=9 (accessed June 5, 2010).

389. Benbrook, C., X. Zhao, J. Yanes, N. Davies, P. Andrews. "New Evidence Confirms the Nutritional Superiority of Plant-Based Organic Foods," State of Science Review, March 2008,

http://www.organic-center.org/science.nutri. php?action=view&report_id=126 (accessed June 5, 2010).

390. Davis, et al. "Changes in USDA Food Composition Data for 43 Garden Crops, 1950 to 1999," *Journal of the American College of Nutrition*, Vol. 23(6): 669–682.

391. Benbrook, C., D. Davis and P. Andrews. "Organic Center Response to the FSA Study," available at http://www.organic-center.org/science.nutri. php?action=view&report_id=157 (accessed June 5, 2010).

392. Worthington, V. 2002. Analyzing data to compare nutrients in conventional versus organic crops. *J Altern Complement Med* Oct;8(5):529–32. PMID: 12470430.

393. Crinnion, W. J. 2010. Organic foods contain higher levels of certain nutrients, lower levels of pesticides, and may provide health benefits for the consumer. *Altern Med Rev* Apr;15(1):4–12. PMID: 20359265.

Györéné, K. G., A. Varga and A. Lugasi. 2006. [A comparison of chemical composition and nutritional value of organically and conventionally grown plant derived foods] *Orv Hetil* Oct 29;147(43):2081–90. PMID: 17297755.

394. Dahlgren, J. G., H. S. Takhar, C. A. Ruffalo, et al. 2004. Health effects of diazinon on a family. *J Toxicol Clin Toxicol* 42(5):579–91. PMID: 15462149.

Takaro, T. K., L. S. Engel, M. Keifer, et al. 2004. Glycophorin A is a potential biomarker for the mutagenic effects of pesticides. *Int J Occup Environ Health* Jul-Sep;10(3):256–61. PMID: 15473078.

Hrelia, P., C. Fimognari, F. Maffei, et al. 1996. The genetic and non-genetic toxicity of the fungicide Vinclozolin. *Mutagenesis* Sep;11(5):445–53. PMID: 8921505.

Weeks, B. S., S. Lee, P. P. Perez, et al. 2008. Natramune and PureWay-C reduce xenobiotic-induced human T-cell alpha5beta1 integrin-mediated adhesion to fibronectin. *Med Sci Monit* Dec;14(12):BR279–85. PMID: 19043362.

Cho, Y. S., S. Y. Oh, Z. Zhu. 2008. Tyrosine phosphatase SHP-1 in oxidative stress and development of allergic airway inflammation. *Am J Respir Cell Mol Biol* Oct;39(4):412–9. Epub 2008 Apr 25. PMID: 18441283.

Goel, A. and P. Aggarwal. 2007. Pesticide poisoning. *Natl Med J India* Jul-Aug;20(4):182–91.PMID: 18085124.

Arcury, T. A., S. R. Feldman, M. R. Schulz, et al. 2007. Diagnosed skin diseases among migrant farmworkers in North Carolina: prevalence and risk factors. *J Agric Saf Health* Nov;13(4):407–18. PMID: 18075016.

Boutsiouki,P. and G. F. Clough. 2004. Modulation of microvascular function following low-dose exposure to the organophosphorous compound malathion in human skin in vivo. *J Appl Physiol* Sep;97(3):1091–7. PMID: 15333628.

Thrash, B., S. Uthayathas, S. S. Karuppagounder, et al. 2007. Paraquat and maneb induced neurotoxicity. *Proc West Pharmacol* Soc 50:31–42. PMID: 18605226.

395. Sheng, J. P., C. Liu, L. Shen. 2009. [Analysis of some nutrients and minerals in organic and traditional cherry tomato by ICP-OES method] *Guang Pu Xue Yu Guang Pu Fen Xi* Aug;29(8):2244–6. PMID: 19839348.

396. Sheng, J. P., C. Liu, L. Shen. 2009. [Comparative study of minerals and some nutrients in organic celery and traditional celery] *Guang Pu Xue Yu Guang Pu Fen Xi* Jan;29(1):247–9. PMID: 19385250.

397. Raigón, M. D., A. Rodríguez-Burruezo, J. Prohens. 2010. Effects of organic and conventional cultivation methods on composition of eggplant fruits. *J Agric Food Chem* Jun 9;58(11):6833–40. PMID: 20443597.

398. Lee, S. H., Y. H. Khang, K. H. Lim, B. J. Kim, J. M. Koh, G. S. Kim, H. Kim, and N. H. Cho. "Clinical Risk Factors for Osteoporotic Fracture: A Population-Based Prospective Cohort Study in Korea." [In eng]. *J Bone Miner Res* 25, no. 2 (Feb 2010): 369-78.

Guadalupe-Grau, A., T. Fuentes, B. Guerra, and J. A. Calbet. "Exercise and Bone Mass in Adults." [In eng]. *Sports Med* 39, no. 6 (2009): 439-68.

399. Donaldson, C. L., S. B. Hulley, J. M. Vogel, R. S. Hattner, J. H. Bayers, and D. E. McMillan. "Effect of Prolonged Bed Rest on Bone Mineral." [In eng]. *Metabolism* 19, no. 12 (Dec 1970): 1071-84.

Krolner, B., and B. Toft. "Vertebral Bone Loss: An Unheeded Side Effect of Therapeutic Bed Rest." [In eng]. *Clin Sci (Lond)* 64, no. 5 (May 1983): 537-40.

Mazess, R. B., and G. D. Whedon. "Immobilization and Bone." [In eng]. *Calcif Tissue Int* 35, no. 3 (May 1983): 265-7.

Ohshima, H. "[Bone Loss and Bone Metabolism in Astronauts During Long-Duration Space Flight]." [In jpn]. *Clin Calcium* 16, no. 1 (Jan 2006): 81-5.

400. Kemmler, W., S. von Stengel, K. Engelke, L. Haberle, and W. A. Kalender. "Exercise Effects on Bone Mineral Density, Falls, Coronary Risk Factors, and Health Care Costs in Older Women: The Randomized Controlled Senior Fitness and Prevention (Sefip) Study." [In eng]. *Arch Intern Med* 170, no. 2 (Jan 25 2010): 179-85.

Kemmler, W., D. Lauber, J. Weineck, J. Hensen, W. Kalender, and K. Engelke. "Benefits of 2 Years of Intense Exercise on Bone Density, Physical Fitness, and Blood Lipids in Early Postmenopausal

Osteopenic Women: Results of the Erlangen Fitness Osteoporosis Prevention Study (Efops)." [In eng]. *Arch Intern Med* 164, no. 10 (May 24 2004): 1084–91.

Engelke, K., W. Kemmler, D. Lauber, C. Beeskow, R. Pintag, and W. A. Kalender. "Exercise Maintains Bone Density at Spine and Hip Efops: A 3-Year Longitudinal Study in Early Postmenopausal Women." [In eng]. *Osteoporos Int* 17, no. 1 (Jan 2006): 133–42.

Kemmler, W., S. von Stengel, J. Weineck, D. Lauber, W. Kalender, and K. Engelke. "Exercise Effects on Menopausal Risk Factors of Early Postmenopausal Women: 3-Yr Erlangen Fitness Osteoporosis Prevention Study Results." [In eng]. *Med Sci Sports Exerc* 37, no. 2 (Feb 2005): 194–203.

Angin, E. and Z. Erden. "[the Effect of Group Exercise on Postmenopausal Osteoporosis and Osteopenia]." [In tur]. *Acta Orthop Traumatol Turc* 43, no. 4 (Aug-Oct 2009): 343–50.

Asikainen, T. M., K. Kukkonen-Harjula, and S. Miilunpalo. "Exercise for Health for Early Postmenopausal Women: A Systematic Review of Randomised Controlled Trials." [In eng]. *Sports Med* 34, no. 11 (2004): 753–78.

401. Borer, K. T. "Physical Activity in the Prevention and Amelioration of Osteoporosis in Women: Interaction of Mechanical, Hormonal and Dietary Factors." [In eng]. *Sports Med* 35, no. 9 (2005): 779–830.

402. Iwamoto, J., T. Takeda, and S. Ichimura. "Effect of Exercise Training and Detraining on Bone Mineral Density in Postmenopausal Women with Osteoporosis." [In eng]. *J Orthop Sci* 6, no. 2 (2001): 128–32.

403. Michalek, J. E., H. G. Preuss, H. A. Croft, P. L. Keith, S. C. Keith, M. Dapilmoto, N. V. Perricone, R. B. Leckie, and G. R. Kaats. "Changes in Total Body

Bone Mineral Density Following a Common Bone Health Plan with Two Versions of a Unique Bone Health Supplement: A Comparative Effectiveness Research Study." [In eng]. *Nutr J* 10 (2011): 32.

404. Borer, K. T. "Physical Activity in the Prevention and Amelioration of Osteoporosis in Women: Interaction of Mechanical, Hormonal and Dietary Factors." [In eng]. *Sports Med* 35, no. 9 (2005): 779–830.

405. Hourigan, S. R., J. C. Nitz, S. G. Brauer, S. O'Neill, J. Wong, and C. A. Richardson. "Positive Effects of Exercise on Falls and Fracture Risk in Osteopenic Women." [In eng]. *Osteoporos Int* 19, no. 7 (Jul 2008): 1077–86.

406. Borer, K. T. "Physical Activity in the Prevention and Amelioration of Osteoporosis in Women: Interaction of Mechanical, Hormonal and Dietary Factors." [In eng]. *Sports Med* 35, no. 9 (2005): 779–830.

407. For more information about Nancy and Kristi, please see the Resources section, page 356.

408. Sinaki, M. "Musculoskeletal Challenges of Osteoporosis." [In eng]. *Aging (Milano)* 10, no. 3 (Jun 1998): 249–62.

Sinaki, M., and B. A. Mikkelsen. "Postmenopausal Spinal Osteoporosis: Flexion Versus Extension Exercises." [In eng]. *Arch Phys Med Rehabil* 65, no. 10 (Oct 1984): 593–6.

Pfeifer, M., M. Sinaki, P. Geusens, S. Boonen, E. Preisinger, and H. W. Minne. "Musculoskeletal Rehabilitation in Osteoporosis: A Review." [In eng]. *J Bone Miner Res* 19, no. 8 (Aug 2004): 1208–14.

Sinaki, M., M. Pfeifer, E. Preisinger, E. Itoi, R. Rizzoli, S. Boonen, P. Geusens, and H. W. Minne. "The Role of Exercise in the Treatment of Osteoporosis."

[In eng]. *Curr Osteoporos Rep* 8, no. 3 (Sep 2010): 138–44.

409. Pfeifer, M., M. Sinaki, P. Geusens, S. Boonen, E. Preisinger, and H. W. Minne. "Musculoskeletal Rehabilitation in Osteoporosis: A Review." [In eng]. *J Bone Miner Res* 19, no. 8 (Aug 2004): 1208–14.

410. Mayhew, P. M., C. D. Thomas, J. G. Clement, N. Loveridge, T. J. Beck, W. Bonfield, C. J. Burgoyne, and J. Reeve. "Relation between Age, Femoral Neck Cortical Stability, and Hip Fracture Risk." [In eng]. *Lancet* 366, no. 9480 (Jul 9-15 2005): 129–35.

411. Sinaki, M., E. Itoi, H. W. Wahner, P. Wollan, R. Gelzcer, B. P. Mullan, D. A. Collins, and S. F. Hodgson. "Stronger Back Muscles Reduce the Incidence of Vertebral Fractures: A Prospective 10 Year Follow-up of Postmenopausal Women." [In eng]. *Bone* 30, no. 6 (Jun 2002): 836–41.

412. Pfeifer, M., M. Sinaki, P. Geusens, S. Boonen, E. Preisinger, and H. W. Minne. "Musculoskeletal Rehabilitation in Osteoporosis: A Review." [In eng]. *J Bone Miner Res* 19, no. 8 (Aug 2004): 1208–14.

413. Kemmler, W., S. von Stengel, K. Engelke, L. Haberle, J. L. Mayhew, and W. A. Kalender. "Exercise, Body Composition, and Functional Ability: A Randomized Controlled Trial." [In eng]. *Am J Prev Med* 38, no. 3 (Mar 2010): 279–87.

Kemmler, W., K. Engelke, S. von Stengel, J. Weineck, D. Lauber, and W. A. Kalender. "Long-Term Four-Year Exercise Has a Positive Effect on Menopausal Risk Factors: The Erlangen Fitness Osteoporosis Prevention Study." [In eng]. *J Strength Cond Res* 21, no. 1 (Feb 2007): 232–9.

414. Specker, B. L. "Evidence for an Interaction between Calcium Intake and Physical Activity on Changes in Bone Mineral Density." [In eng]. *J Bone Miner Res* 11, no. 10 (Oct 1996): 1539–44.

415. Here is a link to one such lab as an example. Neither Lara nor Dr. Wright has any financial connection with this lab: Private MD Labs: http://www. privatemdlabs.com/lab_tests.php?view=all&show =1583&category=17&search=#1583).

416. Hamano, T. "[Bone and Bone Related Biochemical Examinations. Bone and Collagen Related Metabolites. Urinary and Serum Ntx as Bone Resorption Markers]." [In jpn]. *Clin Calcium* 16, no. 6 (Jun 2006): 987–92.

Ju, H. S., S. Leung, B. Brown, M. A. Stringer, S. Leigh, C. Scherrer, K. Shepard, *et al.* "Comparison of Analytical Performance and Biological Variability of Three Bone Resorption Assays." [In eng]. *Clin Chem* 43, no. 9 (Sep 1997): 1570–6.

Here is a link to one of the labs running the NTx. Neither Lara nor Dr. Wright have any financial connection to this lab. Quest Diagnostics: http://www. specialtylabs.com/tests/details.asp?id=4266.

417. Simsek, B., O. Karacaer, and I. Karaca. "Urine Products of Bone Breakdown as Markers of Bone Resorption and Clinical Usefulness of Urinary Hydroxyproline: An Overview." [In eng]. *Chin Med J (Engl)* 117, no. 2 (Feb 2004): 291–5.

Here are links to two of the labs running Pyrilinks-D. Neither Lara nor Dr. Wright has any financial connection to these labs. DiagnosTechs: http://www. diagnostechs.com/Pages/BHPPatientOverview.aspx and Metametrix: http://www.metametrix.com/ test-menu/profiles/health-risk-profiles/bone.

418. Iki, M., T. Akiba, T. Matsumoto, H. Nishino, S. Kagamimori, Y. Kagawa, and H. Yoneshima. "Reference Database of Biochemical Markers of Bone Turnover for the Japanese Female Population. Japanese Population-Based Osteoporosis (Jpos) Study." [In eng]. *Osteoporos Int* 15, no. 12 (Dec 2004): 981–91.

419. Huber, F., L. Traber, H. J. Roth, V. Heckel, and H. Schmidt-Gayk. "Markers of Bone Resorption— Measurement in Serum, Plasma or Urine?" [In eng]. *Clin Lab* 49, no. 5-6 (2003): 203–7.

Here is a link to a lab running the CTX test. Neither Lara nor Dr. Wright has any financial connection to this lab. http://www.privatemdlabs.com/lab_tests.php?view=search_results&show=1473&category=16&search=bone resorption#1473.

420. Here are links to a few labs, but a Google search for this test will bring up many lab options in your area. Lara and Dr. Wright donate to the Vitamin D Council, a 501(c)(3) nonprofit organization, whose mission is to spread reliable information on vitamin D, sun exposure and the vitamin D deficiency pandemic. Neither Lara nor Dr. Wright has any financial connection to ZRT Labs, Mayo Medical Laboratories or Metametrix: http://www.zrtlab.com/vitamindcouncil/ ; http://www.mayomedicallaboratories.com/articles/vitamind/pfriendly.html ; http://www.metametrix.com/test-menu/profiles/vitamins/vitamin-d.

421. Bugel, S. "Vitamin K and Bone Health." [In eng]. *Proc Nutr Soc* 62, no. 4 (Nov 2003): 839–43.

422. Plaza, S. M., and D. W. Lamson. "Vitamin K2 in Bone Metabolism and Osteoporosis." [In eng]. *Altern Med Rev* 10, no. 1 (Mar 2005): 24–35.

Masterjohn, C. "Vitamin D Toxicity Redefined: Vitamin K and the Molecular Mechanism." [In eng]. *Med Hypotheses* 68, no. 5 (2007): 1026–34.

Yamaguchi, M., E. Sugimoto, and S. Hachiya. "Stimulatory Effect of Menaquinone-7 (Vitamin K2) on Osteoblastic Bone Formation in Vitro." [In eng]. *Mol Cell Biochem* 223, no. 1-2 (Jul 2001): 131–7.

Yamaguchi, M., S. Uchiyama, and Y. Tsukamoto. "Inhibitory Effect of Menaquinone-7 (Vitamin

K2) on the Bone-Resorbing Factors-Induced Bone Resorption in Elderly Female Rat Femoral Tissues in Vitro." [In eng]. *Mol Cell Biochem* 245, no. 1-2 (Mar 2003): 115–20.

423. Li, K., R. Kaaks, J. Linseisen, and S. Rohrmann. "Associations of Dietary Calcium Intake and Calcium Supplementation with Myocardial Infarction and Stroke Risk and Overall Cardiovascular Mortality in the Heidelberg Cohort of the European Prospective Investigation into Cancer and Nutrition Study (Epic-Heidelberg)." [In eng]. *Heart* 98, no. 12 (Jun 2012): 920–5.

424. Berkner, K. L., and K. W. Runge. "The Physiology of Vitamin K Nutriture and Vitamin K-Dependent Protein Function in Atherosclerosis." [In eng]. *J Thromb Haemost* 2, no. 12 (Dec 2004): 2118-32.

Cranenburg, E. C., L. J. Schurgers, and C. Vermeer. "Vitamin K: The Coagulation Vitamin That Became Omnipotent." [In eng]. *Thromb Haemost* 98, no. 1 (Jul 2007): 120–5.

Bugel, S. "Vitamin K and Bone Health." [In eng]. *Proc Nutr Soc* 62, no. 4 (Nov 2003): 839–43.

425. Here is one example. Neither Dr. Wright nor Lara Pizzorno has any financial connection to Metametrix: http://www.metametrix.com/test-menu/profiles/vitamins/vitamin-k.

426. Since this is a cutting edge test, only about 4,000 doctors among the 500,000 physicians in the United States know about and use micronutrient testing in their practice. To assist you in locating a doctor, SpectraCell's website (www.spectracell.com) has a FIND A DOCTOR function and also a FIND A DRAW SITE function, where you can plug in your zip code and find a doctor familiar with SpectraCell testing or a place where you can get your blood drawn if you wish to order this test directly. Neither Lara nor Dr. Wright has

any financial connection with SpectraCell Laboratories. http://www.spectracell.com/products/micronutrient-testing-product-specifications/.

427. http://labtestsonline.org/understanding/analytes/pth/tab/test.

428. Ong, G. S., J. P. Walsh, B. G. Stuckey, S. J. Brown, E. Rossi, J. L. Ng, H. H. Nguyen, G. N. Kent, and E. M. Lim. "The Importance of Measuring Ionized Calcium in Characterizing Calcium Status and Diagnosing Primary Hyperparathyroidism." [In Eng]. *J Clin Endocrinol Metab* (Jun 28 2012).

Ong, G. S., J. P. Walsh, B. G. Stuckey, S. J. Brown, E. Rossi, J. L. Ng, H. H. Nguyen, G. N. Kent, and E. M. Lim. "The Importance of Measuring Ionized Calcium in Characterizing Calcium Status and Diagnosing Primary Hyperparathyroidism." [In eng]. *J Clin Endocrinol Metab* 97, no. 9 (Sep 2012): 3138–45.

429. Fraser, W. D. "Hyperparathyroidism." [In eng]. *Lancet* 374, no. 9684 (Jul 11 2009): 145–58.

430. Rude, R. K., and H. E. Gruber. "Magnesium Deficiency and Osteoporosis: Animal and Human Observations." [In eng]. *J Nutr Biochem* 15, no. 12 (Dec 2004): 710–6.

Brown, S. Parathyroid hormone and magnesium: when "normal" is not always a good thing. *The Better Bones Blog* http://www.betterbones.com/blog/post/vitamin-d-parathyroid-hormone-levels-magnesium-deficiency.aspx, accessed 6-20-12.

431. Neither Lara nor Dr. Wright has any connection to Intracellular Diganostics, Inc. http://www.exatest.com/physicians.htm.

432. Here is one example. Neither Lara nor Dr. Wright has any connection to PrivateMD Labs. http://www.privatemdlabs.com/lab_tests.php?view=search_results&show=1559&category=12&search=magnesium#1559.

433. Neither Lara nor Dr. Wright has any financial connection to any of the labs noted here: http://www.optimox.com/pics/Iodine/loadTest.htm.

434. Neither Lara nor Dr. Wright has any financial connection to ZRT Lab: http://www.zrt-lab.com/health-care-consumers/iodine-testing.html?gclid=CNvPrMz__rACFekZQgod9DTJZA.

435. Zimmermann, M. B. "Iodine Requirements and the Risks and Benefits of Correcting Iodine Deficiency in Populations." [In eng]. *J Trace Elem Med Biol* 22, no. 2 (2008): 81–92.

436. http://meridianvalleylab.com/24-hour-urine-hormone-testing-the-gold-standard. (Dr. Wright is the Medical Director of Meridian Valley Lab, which since 1976, has been a world leader in Allergy and Hormone Testing, specializing in Comprehensive 24-Hour Urine Hormone and Metabolite Testing to help doctors use Bio-identical Hormone Replacement Therapy safely and effectively.)

437. Pizzorno, L. and P. Larsen. Ensure Effective Bio-Identical Hormone Replacement: Select the Right Hormone Test for Your Patient. *Longevity Medicine Review*, 2010. For an in-depth comparison of the 24-Hour Comprehensive Urine Hormone test to tests using saliva or blood to evaluate hormone levels.

http://www.lmreview.com/articles/view/select-the-right-hormone-test-for-your-patient-using-bio-identical-hormone-/.

438. Duong, M., J. I. Cohen, and A. Convit. "High Cortisol Levels Are Associated with Low Quality Food Choice in Type 2 Diabetes." [In eng]. *Endocrine* 41, no. 1 (Feb 2012): 76–81.

Vicennati, V., F. Pasqui, C. Cavazza, S. Garelli, E. Casadio, G. di Dalmazi, U. Pagotto, and R. Pasquali. "Cortisol, Energy Intake, and Food Frequency in Overweight/Obese Women." [In eng]. *Nutrition* 27, no. 6 (Jun 2011): 677–80.

London, E., and T. W. Castonguay. "Diet and the Role of 11beta-Hydroxysteroid Dehydrogenase-1 on Obesity." [In eng]. *J Nutr Biochem* 20, no. 7 (Jul 2009): 485–93.

439. Tsigos, C., and G. P. Chrousos. "Hypothalamic-Pituitary-Adrenal Axis, Neuroendocrine Factors and Stress." [In eng]. *J Psychosom Res* 53, no. 4 (Oct 2002): 865–71.

440. Hollowell, J. G., N. W. Staehling, W. D. Flanders, W. H. Hannon, E. W. Gunter, C. A. Spencer, and L. E. Braverman. "Serum Tsh, T(4), and Thyroid Antibodies in the United States Population (1988 to 1994): National Health and Nutrition Examination Survey (Nhanes Iii)." [In eng]. *J Clin Endocrinol Metab* 87, no. 2 (Feb 2002): 489–99.

441. Tarraga Lopez, P. J., C. F. Lopez, F. N. de Mora, J. A. Montes, J. S. Albero, A. N. Manez, and A. G. Casas. "Osteoporosis in Patients with Subclinical Hypothyroidism Treated with Thyroid Hormone." [In eng]. *Clin Cases Miner Bone Metab* 8, no. 3 (Sep 2011): 44–8.

442. O'Reilly, D. S. "Thyroid Hormone Replacement: An Iatrogenic Problem." [In eng]. *Int J Clin Pract* 64, no. 7 (Jun 2010): 991–4.

443. Labrie, F., V. Luu-The, C. Labrie, and J. Simard. "Dhea and Its Transformation into Androgens and Estrogens in Peripheral Target Tissues: Intracrinology." [In eng]. *Front Neuroendocrinol* 22, no. 3 (Jul 2001): 185–212.

444. von Muhlen, D., G. A. Laughlin, D. Kritz-Silverstein, J. Bergstrom, and R. Bettencourt. "Effect of Dehydroepiandrosterone Supplementation on Bone Mineral Density, Bone Markers, and Body Composition in Older Adults: The Dawn Trial." [In eng]. *Osteoporos Int* 19, no. 5 (May 2008): 699–707.

Weiss, E. P., K. Shah, L. Fontana, C. P. Lambert, J. O. Holloszy, and D. T. Villareal. "Dehydroepiandrosterone Replacement Therapy in Older Adults: 1- and 2-Y Effects on Bone." [In eng]. *Am J Clin Nutr* 89, no. 5 (May 2009): 1459–67.

Garnero, P., E. Sornay-Rendu, B. Claustrat, and P. D. Delmas. "Biochemical Markers of Bone Turnover, Endogenous Hormones and the Risk of Fractures in Postmenopausal Women: The Ofely Study." [In eng]. *J Bone Miner Res* 15, no. 8 (Aug 2000): 1526–36.

445. Andrade, S., S. L. Silveira, B. D. Arbo, B. A. Batista, R. Gomez, H. M. Barros, and M. F. Ribeiro. "Sex-Dependent Antidepressant Effects of Lower Doses of Progesterone in Rats." [In eng]. *Physiol Behav* 99, no. 5 (Apr 19 2010): 687–90.

Morita, K., and S. Her. "Progesterone Pretreatment Enhances Serotonin-Stimulated Bdnf Gene Expression in Rat C6 Glioma Cells through Production of 5alpha-Reduced Neurosteroids." [In eng]. *J Mol Neurosci* 34, no. 3 (Mar 2008): 193–200.

Komukai, K., S. Mochizuki, and M. Yoshimura. "Gender and the Renin-Angiotensin-Aldosterone System." [In eng]. *Fundam Clin Pharmacol* 24, no. 6 (Dec 2010): 687–98.

Fronius, M., M. Rehn, U. Eckstein-Ludwig, and W. Clauss. "Inhibitory Non-Genomic Effects of Progesterone on Na+ Absorption in Epithelial Cells from Xenopus Kidney (A6)." [In eng]. *J Comp Physiol B* 171, no. 5 (Jun 2001): 377–86.

Quinkler, M., K. Kaur, M. Hewison, P. M. Stewart, and M. S. Cooper. "Progesterone Is Extensively Metabolized in Osteoblasts: Implications for Progesterone Action on Bone." [In eng]. *Horm Metab Res* 40, no. 10 (Oct 2008): 679–84.

Tremollieres, F., J. M. Pouilles, and C. Ribot. "[Postmenopausal Bone Loss. Role of Progesterone and Androgens]." [In fre]. *Presse Med* 21, no. 21 (Jun 6 1992): 989–93.

Seifert-Klauss, V., and J. C. Prior. "Progesterone and Bone: Actions Promoting Bone Health in Women." [In eng]. *J Osteoporos* 2010 (2010): 845180.

446. Tremollieres, F., J. M. Pouilles, and C. Ribot. "[Postmenopausal Bone Loss. Role of Progesterone and Androgens]." [In fre]. *Presse Med* 21, no. 21 (Jun 6 1992): 989–93.

447. Mansour, D. "The Benefits and Risks of Using a Levonorgestrel-Releasing Intrauterine System for Contraception." [In eng]. *Contraception* 85, no. 3 (Mar 2012): 224–34.

Lopez, L. M., D. A. Grimes, K. F. Schulz, and K. M. Curtis. "Steroidal Contraceptives: Effect on Bone Fractures in Women." [In eng]. *Cochrane Database Syst Rev*, no. 7 (2011): CD006033.

448. Pizzorno, L. and B. Wheeler. Bio-Identical Hormone Replacement: Selecting the Right Hormone Test(s) for Your Male Patient, *Longevity Medicine Review*, 2010, available @ http://www.lmreview. com/articles/view/Selecting-the-Right-Hormone-Tests-for-Your-Male-Patient/ accessed 7-1-2012.

449. Nakamura, K., T. Saito, R. Kobayashi, R. Oshiki, M. Oyama, T. Nishiwaki, M. Nashimoto, and Y. Tsuchiya. "C-Reactive Protein Predicts Incident Fracture in Community-Dwelling Elderly Japanese Women: The Muramatsu Study." [In eng]. *Osteoporos Int* 22, no. 7 (Jul 2011): 2145–50.

http://labtestsonline.org/understanding/analytes/hscrp/tab/test.

450. Many labs run hs-CRP, here is an example. Neither Dr. Wright nor Lara has any financial connection with MetaMetrix. http://www.metametrix.com/test-menu/profiles/health-risk-profiles/cardiovascular.

451. Kuyumcu, M. E., Y. Yesil, Z. A. Ozturk, E. Cinar, C. Kizilarslanoglu, M. Halil, Z. Ulger, *et al.* "The

Association between Homocysteine (Hcy) and Serum Natural Antioxidants in Elderly Bone Mineral Densitometry (Bmd)." [In Eng]. *Arch Gerontol Geriatr* (Jun 6 2012).

452. Bucciarelli, P., G. Martini, I. Martinelli, E. Ceccarelli, L. Gennari, R. Bader, R. Valenti, *et al.* "The Relationship between Plasma Homocysteine Levels and Bone Mineral Density in Post-Menopausal Women." [In eng]. *Eur J Intern Med* 21, no. 4 (Aug 2010): 301–5.

453. Here is one example. Neither Dr. Wright nor Lara has any financial connection with Metametrix http://www.metametrix.com/test-menu/profiles/amino-acids/homocysteine.

454. Jones, S., C. D'Souza, and N. Y. Haboubi. "Patterns of Clinical Presentation of Adult Coeliac Disease in a Rural Setting." [In eng]. *Nutr J* 5 (2006): 24.

"Revised Criteria for Diagnosis of Coeliac Disease. Report of Working Group of European Society of Paediatric Gastroenterology and Nutrition." [In eng]. *Arch Dis Child* 65, no. 8 (Aug 1990): 909–11.

455. Here are two examples: Meridian Valley Lab (Dr. Wright is the Medical Director of MVL, Lara has no financial connection): http://meridianvalleylab.com/allergy-testing-3/allergy-tests-offered/food/gluten-panels; Metametrix: http://www.metametrix.com/test-menu/profiles/immune-function/celiac.

456. Sapone, A., K. M. Lammers, V. Casolaro, M. Cammarota, M. T. Giuliano, M. De Rosa, R. Stefanile, *et al.* "Divergence of Gut Permeability and Mucosal Immune Gene Expression in Two Gluten-Associated Conditions: Celiac Disease and Gluten Sensitivity." [In eng]. *BMC Med* 9 (2011): 23.

457. Neither Dr. Wright nor Lara has any financial connection with EnteroLab. https://www.enterolab.com/default.aspx.

458. Strause, L., P. Saltman, K. T. Smith, M. Bracker, and M. B. Andon. "Spinal Bone Loss in Postmenopausal Women Supplemented with Calcium and Trace Minerals." [In eng]. *J Nutr* 124, no. 7 (Jul 1994): 1060–4.

459. Saltman, P. D. and L. G. Strause. "The Role of Trace Minerals in Osteoporosis." [In eng]. *J Am Coll Nutr* 12, no. 4 (Aug 1993): 384–9.

Gur, A., L. Colpan, K. Nas, R. Cevik, J. Sarac, F. Erdogan, and M. Z. Duz. "The Role of Trace Minerals in the Pathogenesis of Postmenopausal Osteoporosis and a New Effect of Calcitonin." [In eng]. *J Bone Miner Metab* 20, no. 1 (2002): 39–43.

Aaseth, J., G. Boivin, and O. Andersen. "Osteoporosis and Trace Elements - an Overview." [In eng]. *J Trace Elem Med Biol* 26, no. 2-3 (Jun 2012): 149–52.

Klevay, L. M. "Is the Western Diet Adequate in Copper?" [In eng]. *J Trace Elem Med Biol* 25, no. 4 (Dec 2011): 204–12.

460. Clegg, M. S., S. M. Donovan, M. H. Monaco, D. L. Baly, J. L. Ensunsa, and C. L. Keen. "The Influence of Manganese Deficiency on Serum Igf-1 and Igf Binding Proteins in the Male Rat." [In eng]. *Proc Soc Exp Biol Med* 219, no. 1 (Oct 1998): 41–7.

461. Strause, L., P. Saltman, K. T. Smith, M. Bracker, and M. B. Andon. "Spinal Bone Loss in Postmenopausal Women Supplemented with Calcium and Trace Minerals." [In eng]. *J Nutr* 124, no. 7 (Jul 1994): 1060–4.

462. Calabrese, E., C. Sacco, G. Moore, and S. DiNardi. "Sulfite Oxidase Deficiency: A High Risk Factor in So2, Sulfite, and Bisulfite Toxicity?" [In eng]. *Med Hypotheses* 7, no. 2 (Feb 1981): 133–45.

463. Reffitt, D. M., N. Ogston, R. Jugdaohsingh, H. F. Cheung, B. A. Evans, R. P. Thompson, J. J. Powell, and G. N. Hampson. "Orthosilicic Acid Stimulates Collagen Type 1 Synthesis and Osteoblastic

Differentiation in Human Osteoblast-Like Cells in Vitro." [In eng]. *Bone* 32, no. 2 (Feb 2003): 127–35.

464. Macdonald, H. M., A. C. Hardcastle, R. Jugdaohsingh, W. D. Fraser, D. M. Reid, and J. J. Powell. "Dietary Silicon Interacts with Oestrogen to Influence Bone Health: Evidence from the Aberdeen Prospective Osteoporosis Screening Study." [In eng]. *Bone* 50, no. 3 (Mar 2012): 681–7.

Jugdaohsingh, R., K. L. Tucker, N. Qiao, L. A. Cupples, D. P. Kiel, and J. J. Powell. "Dietary Silicon Intake Is Positively Associated with Bone Mineral Density in Men and Premenopausal Women of the Framingham Offspring Cohort." [In eng]. *J Bone Miner Res* 19, no. 2 (Feb 2004): 297–307.

465. Heaney, R. P., R. R. Recker, J. Grote, R. L. Horst, and L. A. Armas. "Vitamin D(3) Is More Potent Than Vitamin D(2) in Humans." [In eng]. *J Clin Endocrinol Metab* 96, no. 3 (Mar 2011): E447–52.

Logan, V. F., A. R. Gray, M. C. Peddie, et al. Long-term vitamin D3 supplementation is more effective than vitamin D2 in maintaining serum 25-hydroxyvitamin D status over the winter months. British Journal of Nutrition, Available on CJO doi:10.1017/S0007114512002851;accessed 7-26-12 @ http://journals.cambridge.org/action/displayAbstract?fromPage=online&aid=8637888&fulltextType=RA&fileId=S0007114512002851.

466. Shearer, M. J., X. Fu, and S. L. Booth. "Vitamin K Nutrition, Metabolism, and Requirements: Current Concepts and Future Research." [In eng]. *Adv Nutr* 3, no. 2 (Mar 2012): 182–95.

467. Ohrvik, V. E. and C. M. Witthoft. "Human Folate Bioavailability." [In eng]. *Nutrients* 3, no. 4 (Apr 2011): 475–90.

Wien, T. N., E. Pike, T. Wisloff, A. Staff, S. Smeland, and M. Klemp. "Cancer Risk with Folic Acid Supplements: A Systematic Review and Meta-Analysis." [In eng]. *BMJ Open* 2, no. 1 (2012): e000653.

Figueiredo, J. C., M. V. Grau, R. W. Haile, R. S. Sandler, R. W. Summers, R. S. Bresalier, C. A. Burke, G. E. McKeown-Eyssen, and J. A. Baron. "Folic Acid and Risk of Prostate Cancer: Results from a Randomized Clinical Trial." [In eng]. *J Natl Cancer Inst* 101, no. 6 (Mar 18 2009): 432–5.

468. Bailey, R. L., J. L. Mills, E. A. Yetley, J. J. Gahche, C. M. Pfeiffer, J. T. Dwyer, K. W. Dodd, *et al.* "Unmetabolized Serum Folic Acid and Its Relation to Folic Acid Intake from Diet and Supplements in a Nationally Representative Sample of Adults Aged > or =60 Y in the United States." [In eng]. *Am J Clin Nutr* 92, no. 2 (Aug 2010): 383–9.

469. Thomas, P. and M. Fenech. "Methylenetetrahydrofolate Reductase, Common Polymorphisms, and Relation to Disease." [In eng]. *Vitam Horm* 79 (2008): 375–92.

Ward, M., C. P. Wilson, J. J. Strain, G. Horigan, J. M. Scott, and H. McNulty. "B-Vitamins, Methylenetetrahydrofolate Reductase (Mthfr) and Hypertension." [In eng]. *Int J Vitam Nutr Res* 81, no. 4 (Jul 2011): 240–4.

470. Wilson, C. P., M. Ward, H. McNulty, J. J. Strain, T. G. Trouton, G. Horigan, J. Purvis, and J. M. Scott. "Riboflavin Offers a Targeted Strategy for Managing Hypertension in Patients with the Mthfr 677tt Genotype: A 4-Y Follow-Up." [In eng]. *Am J Clin Nutr* 95, no. 3 (Mar 2012): 766–72.

471. Ahmadieh, H. and A. Arabi. "Vitamins and Bone Health: Beyond Calcium and Vitamin D." [In eng]. *Nutr Rev* 69, no. 10 (Oct 2011): 584–98.

Zhang, J., R. G. Munger, N. A. West, D. R. Cutler, H. J. Wengreen, and C. D. Corcoran. "Antioxidant Intake and Risk of Osteoporotic Hip Fracture in Utah: An Effect Modified by Smoking Status." [In eng]. *Am J Epidemiol* 163, no. 1 (Jan 1 2006): 9–17.

Ima-Nirwana, S. and S. Suhaniza. "Effects of Tocopherols and Tocotrienols on Body Composition and Bone Calcium Content in Adrenalectomized Rats Replaced with Dexamethasone®." [In eng]. *J Med Food* 7, no. 1 (Spring 2004): 45–51.

Norazlina, M., S. Ima-Nirwana, M. T. Abul Gapor, and B. Abdul Kadir Khalid. "Tocotrienols Are Needed for Normal Bone Calcification in Growing Female Rats." [In eng]. *Asia Pac J Clin Nutr* 11, no. 3 (2002): 194–9.

Norazlina, M., P. L. Lee, H. I. Lukman, A. S. Nazrun, and S. Ima-Nirwana. "Effects of Vitamin E Supplementation on Bone Metabolism in Nicotine-Treated Rats." [In eng]. *Singapore Med J* 48, no. 3 (Mar 2007): 195–9.

Ahmad, N. S., B. A. Khalid, D. A. Luke, and S. Ima Nirwana. "Tocotrienol Offers Better Protection Than Tocopherol from Free Radical-Induced Damage of Rat Bone." [In eng]. *Clin Exp Pharmacol Physiol* 32, no. 9 (Sep 2005): 761–70.

Shuid, A. N., Z. Mehat, N. Mohamed, N. Muhammad, and I. N. Soelaiman. "Vitamin E Exhibits Bone Anabolic Actions in Normal Male Rats." [In eng]. *J Bone Miner Metab* 28, no. 2 (Mar 2010): 149–56.

Hamidi, M. S., P. N. Corey, and A. M. Cheung. "Effects of Vitamin E on Bone Turnover Markers among Us Postmenopausal Women." [In eng]. *J Bone Miner Res* 27, no. 6 (Jun 2012): 1368–80.

Nizar, A. M., A. S. Nazrun, M. Norazlina, M. Norliza, and S. Ima Nirwana. "Low Dose of Tocotrienols Protects Osteoblasts against Oxidative Stress." [In eng]. *Clin Ter* 162, no. 6 (2011): 533–8.

Nazrun, A. S., M. Norazlina, M. Norliza, and S. I. Nirwana. "The Anti-Inflammatory Role of Vitamin E in Prevention of Osteoporosis." [In eng]. *Adv Pharmacol Sci* 2012 (2012): 142702.

Pizzorno, L. Beyond α-Tocopherol: A Review of Natural Vitamin E's Therapeutic Potential in Human Health and Disease: Part I http://www.lmreview.com/articles/view/beyond-tocopherol-a-review-of-natural-vitamin-es-therapeutic-potential-in-human-health-and-disease-part-I/.

Pizzorno, L. Beyond α-Tocopherol: A Review of Natural Vitamin E's Therapeutic Potential in Human Health and Disease: Part IIhttp://www.lmreview.com/articles/view/beyond-tocopherol-a-review-of-natural-vitamin-es-therapeutic-potential-in-human-health-and-disease-part-II/.

472. Griel, A. E., P. M. Kris-Etherton, K. F. Hilpert, G. Zhao, S. G. West, and R. L. Corwin. "An Increase in Dietary N-3 Fatty Acids Decreases a Marker of Bone Resorption in Humans." [In eng]. *Nutr J* 6 (2007): 2.

473. Tartibian, B., B. Hajizadeh, J. Kanaley, et al. Long-term aerobic exercise and omega-3 supplementation modulate osteoporosis through inflammatory mechanisms in post-menopausal women: a randomized, repeated measures study. Nutrition & Metabolism 2011, 8:71 doi:10.1186/1743-7075-8-71 http://www.nutritionandmetabolism.com/content/8/1/71/abstract.

474. http://www.progressivelabs.com/product.php?productid=2.

http://www.progressivelabs.com/product.php?productid=1.

475. Lara writes blogs on the breaking research related to bone health which are posted on AlgaeCal's website. Dr. Wright has no connection with AlgaeCal®. http://www.algaecal.com/.

476. Neither Dr. Wright nor Lara Pizzorno has any financial connections with any of the following companies:

- NowFoods:http://www.nowfoods.com/Supplements/Products-by-Category/Minerals/M004240.htm

- Natural Factors: http://naturalfactors.com/ca/en/ products/detail/4389/healthy-bone-factors.

- Advanced Bionutritionals: http://www. advancedbionutritionals.com/Special-Offers/ Ultimate-Bone-Suport-ABBONEPPC.htm?gclid =CLjTz07677ACFQkaQgodlkHlvQ.

- Thorne: http://www.thorne.com/Products/Musculo- skeletal-Health/Bone_Support/prd~SG823.jsp.

- Life Extension Foundation: http://www.lef.org/ search/?q=bone%20support.

- Carlson Labs: http://www.carlsonlabs.com/p-5-nu- tra-support-bone.aspx.

- NBI: http://www.nbihealth.com/t-bone-health-sup- plements.aspx.

- Swanson: http://www.swansonvitamins.com/ JR046/ItemDetail.

- Nutricology/Allergy Research: http://www.nutricol- ogy.com/.

About the Authors

Lara Pizzorno, MA, LMT, is the managing editor for *Longevity Medicine Review* and senior medical editor for SaluGenecists, Inc. She is co-author of *Natural Medicine Instructions for Patients*, co-author of *The Encyclopedia of Healing Foods*, and editor of *The World's Healthiest Foods: Essential Guide for the Healthiest Way of Eating*.

Jonathan V. Wright, MD, is the founder and medical director of Tahoma Clinic in Renton, Washington. With degrees from Harvard and the University of Michigan, Dr. Wright has been at the forefront of natural biomedical research and treatment since 1973 and has written many best-selling books including *Your Stomach*, also published by Praktikos Books.

Index

#

A

C

F

N

U

V